Social Issues and Party Politics

After the landslide election of a new Labour government in May 1997, what are the key social policy issues and problems which the new government needs to address?

By looking at the manifestos of the main parties and the way each issue figured in the 1997 election campaign and the early days of the new government, *Social Issues and Party Politics* presents a convincing and incisive analysis of current social policy approaches and inherited problems. It identifies the deep social questions which will need to be addressed if Labour is to deliver on its promise of a new Britain.

With a central theme of social policy, the chapters discuss the management and financing of welfare in contemporary Britain, the delivery of key services in health, education, criminal justice, housing, social services, pensions and other areas of social security. These issues are looked at from different angles, including the view from Scotland, Northern Ireland and Wales, and from a Green perspective.

Helen Jones is Lecturer in Social Policy at Goldsmiths College, London. **Susanne MacGregor** is Professor of Social Policy at Middlesex University.

Social Issues and Party Politics

Edited by Helen Jones and
Susanne MacGregor

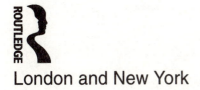

London and New York

First published 1998
by Routledge
11 New Fetter Lane, London EC4P 4EE

Simultaneously published in the USA and Canada
by Routledge
29 West 35th Street, New York, NY 10001

Typeset in Times by
Ponting–Green Publishing Services, Chesham,
Buckinghamshire
Printed and bound in Great Britain by
MPG Books Ltd, Bodmin

British Library Cataloguing in Publication Data
A catalogue record for this book is available from the
British Library

Library of Congress Cataloging in Publication Data
Social Issues and Party Politics/edited by Helen Jones and
    Susanne MacGregor.
        Includes bibliographical references
        1. Great Britain–Social policy–1979– .
    2. Great Britain–Politics and government–1997– .
    3. Political parties–Great Britain.
    I. Jones, Helen, 1954– . II. MacGregor, Susanne.
    HN383.5.S56   1998
    361.6'1'0941–dc21   97–45136

ISBN 0–415–17427–9 (hbk)
ISBN 0–415–17428–7 (pbk)

Contents

List of figures and tables   vii
Notes on contributors   viii
Preface   xi

1 **The road to 1997**   1
   Helen Jones

2 **Managing the welfare state**   24
   Tony Butcher

3 **Taxing and spending the people's money**   39
   Susanne MacGregor

4 **Jobs, unemployment and the European Union**   56
   Valerie Symes

5 **'Education, education, education'**   74
   Miriam E. David

6 **The people's health**   91
   Helen Jones

7 **New partnerships for social services**   106
   Susan Balloch

8 **Home truths**   121
   Mark Liddiard

9 **Poverty and social security in a changing Britain**   139
   Carey Oppenheim

10 **Paying for pensions**   155
    Barbara Waine

11 Criminal justice: security, social control and the
    hidden agenda   168
    Frances Heidensohn

12 The greenest election ever?   181
    Sue Barber

13 The view from Scotland   194
    Richard Parry

14 The view from Northern Ireland   214
    Eithne McLaughlin

15 The view from Wales   233
    Michael Sullivan

16 A new deal for Britain?   248
    Susanne MacGregor

    Index   273

Figures and tables

FIGURES

3.1	Current spending	41
3.2	Current taxation	41

TABLES

9.1	Perception of the level of poverty, 1994	141
9.2	Social security benefits as priorities for extra public spending, 1995	141
13.1	Vote figures in Scotland, 1992–97	195
13.2	Polls of Scottish voters on constitutional options, 1997	196
13.3	Most important issues in voting decisions of Scottish electorate	200
13.4	The main social policies in the SNP manifesto	202
13.5	The main issues in Scotland	205
13.6	Scotland campaign polls, 1997	210
13.7	Conservative Scottish seat losses in 1997 General Election	211

Contributors

Susan Balloch is Director of Policy at the National Institute for Social Work. She joined the Institute in 1993 to manage a survey of the Social Services Workforce. Previously she lectured in social policy at Goldsmiths College, University of London and helped develop local authority anti-poverty strategies at the Association of Metropolitan Authorities.

Sue Barber lectures in social policy at Middlesex University. Her current research looks at sustainable development in cities. In 1997, she was joint co-ordinator of the UNED/UK – Gender21 Round Table on Women and Sustainable Development for 'Earth Summit 2'. She is an associate of the Mega-Cities Network and former UK representative of WIDE (Women in Development Europe).

Tony Butcher is Senior Lecturer in Government and Head of Department of Social Policy and Politics at Goldsmiths College, University of London. He is the author of *Delivering Welfare: The Governance of the Social Services* (Open University Press 1995) and co-author of *The Civil Service Today* (2nd edn, Blackwell 1991).

Miriam E. David is Dean of Research at the London Institute. Her most recent publication is *Educational Reforms and Gender Equality in Schools* (with Madeleine Arnot and Gaby Weiner) (1996, Equal Opportunities Commission, research discussion series). She is co-editor, with Dr Dulcie Groves, of *The Journal of Social Policy* and an executive editor of the *British Journal of the Sociology of Education*.

Frances Heidensohn is Professor of Social Policy, Goldsmiths College, University of London. She has researched and written extensively on crime, criminal justice and gender. Her publications include *Women and Crime* (Macmillan 1996), *Crime and Society* (Macmillan 1989) *Women in Control?* (Oxford University Press 1992).

Helen Jones lectures in Social Policy at Goldsmiths College, University of London. Her publications include *Health and Society in Twentieth-Century Britain* (Longman 1994). She has edited *Towards a Classless Society?* (Routledge 1997), and co-edited with John Lansley, *Social Policy and the City* (Avebury 1995), and with Jane Millar *The Politics of the Family* (Avebury 1996).

Mark Liddiard is a Lecturer in Social Policy at the University of Kent at Canterbury. To date, most of his research has been in the field of youth homelessness, and he is co-author, with Susan Hutson, of *Youth Homelessness: The Construction of a Social Issue* (1994), published by Macmillan. However, his current research has shifted in focus towards arts and cultural policy, with a particular interest in museums and the mass media.

Susanne MacGregor is Professor of Social Policy at Middlesex University. She has a long-standing interest in the politics of social policy, beginning with her book *The Politics of Poverty* (Longman 1981). Her most recent books are *The Other City: People and Politics in New York and London*, co-edited with Arthur Lipow (Humanities 1995) and *Transforming Cities: contested governance and new spatial divisions*, co-edited with Nick Jewson (Routledge 1997). Her current research focuses on social problems, social policy and social exclusion in the city.

Eithne McLaughlin is the Professor of Social Policy at the Queen's University Belfast. She previously held posts at the universities of York and Ulster. Her research interests cover unemployment, labour supply and social security, equal opportunity, and informal and community care.

Carey Oppenheim, currently on secondment to the Institute of Public Policy Research, is a senior lecturer in social policy at South Bank University. She worked previously for the Child Poverty Action group. She has written widely on poverty and social security. Recent publications include *Poverty: The Facts* (with Lisa Harker) (Child Poverty Action Group 1996), and *An Inclusive Society: Tackling Poverty* (Institute for Public Policy Research, 1998).

Richard Parry is Senior Lecturer in Social Policy at the University of Edinburgh and has researched and published in the field of

Scottish government, privatization and European social policy. He and Nicholas Deakin have recently been researching on the Treasury and Social Policy as part of the ESRC Whitehall programme.

Michael Sullivan is Reader and Head of Social Policy at the University of Wales, Swansea. He has written extensively on the politics and history of the welfare state. He is the author of *The Politics of Social Policy* (1992) and *The Development of the Welfare State* (1996) among numerous other books, chapters and articles.

Valerie Symes is a lecturer in economics at Goldsmiths College, University of London. Her recent publications include *Unemployment in Europe* (Routledge 1995) and as a contributor and co-author, *The Future of Europe* (Macmillan 1997). She has recently co-ordinated research on evaluating policies for the long-term unemployed in six European countries.

Barbara Waine is Principal Lecturer in Social Policy and Administration at Middlesex University. She has published on pensions, employment in higher education and public sector management. Her most recent book is *Managing the Welfare State: the Politics of Public Sector Management* (with Tony Cutler) (Berg 1994, updated 2nd edn 1997).

Preface

After the landslide election of a new Labour government in May 1997, what does the future hold for social policy? What does the new government intend to do? How do Labour promises compare with those of other political parties? What are the key issues and problems which the new government needs to address? The essays in this volume aim to provide some answers to these important questions.

The new government is offering a reinvention of Britain within which a reinvention of social policy will play a major part. But historical awareness tells us that underlying whatever new designs may be created, there are social, political, cultural, and economic forces at work and institutional and attitudinal factors which limit how much can be achieved. To say this is not to be negative, cynical or pessimistic about change but to argue for careful, reasoned and well-informed accounts of the context in which policy aims to intervene and an understanding of what has been tried before and what can be done.

The book was first conceived in the early days of 1997. All the contributors followed closely the days running up to the election, the campaign itself and the early days of the new government. The chapters in the collection are therefore informed by this scrutiny of the party political and public debates on social policy in these months. The authors set their review of this watershed election in the context of what has gone before, providing a unique perspective from expert analysts on the problems with which policy has to grapple and the choices that have to be faced.

Chapter 1

The road to 1997

Helen Jones

THE SUN SHINES ON BLAIR

On 17 March John Major, and on 2 May Tony Blair, provided the 1997 General Election with a symbolic stage-managed symmetry. John Major, following a format he instigated in 1992, stood alone and isolated in Downing Street to announce 1 May as Polling Day. He used the occasion to launch the formal campaign (a phoney one had been underway for at least a year) with a party-political plea for the Conservatives. Six and a half weeks later Tony Blair walked up Downing Street (the formality and separation from the people of an official car abandoned) with a youthful and apparently happy family to the cheers and flag-waving of hand-picked party workers. These strong and contrasting images – of John Major, formal and isolated from party and people and Tony Blair, informal and surrounded by loyal supporters – were present throughout the campaign. Both parties put enormous effort into trying to control the media's presentation of their leaders. Labour succeeded, but the Conservatives failed miserably, not least because the bulk of newspapers were no longer, as in previous General Elections, the willing accomplices of the Conservative Party.

The way in which the parties presented their leaders and aimed to control the media affected the conduct of the campaign which some commentators believed signalled the growing 'Americanisation' of British elections with a more presidential style campaign, focusing on the leader, not the party. A live TV debate between candidates for the Presidency is an accepted event in American elections. Negotiations (conducted in private between Lord Irvine for Labour and Michael Dobbs for the Conservatives and slogged out in public between Peter Mandelson and Brian Mawhinney) to present a live

TV debate between John Major and Tony Blair became a part of the campaign, foundering largely on the 'Paddy problem', that is, what role Paddy Ashdown, leader of the Liberal Democrats, should play. The Conservatives paid a man to dress up in a yellow chicken suit with a placard 'Chicken Blair Won't Debate' to chase Blair until he agreed to a live TV debate. (This was another echo of the 1992 presidential campaign.) The chicken spawned a whole zoo of animals posing for photographers, but it did little to leaven the Conservatives' gloom.

The media itself became part of the election news, not only over the negotiations for the TV debate but also, when the *Sun* declared early on in the campaign for Labour, with the *Guardian*'s exposé of sleaze, and when the BBC's war correspondent, Martin Bell, stood as the Independent anti-corruption candidate to fight Tatton against Neil Hamilton. There was, too, a showbizz air to the campaigns with the parties trying to outdo each other by claiming the support of 'personalities'. After the disastrous Sheffield rally of 1992, however, Labour trod warily in ensuring that showbizz support did not tarnish Tony Blair's carefully crafted prime ministerial image, or become triumphalist. Major's and Blair's touch of glamour came from their wives who closely shadowed them around the country.

Throughout the campaign the sun shone on Blair both literally and metaphorically. Opinion polls, even when they wobbled, gave Labour a long lead, as indeed they had done continuously for over four years. Notwithstanding this lead, Labour had learnt the lessons of 1992 and took nothing for granted. Blair and the Labour Party leadership repeatedly warned against complacency and focused their campaign, like the Conservatives, on the key marginals, roughly ninety seats, they would need to win, to form a government. Labour rarely attacked the Liberal Democrats, in order to encourage tactical voting against Conservative candidates (which paid off).

While all three parties targeted an exclusive number of constituencies, the voters they targeted were all inclusive. Both Conservatives and Labour presented themselves as the 'one nation' party. For the Labour Party this was part of its modernised image of catering for all sections of society but no sectional – particularly trade union – interests. The Conservatives tried to counter Labour's claims by spreading scare stories about the ghost of trade union power ready to rise from the grave where it had been buried by Mrs Thatcher. That this message was not taken seriously was largely due to the voters' lack of trust in the Conservative Party.

Voters' trust in the Conservatives had evaporated as a result of the Government's withdrawal from the Exchange Rate Mechanism (ERM) in September 1992, and rises in taxes. Good economic figures which appeared during the campaign did nothing to restore voters' faith in the ability of the Conservatives to manage the economy. Research into the links between voting behaviour and the economy from 1983 onwards suggested that voters were affected by the state of the economy over the whole life of a Parliament, not just in the run-up to an election. Voters treated the good economic news with scepticism; they did not think it would last, and anyway there was more faith in Labour's ability to manage the economy competently than there was in the Conservatives' (quoted in *The Independent*, 27, 30 March 1997). The Conservatives had, moreover, lost the trust of the nation as one aspect of corruption after another hit the news stands. The scandals were remorseless and continued throughout the campaign. The Labour Party exploited this lack of trust to the full, basing its whole campaign around the issue. John Prescott, Deputy leader of the Labour Party, who toured marginals in a bus, the 'Prescott Express', handed out cards with Labour's pledges; he explained 'We're hoping it will help build trust' (*Independent*, 27 March 1997).

Sleaze dominated the campaign and meant that both Conservative and Labour parties conducted largely negative campaigns. Only the Liberal Democrats campaigned positively on their policies, focusing on health and education. It was more difficult for Labour and Conservatives to highlight their policies because they appeared so close on many key issues. They wanted to provide the media with sound bites for the evening TV news, not expound the subtlety of their policies. On 20 January 1997, Gordon Brown, Shadow Chancellor, had ruled out rises in the basic rate of income tax for the life of the Parliament and the two main parties pledged themselves to the same spending targets for two years. Labour sought to reassure voters that their trust in the newly modernised Labour Party was well-founded and that Labour was 'fit to govern'. It was difficult for the Conservative campaign managers to focus on policies because sleaze and divisions within the party, particularly over the EU, stayed to the forefront of the campaign. While no-one accused Major of corruption, it rebounded to his disadvantage because he was unable to stamp it out, and contradictory reports appeared in the Press as to whether senior Conservatives really supported those accused of sleaze, or whether they were furious and wanted them to stand down immediately. So, the image of the Conservative Party was not only of sleaze but also of dithering, confusion and splits. Whereas Labour played to its strengths, the Conservatives somewhat oddly gave a great deal of attention to Europe, and according to Nicholas Jones this both surprised Labour and meant that Labour did not devote as much attention as it would have liked to health, and law and order (Jones, N. 1997: 234). There were good reasons for Labour avoiding too much dissection of these policies, however, because of incompletely-thought-out positions, and similarities with Conservative policies.

THE COURSE OF THE CAMPAIGN

On Monday 17 March, following a Cabinet meeting and an audience with the Queen, John Major announced 1 May as Polling Day. Standing outside No. 10, he fielded questions from the assembled journalists and in effect turned his announcement into an election broadcast. He needed the head start. The Conservatives were roughly 20 points behind Labour in the opinion polls, and had trailed badly for years. The Conservatives assumed that the longest campaign since 1918 would work to their advantage: with plenty of time for them to get their message across that the economy was booming, and for Labour to trip up. If they had been able to win in 1992 with a recession, and record bankruptcies and home repossessions, then surely the improving economy – as judged by falling unemployment, growth of roughly 2.5 per cent, consumer spending rising by 3 per cent a year, and the service sector compensating for the stagnating manufacturing sector – would be to their advantage? This assumption was challenged during the election by those who argued that voters' memories went back across the life of the whole Parliament, and that improvements in the economy might make people more willing to step into the unknown and trust Labour.

A willingness to trust Labour and widespread mistrust of the Government was fuelled when it emerged that Parliament was to be prorogued the following Friday, the very day Sir Gordon Downey, Parliamentary Commissioner for Standards, was due to present his report to the Standards and Privileges Committee on allegations that Mohamed al Fayed had bribed MPs to ask questions as part of a campaign orchestrated by Ian Greer, the political lobbyist, to discredit 'Tiny' Rowland of Lonhro. This meant that two former Conservative ministers, Neil Hamilton, MP for Tatton, and Tim Smith, MP for Beaconsfield along with a former Whip, Michael

Brown, MP for Cleethorpes, and Sir Andrew Bowden, MP for Brighton Kemptown, could all stand for Parliament, if adopted by their constituency associations. The task for the Conservatives was now made even harder. Sleaze and Conservative divisions over Europe would dominate the campaign.

Major tried to dampen the sleaze issue in the first few days by claiming that he had not knowingly kept a minister at the heart of the cash for questions affair in his government, but this was rejected by Labour who tried to drag Major into the issue and while this was not successful, sleaze did overshadow the Conservatives' launch of their poster 'Britain's Booming'. When John Redwood announced that for the Conservatives to win they had to show how education, health, and law and order would improve under another Conservative administration, and to explain how the Conservatives had followed the right economic policy over the previous three years, the task was to prove almost impossible because of the difficulty for the Conservatives to 'show' or 'explain' when there was so much disbelief in them.

The Conservative strategy rested largely on John Major. His winning soapbox style in 1992, when he was seen among, and of, the people was immediately revived. The raw and simple style of Major was meant to contrast with the slick (some thought smarmy) image of Tony Blair, born with a silver rosette in his mouth. On the day John Major called the election he stepped onto his soapbox, and Mrs Thatcher stepped out of her Belgravia office with dire warnings of the dangers of electing Tony Blair: '"New Labour" is cunningly designed to conceal a lot of old socialism. Don't be taken in' (*Independent*, 18 March 1997). This warning served a dual purpose: it distanced Mrs Thatcher from the rumours that she had said that Blair would not 'let Britain down', and it took up the theme which the Conservatives were now going to plug, that Labour represented a new danger. Initially the Conservatives had hoped to campaign on their economic record but with no evidence that economic recovery would swing voters back to them, alternative and additional messages were required (*Daily Telegraph*, 17 March 1997).

An early indication of Labour's cautious style came when it emphasised that voting Labour would be quite safe as a Labour Administration would provide elements of continuity under a revitalised government (*Daily Telegraph*, 18 March 1997). Certainly, Labour's announcements that there would be new cabinet subcommittees to give horizontal integration to policy, and that it would prioritise employment for young people were hardly likely to frighten the shires (*Financial Times*, 19 March 1997).

It was also clear from the outset that the leadership package included the wives. On the evening of 19 March, Norma Major and Cherie Booth were both present, along with Diana, Princess of Wales, at the Gold Awards for Courage at the Savoy. Photos of the two wives, comments on what they allegedly did and did not say to each other, and how they behaved towards each other attracted newspaper coverage the next day. The event provided two further pointers to the campaign.

First, to a certain extent, the campaign became a 'glamour' event, with media, sporting and business personalities coming out for the parties. Supporters of the Conservatives included Geri of the Spice Girls; Lord Lloyd-Webber; Sir Cliff Richard; Frank Bruno; Michael Atherton; David Platt; David Seaman; Earl Attlee, grandson of the former Labour Prime Minister; Ian Gibson, Chief Executive of Nissan; and Baroness (P.D.) James. Labour supporters included Mel C. of the Spice Girls; Stephen Fry; Sir Terence Conran; Bianca Jagger; the Chief Rabbi, Jonathan Sacks; Lord Attenborough; Gerry Robinson, chairman of Granada Group; Alec Reed, founder of Reed Employment Agency; Lord Douro, chairman of Sun Life; and Jeremy Hardie, chairman of W.H. Smith (*Independent*, 18 March 1997). The support of leading business people was especially helpful for Labour.

Second, the two leaders' wives were the only two women to receive continuous media coverage throughout the campaign. Mrs Thatcher popped up from time to time, and Christine Hamilton had a number of walk-on parts. None of the parties pushed their female politicians into the limelight or gave them lead roles in the campaign. The campaign was a boys' own story.

During the first week of the campaign, Parliament was still sitting so there was the campaign in the House of Commons as well as the beginnings of activity in the country. At Prime Minister's Question Time, Blair and Major traded blows over the NHS much as they had done for the previous three years (*Financial Times*, 19 March 1997). Peter Lilley launched a £1 billion benefits pledge, the Family Benefits Guarantee, which the Conservatives claimed was further evidence that they were the party of the family. Lilley undermined this claim by laying new regulations before Parliament to cut housing benefit and funeral grants for the poorest families (*Guardian*, 22 March 1997).

During Week 2, when Parliament had been prorogued and the

campaign really got under way around the country, both parties appeared edgy. Tony Blair urged his party not to be complacent and to reassure the country that it was safe to vote Labour. There was concern in the Blair camp that the sleaze issue would not help Labour in the end because voters (including potential Labour ones) would be turned off politicians and not vote. The Conservatives were also nervy. They twice changed a prearranged Press conference at the last minute to go with a different issue. This gave the impression that they were panicking. So, Conservative messages, such as the dangers of Labour's policy towards the trade unions, got lost in poor presentation.

One piece of negative news about the Conservatives followed hard on the next. Tim Smith resigned under pressure from local Conservatives from the third safest Conservative seat in the country, despite having support from Major, Heseltine and Portillo the previous week, a fact which seemed to underline how out of touch senior Conservatives were with the mood of the country; John Redwood published a book which was off-message on Europe and a single currency; George Gardiner, right-wing Euro-sceptic, was deselected by his constituency and slunk off to join the Referendum Party; and the *Sun* published pictures of Piers Merchant, a Conservative MP, which purported to show him kissing a 17-year-old girl, with allegations of an adulterous affair. Allan Stewart, a Scottish Conservative MP, and Sir Michael Hirst, a senior Scottish Conservative, both resigned amid whispering campaigns about their private lives. Negotiations over the TV debate broke down among recriminations from which neither party emerged particularly well. Only Paddy Ashdown, whose role had been at the centre of the dispute, emerged with any credibility as he set himself apart as the practical man with practical answers.

Week 2 ended with the Labour candidate in Tatton announcing that he was standing down to give a free run to an Independent anti-corruption candidate, and Labour hoped that the Liberal candidate would also stand down, which he duly did. The search for an Independent candidate led to names such as Frances Lawrence, Judge Stephen Tumim, David Attenborough, Richard Branson, Glen Hoddle, Joe Kinnear (manager of Wimbledon FC) and Chelsea Clinton being put forward, in varying degrees of seriousness.

Week 3, as all other weeks during the campaign, began badly for the Conservatives. Over the weekend there had been allegations that fellow Conservatives had stitched-up Sir Michael Hirst; Neil Hamilton had released transcripts of his evidence to Downey, which was a breach of Parliamentary privilege; and Piers Merchant's Beckenham constituency had refused to deselect him, so flying in the face of John Major's wishes. Frederick Forsyth's likening of the single currency to the Holocaust made the right-wing of the Conservative Party look obscene with no sense of proportion. Further Conservative splits were signalled by a break-away rump of disaffected ex-Conservative Association executives.

There were two hiccups for Labour. Blair likened the proposed Scottish Parliament to a parish council, which outraged the Scots, and the *Daily Mail* claimed that all the trade union leaders had taken a vow of silence for the duration of the campaign so as not to embarrass Labour. Labour's Excalibur (computerised) rebuttal system was in action as soon as the claim had been made; the union leaders fell over themselves to refute any such self-denying ordinance. Less remarked on were the notable absences from the campaign of the Party's leftwingers, Tony Benn, Diane Abbott and Ken Livingstone, none of whom could be described as media-shy.

During Week 3 the main parties launched their manifestos. The Conservatives made a pitch for the 'traditional' family vote. The centre piece of the manifesto was a £1.2 billion tax break for some married couples or dependent relatives – calculated to be worth £900 a year – and plans for a respite care programme to help those caring for elderly relatives to take a break from caring. The newspapers usually sympathetic to the Conservatives (*The Times, Daily Mail, Daily Express* and *Evening Standard*) gave the manifesto a mixed, and on the whole, luke-warm reception. Only the *Daily Telegraph* gave whole-hearted support. Labour undertook a spoiling operation by releasing photocopies of Blair's handwritten ten pledges, a personal contract with the people.

The Labour manifesto, launched the day after the Conservatives, was presented with the heralded ten-point commitment covenant, the main points of which covered education, crime, the NHS, jobs, taxes and the economy. 'Cautious improvements' was the message. Blair homed in on the theme of trust when he challenged the voters to hold Labour to its pledges so that at the next election Labour could say 'Trust us again, because we keep our promises'.

The following Week 4 was dominated by the news that Tatton Conservatives had reselected Neil Hamilton as their candidate and that Martin Bell, the white-suited BBC war correspondent, was to stand as the anti-corruption Independent candidate. John Major and

Brian Mawhinney refused to interfere in Tatton on the grounds that the Conservative Party constitution did not allow for centralised control of local associations. This may, however, have been as much a reflection of Major's weak leadership as the nature of Conservative Party organisation. (At the 1950 General Election Churchill and Lord Woolton, the Party chairman, stopped Andrew Fountaine, the Conservative Party candidate in Chorley, and an extremist who later co-founded the National Front, from standing as the official Conservative Party candidate. He was forced to stand as an Independent Conservative – *Times*, 22 September 1997.)

Journalists flocked to Tatton and recorded the first skirmish between the Hamiltons and Bell, which the former won. The emergence of Bell's daughter and her friends to support him added a whiff of glamour. The other news during the week was far more serious and less attractive to the parties and the media. The Council of Churches (1997) report on inequality did not find favour with Conservatives who had been in Government while inequality had increased, or among Labour spin doctors and leaders who knew very well that they would not be increasing spending on the poor. Radical attacks on inequality were no part of the Labour script. The parties squirmed further as the Institute for Fiscal Studies attacked the unrealistically low spending plans of the parties, and as charities appeared to gang up against them.

The only bright moment of the week for the Conservatives came with Labour's slippery response to questions about the scope of its windfall tax and its air-traffic control policy. The Press reported disagreements between Blair and Brown over how much money should be raised from a windfall tax on privatised utilities and which companies should carry the heaviest burden. Blair allegedly wanted a more limited tax than Brown did (*Financial Times*, 10 April 1997). There also appeared to be confusion within the Labour Party over its attitude towards further privatisation. Reports that the Party was considering plans to sell off the Post Office and air-traffic control prompted questions but not answers as to whether Labour was committed to further privatisation or not.

Week 5 proved difficult for both main parties. Election fatigue set in among the tabloids which were more interested in covering news of the pop singer Liam Gallagher's love life with Patsy Kensit, and allegations of Will Self taking heroin on the Prime Minister's plane.

Voters found it hard to distinguish between the two parties' policies, and the distinction was not helped by John Major and Tony

Blair both trying to revitalise the campaign by focusing on their policies, for both used the language of 'one nation'. Only the Liberal Democrats seemed to have a distinctive and radical line, underlined by Vanessa Redgrave, long-time far-left campaigner, announcing that she would vote Liberal Democrat.

At the beginning of the week Blair tried to focus on education and set out a twenty-one point policy initiative, poo-pooed by Major who launched a personal attack on Blair for his 'hypocrisy' over education. This attack on Labour's moral fibre and credibility was central to the Conservative campaign which had to undermine Labour's central tenet of trust.

Neither Labour nor Conservatives had a good week. Labour were embarrassed by John Prescott's alleged comments, reported in the *Sunday Times*, that a minimum wage would lead to a rise in unemployment, but it was not possible to say so publicly. Journalists were furious when they discovered that they were subsidising Labour's battle bus through the hotel bills they received; and the use of a bulldog in an advertisement which initially went down well had to be withdrawn when it was criticised as a British National Party symbol and therefore racist. Labour's consolation was that the Conservatives had a worse week. Most seriously, Angela Rumbold, a vice-chair of the Conservative Party who was fighting the highly marginal seat of Mitcham and Morden, came out against a single currency. Worse was to follow when Major refused to sack John Horam, a health minister, for flying in the face of agreed Government policy on the issue. This failure to act swiftly and decisively made Major look weak and it drew attention to the divisions in the Party. Division was compounded by apparent desperation when Major pleaded 'Like me or loathe me, but do not bind my hands on Europe'. The Party had to apologise for a candidate's leaflet which linked Labour with Sinn Fein; John Major's plans for a grammar school in every town melted away in a muddle; the Government failed to respond convincingly to allegations that it had inflated the job figures; and a poster of a tiny Blair sitting like a ventriloquist's dummy on Chancellor Kohl's lap went down badly.

In the last full week of campaigning the Conservatives tried to divert attention away from Europe and towards education, the constitution and the economy, but with little success as Clarke and Howard publicly disagreed over the EU and a single currency. Jacques Santer, President of the European Commission helped no party when he warned that there was no going back on further

European integration. Despite its divisions over Europe, the Conservatives did seem to be catching an anti-EU mood and opinion polls reported a shrinking Labour lead. John Major effectively linked the constitutional issues of Scottish devolution and the EU. Senior Conservatives, nevertheless, already appeared to be manoeuvring into position for the leadership contest expected to follow their 1 May defeat: 'Dorrelling away pretending to hold views that they don't' (quoted in the *Guardian* 21 April 1997). The question mark hanging over 1 May was now not who would win but whether the IRA would attempt to undermine the democratic and constitutional process by causing chaos through hoax phone calls or bombs.

Despite claims that they wanted a more positive campaign, Labour produced a remorselessly negative TV advert with the message that if the Conservatives were re-elected they would fiddle as Rome burnt. To the strains of 'Land of Hope and Glory' pictures of laughing Cabinet ministers were intercut by muggings, car thefts and empty hospital wards. The Conservatives tried to embarrass Labour by leaking its War Book which set out where Labour and Conservatives were both strongest and weakest and how Labour would counter-attack. Blair conveniently produced a populist diversion by promising to channel some of the mid-week lottery money to innovative projects in health and education.

Blair returned to the themes of modernisation and stakeholding which he had been developing throughout the 1990s. Generally, Blair avoided complex ideas such as stakeholding and communitarianism during the campaign, instead focusing on easily understood themes. This was part of the 'soundbite not exposition' strategy.

The Conservatives must have been desperate when they revived their 1992 tactic by claiming that voters would pay £640 a year extra tax after two years of Labour: Labour's rebuttal system was in operation even before Major had got the words out. Yet, the Conservatives failed to exploit the most obvious weak point of Labour, their lack of ministerial experience.

The Conservative camp appeared dispirited as squabbles within the Party were reported more than arguments between Conservatives and the other parties. Labour of course had its disagreements, as can be seen by the see-sawing strategy of going from positive to negative campaigning, but as the parties entered the home straight Labour's lead in the marginals began to look invincible and people began to believe the unbelievable: forecasters were already talking of a Labour landslide. Blair, who had been careful not to make any unrealistic promises, now claimed 'I'm going to be a lot more radical in government than many people think' (*Observer*, 27 April 1997).

A nasty spat between Labour and Conservatives over the former's claims that the Conservatives wanted to get rid of the state pension led Major to call Blair 'absolutely contemptible', but the story lasted three days and then fizzled out. Major's final gesture was to fly to the four corners of the UK, with the message '72 hours to save the Union'. No-one seemed to heed his warning. The drama of the final few days campaigning was nothing compared with the result.

As the polls closed on 1 May and the country sat down to the night's viewing, exit polls predicted a Labour landslide. Until the result in Birmingham Edgbaston – the first seat to fall to Labour and sixty-seventh on its hit-list – was declared no-one, least of all the Labour leadership, believed the seismic landslide. Pictures of Blair and Alistair Campbell anxiously pacing in Blair's constituency house belied the enormity of what was unfolding in front of millions of bleary eyes. Portillo's defeat confirmed the Conservative Party's meltdown.

The country experienced a political earthquake. It was Labour's biggest win ever and the biggest swing to Labour since 1945. Tony Blair was the youngest Prime Minister since 1812. Three-quarters of the House of Commons was either Labour or Liberal Democrat. Not since the 1920s had the Liberals done so well. Not since 1832 had the Conservatives done so badly. Conservative defeats included seven members of the Cabinet (Defence Secretary, Michael Portillo; Foreign Secretary, Malcolm Rifkind; Scottish Secretary, Michael Forsyth; President of the Board of Trade, Ian Lang; Chief Secretary to the Treasury, William Waldegrave; Leader of the House, Tony Newton; and Chancellor of the Duchy of Lancaster, Roger Freeman), thirteen junior ministers and various senior backbenchers including David Mellor who had to contend with Jimmy Goldsmith, leader of the Referendum Party, standing in his Putney constituency. Huge swings occurred, 17.5 per cent against Portillo in Enfield Southgate, 19 per cent in Croydon North and 18 per cent in Wimbledon. All Conservative MPs were obliterated in Wales and Scotland. Martin Bell trounced Hamilton by 11,000 votes.

Anthony King argued that the scale of the landslide was due to a substantial increase in Labour's vote (43 per cent compared with 35 per cent in 1992), the collapse of the Conservative vote (from 43 per cent in 1992 to 31 per cent in 1997), but most importantly, the percentage of the population who voted Labour or Liberal Democrat in the marginals (King 1997).

By the final count Labour had 418 seats (146 gains) and 43 per cent of the vote. The Conservatives had 165 seats (178 losses) and 31 per cent of the vote. The Liberal Democrats had 46 seats (30 gains and 2 losses) and 17 per cent of the vote. The Scottish Nationalists had 6 seats (3 gains) and Plaid Cymru 4 seats (no change). The Ulster Unionists had 10 seats (1 gain). The Democratic Unionists had 2 seats (2 losses). UK Unionists had 1 seat (1 gain). The SDLP had 3 seats (1 loss); Sinn Fein had 2 seats (2 gains). The total was completed by 1 Independent MP (1 gain) and the non-partisan Speaker's seat (*Daily Telegraph*, 3 May 1997). There were twice as many women in the new Parliament as in the old one. The country elected 120 women, 100 of them Labour, representing both safe and marginal seats. Five women subsequently sat in Blair's first Cabinet.

A NEW DEPARTURE?

The course of the campaign and the outcome raise important issues about the way in which the new Labour Government develops its social policies. What was the balance of influences on New Labour when it entered Office on 2 May 1997? What influence did American electioneering techniques have on the Party's relationship with the people; and what was the balance of influences – from eighteen years of Conservative Government as opposed to the Party's own history – on its policy agenda when it entered Office?

There are a number of similarities between the American 1992 presidential campaign and the 1997 General Election. The conduct of the campaign is the most striking similarity. One of Labour's media advisors, Philip Gould, had worked on Clinton's campaign. Both Gordon Brown and Ed Balls, his economics advisor, had contacts in the USA and learnt from US campaign techniques. In 1993 Brown and Blair met Stan Greenberg who had worked as a pollster and aide for Clinton, and they continued to keep in contact. Greenberg had developed the use of small focus groups on whom to try out policies in the USA and he introduced the same techniques for Labour and helped to shape Labour's image. Gordon Brown and Ed Balls had kept in contact with Robert Reich, Clinton's Labor Secretary. The Conservatives too had adapted American techniques (*Daily Telegraph*, 2, 3 April 1997). The late Jimmy Goldsmith, sometimes described as the 'loose cannon' Referendum Party leader, could be paralleled with Ross Perot. Clinton targeted the states he would need to win for overall victory, and all three parties in Britain focused on their key seats. Clinton went for the white suburban middle-class vote, Blair for comfortable middle England. Control of the media was the main aim of the spin doctors and while both Democrats and Labour did this successfully up to and during the campaign, as soon as they were victorious, media control appeared less easy. Clinton's honeymoon was short-lived as he received unfavourable press coverage over the failed nomination of Zoe Baird as Attorney General, his $200 hair cut and his support for homosexuals in the military. Media hostility to his media anchorman George Stephanopoulos spilled over in the same way as it did against Peter Mandelson in Britain. The Republicans had no overarching theme whereas the Democrats focused on economic decline, trust and corruption. Both American and British voters were concerned about health, education and the management of the economy. In both America and Britain there had been an overall shift to the Right in domestic policies. In both countries there was a strong desire for change. In contrast to the USA where Bush attempted to label Clinton a 'tax and spend' candidate in the mould of previous Democrat presidents, no such charge against the Labour Party was credible because it had promised not to raise the basic rate of income tax and to keep spending within the Conservatives' target for two years. In fact, Labour imitated the technique of blocking-off all the negatives, on taxation, on its relationship with the trade unions, and on a single currency (by promising a referendum). It was not, moreover, possible to level charges against the way any of the party leaders conducted their private lives, whereas Clinton's allegedly womanising lifestyle was used against him (for the American campaign see Caesar and Busch 1993; Maltese 1994).

So, there were clearly American influences on the way Labour conducted its campaign, even though the TV debate did not take place. The Blairs, moreover, upstaged the Queen at the opening of Parliament when they walked down to the Palace of Westminster from Downing Street, for all the world a presidential couple. Blair's massive victory and closeness to ordinary people was in sharp contrast to an unelected head of state arriving in a carriage to open Parliament and deliver a speech written by the elected Government. (The contrast was of course reinforced by their public reactions to the tragic death of Diana, Princess of Wales less than four months later.) The influence of American electioneering and media techniques should not however detract from the strong continuities in the way in which Labour adapted to the demands of the 1990s.

PREVIOUS GENERAL ELECTIONS

From the early 1920s when the Labour Party was first a serious contender for government it has struggled against internal divisions and with having to prove itself 'fit to govern'. That the manner in which power will be exercised has often proved as important as the policies to be pursued in power has meant that it is not unusual for social issues to play a secondary role in General Election campaigns. The tone and values identified with political parties have played a more important role than the policies of parties. Social policies have often appeared similar with differences more apparent with hindsight or with careful policy analysis, which does not usually take place during a campaign. Influence over communication techniques has played an important part in general elections this century as parties have see-sawed in their abilities to best exploit new techniques, through radio, film, television, advertising agencies and most recently, information technology.

In the early 1920s the most striking policy similarities were between the Asquithian Liberals and Labour, although there was little difference between any of the parties over social policy. The challenge to the Labour Party was to overcome the jibe of Winston Churchill and Lord Birkenhead that Labour was 'unfit to govern'. As well as policy similarities, all the parties were attempting to associate themselves with the image of stability, moderation and common sense (Cowling 1971). J.R. Clynes, one of Labour's most senior politicians, made a pitch for the business and commercial vote, not seen as Labour's natural allies, as well as for the working-class vote. In both 1923 (successfully) and 1924 (unsuccessfully) the Labour Party had to contend with the Conservatives 'red scare' tactics. In 1924 and in 1931, when the Conservatives offered stability, the voters responded. Neither in the 1920s nor in the 1930s did the parties present the voters with radically different social policies.

The General Election in 1945 gave Labour its first majority. The swing to Labour had begun well before the election. If there had been an election in 1940 it is unclear who would have won; certainly from 1942 the mood of the country swung behind Labour. There was a backlash against the Conservatives, while Labour's policies of greater state intervention and an alleviation of poverty were widely approved. The popularity of the Soviet Union rebounded to Labour's favour even though in the past it had distanced itself from the Soviet regime. At the election the policies offered by the parties differed little on the surface, but there was far greater trust in the Labour Party to honour its pledges. Social issues, in particular housing, were uppermost among voters' concerns. Between 1945 and 1951 the comparative strength of the parties' organisations changed. In 1945 the Conservative Party machine had run-down far more dramatically than the Labour Party organisation from its pre-war strength. After its dramatic defeat the Conservatives rebuilt the Party organisation, and accepted Keynesian economics and Labour's state welfare policies. Throughout the 1950s the parties' differences on social policies barely registered with voters although overall the Conservatives enjoyed an image of greater competence (Butler and Rose 1960).

Again, in the 1960s, policy differences were difficult to detect. Some parallels can be drawn between 1964 and 1997. In 1964 the Conservatives had ruled for thirteen years, there was a sense that it was time for a change and the Conservative Government had been damaged by the scandal of the Profumo affair. Labour had been dogged by damaging internal squabbles at the turn of the decade, but since then there had been concerted efforts to 'modernise' the Party. Policies had been updated and disassociated from dogma; in an effort to counter the trend towards the declining working-class industrial base of the Labour Party it had attempted to forge new links with the professional classes and with young people, so presenting itself as a more classless and up-to-date party than either the current Conservatives or Labour in the past. It had updated its use of publicity and propaganda and begun to exploit survey techniques more effectively (Butler and King 1965). As in 1997, when the social policies of the Labour Party were very different, the style of presentation was all-important.

In 1970 and in the two 1974 elections, voters were presented with the parties undermining the others' credibility, and in February 1974 the need for strong government in the face of economic crisis and the miners' strike was emphasised by the Conservatives (Butler and Kavanagh 1974, 1975). Again in 1979, it was less the details of policies which were put forward by the winning party than the importance of the tone and values with which it was associated. The conduct of government and the management of the economy were all-important. Mrs Thatcher gave few policy hostages to fortune. Other than selling off council houses it was unclear in May 1979 how the social policy agenda would develop.

SOCIAL POLICIES 1979–97

Mrs Thatcher's policies were based on the assumption that state welfare encourages a dependency by individuals on the state and discourages a sense of individual and family responsibility. Business methods, she believed, needed to be injected into all aspects of life, and most pertinently for our current discussion, welfare provision, and this could only be done through a reduction in direct taxes, and a reduction in state, in particular local authority, welfare provision. There should be competition to provide the best welfare services to clients who could pick and choose the services they required. A society run purely on business lines inevitably had winners and losers, and of this 1980s Conservatives approved. The growth in inequality, most notably income inequality, but other aspects of inequality also, was something to be welcomed; after all, no-one suggested that all businesses should or could be equally profitable, so too with individuals. Such thinking denoted a distinctive break with the welfare state as it developed for a generation after the Second World War, but the foundations for such thinking to be politically acceptable had been laid in the 1970s when inflation, overmighty unions and an unwieldy bureaucratic welfare state led those on both Left and Right to believe they were witnessing a crisis in the welfare state. While they might not have been agreed on prescriptions they did seem agreed on the disease. A restructuring of the economy was already underway as a result of changes in the global market, and this was given a boost by Conservative governments of the 1980s. Indeed, the most radical policies of governments in the 1980s lay in the economic and industrial field. Yet, just as government was withdrawing from certain areas so it was increasingly intervening in other areas of society. Both the economy and the state were being restructured.

Inevitably there was some fall-out for social policies: the sale of council houses and increased powers of the police are the most obvious, but a major restructuring of the institutions delivering welfare services only came at the end of Mrs Thatcher's tenure, and indeed were only properly implemented under her successor John Major. While implementing those policies already on stream, a change in priorities can be detected under Major. The deeply unpopular poll tax was withdrawn, and in 1993 Major launched his Citizen's Charter which in spirit at least flew in the face of Mrs Thatcher's philosophy. For her, citizens' power lay in the way they made their choices in the market, not in protective consumer measures. The impact, however, of this shift was barely perceptible: inequalities continued to increase; structural shifts continued in welfare provision; and the fundamental problems of resourcing welfare in a changing society were not addressed let alone tackled. By the mid-1990s the failure of government to grasp these nettles was widely recognised and the willingness of the population to trust the government to address the problems with competence was dwindling.

THE CONSERVATIVE PARTY'S CHANGING FORTUNES

No sooner had John Major led his party to victory in April 1992 than his Government began to fall apart and like Humpty Dumpty nothing could put it back together again. In September 1992 Britain withdrew from the ERM and the image of a government floundering around unable to cope with a situation for which it was in part responsible – a previous Conservative Government under Mrs Thatcher had chosen to join the ERM – led to a massive loss of confidence in the Government. A sterling crisis under a Conservative Government was a new experience. Opinion polls which showed Labour out in front were confirmed in 1994 when the Conservatives gained 27 per cent of the votes cast in the local elections and 28 per cent in the European elections, a performance which put them on a par with the Liberal Democrats.

The Party's problems went from top to bottom. As well as appearing incompetent at running the economy, pit closures made the Government appear indifferent to the social problems in the country. Although John Major was one of the Party's assets, his image was a very mixed one. His rhetoric of wanting to create a classless society and a nation at ease with itself did not fit with a substantial section of the electorate's opinion of the state of the country or with the policies his Government pursued (Jones, H. 1997). While not himself linked with sleaze and immorality he appeared indifferent or unable to stamp out corrupt practices. His leadership appeared weak and dithering and although he tried to stamp his authority on the Party it was never entirely convincing, and this was confirmed by his taped off-the-record comment that he had three bastards (assumed to be Peter Lilley, Michael Portillo and John Redwood) in the Cabinet. In July 1993 the Government was defeated in the House of Commons over its European policy and the deep divisions over the Party's stance towards Europe remained unresolved. The Party organisation failed to keep pace with developments in IT and communications and the traditional constituency support for the Party was weak with fewer members and relatively few young ones; in 1994 the average age of Party members was 62. The Conservatives' failure to keep in touch with the mood of the country was partly due to its own policy of running-down local government, which had the knock-on effect of weakening the role of local Conservative politicians and the Party at the local level.

Although the economy improved after the recession of the early 1990s the country had little faith in these improvements being sustained and the 'feel good factor' never returned. Efforts to revitalise the Government backfired. The 'back to basics' call which was widely interpreted as referring to personal morality, although in fact this was never made explicit, made the Party seem hypocritical when too many ministers were found to have personal lives which did not live up to the rhetoric (see Evans and Taylor 1996 on the Conservatives). The Conservative Party's weaknesses stood in ever-sharper contrast to the new image emerging of the Labour Party with its modernised and youthful organisation and policies, dominated by men with an aura of incorruptibility.

LIFT-OFF WITH LABOUR

Labour inevitably gained from the unpopularity of the Conservatives, but this does not in itself explain Labour's landslide victory. It was also due to tactical voting and the organisational and policy changes which had begun in 1983 under Neil Kinnock, continued haltingly by John Smith, and pursued single-mindedly by Tony Blair. As argued above, the Labour Party has evolved throughout the twentieth century; it has constantly had to adapt to electoral and policy challenges. Indeed, all parties have had to adapt to survive. The careful balancing of principles and pragmatism is an on-going adjustment. After 1945 the Conservatives adapted to Keynesianism and the welfare state; the Labour Party has now adapted to market economics and Thatcherite values. The first post-war consensus was built on the Labour Party's terms, the second one on the Conservatives' terms. So, to see the current Labour Party as a 'new' party is to misunderstand where Labour has come from and how it pulled off the stunning victory of 1 May.

To stereotype the Labour Party as a bureaucratic, trade union dominated dinosaur until it was overhauled by Tony Blair is to focus on a relatively short period of its history. Blair's focus on values rather than specific pieces of policy is in line with the early Labour Party which was dominated by an ethical socialism. Labour's close association with state bureaucracy developed in the 1930s; it is most clearly identified with Labour in the 1940s and again with the Left-dominated party of the early 1980s. In the 1940s Labour's policies of nationalisation and building up a state bureaucracy, especially in the welfare field, was at the cutting edge of politics. The need to broaden the electoral base of Labour and develop its policies was taken up by Harold Wilson in the 1960s when the Party was again associated with youth, modernisation and technology. To see Blair's organisational and policy upheavals as a new departure in terms of strategy is misleading.

By the 1980s a new wave of reforms was inevitable if the Labour Party was ever to win power again. The electoral base had moved on again since the 1960s, the economy had been restructured, new social issues had emerged while old social problems had intensified. The old powers of local authorities, trade unions and manufacturing producers had gone. A life cycle in which certain activities were associated with particular age groups had disappeared and become more fluid, and social policies needed to respond to this change. The defeat of 1992 taught the Party a number of important lessons: to take nothing for granted; to control the media; to remove from the policy commitments anything which could frighten floating voters (particularly the possibility of higher income taxes and a revival of trade union power); and to appeal to a broad swathe of voters, not solely composed of a rainbow alliance of sectional interests (see Adelman 1996; Davies 1992 on Labour).

Since 1983 the Labour Party had been rethinking and adapting to changing circumstances. Foote provides the best analysis of the evolution of Labour's political thought. He shows that from 1983 onwards there was a gradual rejection of corporate socialism. In its place Kinnock tried to revive old Labour values of community and political democracy with an emphasis on an enabling, not a bureaucratic, state. He also tried to provide a clear moral alternative to Mrs Thatcher's cold-blooded free-market strategy. These values continued to be emphasised by Tony Blair and Gordon Brown. Blair's vision of community assumed common interests and objectives, and relied heavily on the notion of partnership with everyone having a stake in society. Brown highlighted the relevance of these values to a dynamic economy for the twenty-first century by underlining the role of an enabling state in developing lifelong education and skills so that individuals could take personal responsibility for their lives in the market place and thus avoid poverty. The enabling state was also one which had undergone constitutional reform so that all aspects of society would be modernised (Foote 1997). The process of modernisation began with the Labour Party itself.

The two defining moments in Labour's road to victory came in the Autumn of 1994 at the Annual Labour Party Conference when Blair announced plans to rework Clause 4 and in January 1997 when Brown announced that Labour would not raise the basic rate of income tax. There was also much activity behind the scenes which was building a Party machine to take on the Conservatives. Labour wooed the tabloids and business. In October 1995 it bought the Excalibur software package in which huge amounts of information could be stored and retrieved instantly, thus offering the possibility of instant rebuttal to anything the Conservatives might throw at them. It also meant that all those in the Party could be closely monitored and prevented from going off-message. Media, research and campaigning teams were integrated at Millbank Towers (Jones, N. 1997: 20–9). Adaptations of electioneering techniques, including new means of controlling the media, which have dominated discussion of new Labour, should not detract from the need to place social policies during Blair's first term in the context of policy developments up to the point at which Labour entered Office and began to set its own agenda. This book provides that context.

The key new Labour values of modernisation, stakeholding, opportunity, personal responsibility and financial independence, efficiency, trust, partnership and communitarianism are behind many of the policies advocated by Labour. The policies, as the following chapters show, display strong continuities with the preceding Conservative governments. Common themes in policies which have been carried over include consumerism, value for money, standards, competition and choice, flexibility and deregulation, and financial stringency in resourcing. These themes, however, are now mixed with other ones which were not prioritised by the Conservatives. The new Government is recognising that socioeconomic deprivation excludes sections of society from the opportunity to be financially independent and secure, to share in the common good life, and to enjoy a genuine stake in society. The Government is placing far greater emphasis on life-long learning and skills for life. Above all, Labour, by emphasising the need for trust during the campaign, has staked a great deal not only on the policies it pursues but also the manner in which it pursues them.

Focusing on values rather than specific policies had the advantage of not alienating any voter who did not like a particular policy. Thus, as the following chapters show, Labour presented its policies in terms of the Party's core values.

Avoiding detailed policy discussion had the disadvantage of not offering clear blue water between the Labour and the Conservative Party. It meant that issues other than specific policies had to be addressed at the election. The Conservative Party, however, played into the hands of Labour, as it was especially vulnerable to charges that its values had been corrupted as stories of sleaze and broken election promises regularly hit the headlines. Labour made a double gain by focusing on its values and undermining the way in which the Conservative Party operated, which Labour characterised as being corrupt and dishonest, with a selfish and irresponsible disregard for the social fabric of society. Fear of a future under the Conservatives was made as much of as the Conservatives' record. When the Conservative record was tackled it was the corruption not the policies which were focused on because, of course, as a number of the following chapters show, Labour had incorporated key aspects of Conservative social policies into its own programme.

On 1 May 1997 the potential for radical reform was certainly present. The desire for change and the overwhelming importance of social issues to voters meant that there was an expectation that the election would be a watershed. An ICM recall survey on Polling Day asked respondents who had voted Labour why they had done so. The main reason given by 40 per cent was that it was time for a change; 39 per cent explained that they were mainly influenced by health and welfare state policies. 36 per cent said that the issue of education was most important to them. Only 19 per cent said that they voted Labour because they always supported the Party (quoted in the *Guardian* 3 May 1997). The development of social policies under Labour will be crucial to an assessment of the extent to which 1 May was the watershed which many hoped for when they responded to the Labour Party's call to trust it to govern. Only time will tell the extent to which new Labour can build a new Britain on foundations laid by both the Conservatives and its own traditional values.

REFERENCES

The section on the course of the campaign is based on a daily reading of the broadsheets and a selection of the tabloids.

Adelman, P. (1996) *The Rise of the Labour Party, 1880–1945*, London: Longman (first published 1972).

Butler, D. and Kavanagh, D. (1974) *The British General Election, February 1974*, London: Macmillan.

—— (1975) *The British General Election, October 1975*, London: Macmillan.

Butler, D. and King, A. (1965) *The British General Election of 1964*, London: Macmillan.

Butler, D. and Rose, R. (1960) *The British General Election of 1959*, London: Macmillan.

Caesar, J. and Busch, A. (1993) *Upside Down and Inside Out: The 1992 Elections and American Politics*, Lanham, Maryland: Littlefield Adams Quality Paperbacks.

Council of Churches (1997) *Unemployment and the Future of Work*, London: Council of Churches.

Cowling, M. (1971) *The Impact of Labour*, Cambridge: Cambridge University Press.

Davies, A.J. (1992) *To Build A New Jerusalem: The British Labour Movement from the 1880s to the 1990s*, London: Michael Joseph.

Evans, B. and Taylor, A. (1996) *From Salisbury to Major: Continuity and Change in Conservative Politics*, Manchester: Manchester University Press.

Foote, G. (1997) *The Labour Party's Political Thought: A History*, London: Macmillan, 3rd edn, first published by Croom Helm London in 1985.

Jones, H. (1997) (ed.) *Towards a Classless Society?*, London: Routledge.

Jones, N. (1997) *Campaign 1997: How the General Election was Won and Lost*, London: Indigo.

King, A. (1997) 'Tactical voting turned loss into a rout', *Daily Telegraph* 3 May 1997.

Maltese, J.A. (1994 edn) *Spin Control*, Chapel Hill: University of North Carolina Press (first published 1992).

Chapter 2

Managing the welfare state

Tony Butcher

The organisational arrangements for the delivery of social services have been a key theme in social policy developments since the election of the first Thatcher Government in 1979. The Thatcher and Major administrations launched a series of radical initiatives in the organisation and management of the welfare state. These developments challenged the traditional public administration model of welfare delivery – with its emphasis on efficient and impartial bureaucracy, the central role of professionals and the concept of public accountability – which had been associated with the post-war welfare state. A new paradigm emerged – sometimes described as 'the new public management' – which emphasised a more managerialist and consumerist approach to the organisation of the public sector. (See Butcher 1995 for a fuller discussion of both the public administration model and developments prior to 1997.)

By the mid-1990s, there was a growing consensus on the application of the doctrines of the new public management to the organisation and management of the state (Farnham and Horton 1996: 259). These ideas were reflected in the plans for managing the welfare state advanced by the two major political parties during the 1997 election campaign. However, before examining these proposals, it is necessary to review the developments of the Thatcher and Major years.

MANAGING THE WELFARE STATE UNDER THE THATCHER AND MAJOR GOVERNMENTS

The 1980s and 1990s saw the emergence of a number of new ideas on the organisation and management of the welfare state. These developments were part of a wider movement from the traditional bureaucratic model of public administration to the 'new public management', the central doctrines of which consist of an emphasis on value for money; clear standards and measures of performance; the disaggregation of large bureaucratic organisations; the promotion of greater competition through the use of market-type mechanisms; and the customer orientation (see, for example, Hood 1991: 4–5).

One manifestation of the new public management during the period of the Thatcher and Major Governments was the increased emphasis on obtaining value for money in the public sector. Within central government departments, the Rayner scrutinies introduced by the first Thatcher Government were concerned with uncovering inefficiency and waste, while the Financial Management Initiative, launched in 1981, involved moves towards delegated authority and accountable management. The first Thatcher Government also created the Audit Commission, with responsibility for ensuring value for money in local authorities. The development of such initiatives as cost improvement programmes, the Resource Management Initiative and general management were directed at improving efficiency in the National Health Service.

Another key element in attempts to improve the efficiency of the delivery agencies of the welfare state was the introduction of a more performance-based culture as characterised by the setting of targets and the introduction of performance measurement. Performance indicators became an important feature of the new managerialism. The setting of targets was central to the operations of the Benefits Agency, Employment Service and other Next Steps agencies responsible for the delivery of social security benefits. As a result of the Major Government's Citizen's Charter, local authorities were required to measure their performance in such areas as housing accommodation and the provision of personal social services against indicators drawn up by the Audit Commission. Since 1992 state schools have had to publish annual statistics on examination results. Performance indicators also became an important element in the management of the NHS, enabling comparisons to be made between different health authorities. This increased emphasis on results-oriented organisations was further manifested in such initiatives as the use of performance-related pay across the public sector.

There was also an emphasis on market-type mechanisms, involving contracting out and competition. The use of the contractual approach in the public services – entailing the separation of the responsibility for deciding the type of service required from the responsibility for delivering it – characterised several reforms in the management of the welfare state during the 1980s and early 1990s (Harden 1992: 14). Thus the Next Steps programme, introduced in 1988 by the Thatcher Government and developed by the Major Administration, separated the executive and policy-making roles of central government departments. The programme resulted in the creation of a range of semi-autonomous executive agencies, such as the Benefits Agency, the Employment Service and the Child Support Agency, responsible for the delivery of social and other services. Next Steps agencies have framework documents, annual business plans and medium-term corporate plans which form 'contracts' between ministers and the agency chief executives, specifying agency objectives, finances and freedoms. The development of this 'management by contract' was followed in the early 1990s by a move to 'management of contract', with the Major Government's market testing initiative requiring the Benefits Agency and other executive agencies to test the cost of providing services in-house against the cost of purchasing them from the private sector (Greer 1994: 59–80). The introduction of compulsory competitive tendering (CCT) in both local government and the NHS during the 1980s was another manifestation of the separation of the purchaser and provider functions. The use of contract was also a feature of the Conservatives' NHS reforms in the early 1990s, which created an 'internal market' in health care, in which district health authorities and fundholding GPs purchased health care services from NHS trusts, other directly managed units and the private sector.

Another central principle of the new public management is its emphasis on the needs of the consumers of public services – the customer orientation. Several pieces of legislation in the late 1980s – notably the Education Reform Act of 1988 and the Housing Act of the same year – attempted to provide the consumers of social services with greater choice. However, the centrepiece of Conservative government attempts to empower the consumer was the Citizen's Charter introduced by the Major Government in 1991. The Charter highlighted the need for the provision of more information about public services through the publication of service standards and details of performance, as well as stressing the importance of consultation, helpful staff and well publicised and easily available complaints procedures. The main delivery agencies of the welfare state – Next Steps agencies, local authorities and the institutions of the NHS – were all required to pay more attention to the position of the users of public services. The publication of the Charter was followed by the launching of a number of individual service charters for various groups, including the parents of school-age children, NHS patients, council house tenants, job seekers and those receiving social security benefits.

A number of organisational changes in the institutions of the welfare state – involving the disaggregation of large monolithic welfare bureaucracies – also took place under the Thatcher and Major administrations. At the national level, the Next Steps programme created semi-autonomous executive agencies responsible for the delivery of social and other services. The initiative transformed the structure – as well as the culture – of the two central government departments responsible for the delivery of social security benefits. By 1997, nearly all of the staff of the giant Department of Social Security worked in semi-autonomous executive agencies such as the Benefits Agency and the Child Support Agency. The day-to-day delivery of the social security benefits administered by the Department for Education and Employment was in the hands of another Next Steps agency, the Employment Service.

At the sub-national level, the organisation of the three major social services traditionally delivered by local authorities was also dramatically affected. The role of many local education authorities – seen by critics as bureaucratic and self-interested – as direct deliverers of education was downgraded as a result of the encouragement of state schools to opt out of local education authority control and acquire grant maintained status with funding coming directly from central government. Local education authorities also lost responsibilities to further education corporations and city technology colleges. In the field of council housing, the 'right to buy' legislation of the 1980s reduced the role of local housing authorities – seen by the Conservative Government, like local education authorities, as being dominated by bureaucratic and professional self-interests – by requiring them to sell off much of their housing stock. Government policy subsequently emphasised the importance of housing associations in the development and provision of social housing, and a large number of local housing authorities transferred housing stock to local community housing associations through the large-scale voluntary transfer scheme. Housing Action Trusts, with government appointed boards, were set up in parts of the country to take over and renovate selected council estates. Local authority social service departments were also affected. Responding to the recommendations of the 1988 Griffiths Report, Conservative government policy in the 1990s was to require social services departments to make greater use of the private and voluntary sectors in the provision of community care (Griffiths 1988).

The organisation of the other major sub-national delivery agency of the welfare state – the NHS – also underwent radical reform, with the introduction in 1991 of the purchaser–provider split as part of the Conservative government's internal market system. A central component of this new system was the opportunity for hospitals and other provider units to apply to opt out of management by local health authorities and become self-governing NHS trusts. Run by boards of directors appointed by, and directly accountable to, the Secretary of State for Health, trusts were given considerable managerial freedoms, including the power to employ their own staff and to borrow money. By 1997, trusts delivered almost all hospital and community health services.

Thus the transformation of the organisation and management of the social services – at the national and sub-national levels – was a key feature of social policy during the Thatcher and Major years. Although not taken up by politicians and the media during the 1997 campaign, the management of the welfare state was an important element in Conservative and Labour plans for social policy, both in the manifestos and in policy announcements in the period leading up to the election. We can identify three key issues in these plans: the debate on the role of elected local authorities in the welfare state; the consensus on the need to improve the management and efficiency of delivery agencies; and the recognition of the importance of the customer orientation in the delivery of social services.

LOCAL GOVERNMENT AND THE DELIVERY OF WELFARE

Conservative plans for local government involved the continuation of the restructuring process which had taken place under the Thatcher and Major Governments. The Conservative Party's vision of the role of local government was that of the 'enabling local authority'. Local authorities should no longer be the direct providers of services, but should concentrate on setting priorities, deciding standards and finding the best ways of providing services. As the Conservatives stated in their election manifesto, local authorities 'can enable things to happen rather than necessarily running them themselves' (Conservative Party 1997: 30).

Thus it was the clear intention of the Conservatives to continue with the downgrading of local education authorities, the manifesto stating that the ultimate objective was 'that all schools should take full responsibility for the management of their own affairs' (Conservative Party 1997: 23). A central plank in this policy of diminishing the role of local education authorities was to build upon earlier legislation which had encouraged the creation of grant maintained schools. The manifesto reaffirmed that state schools would be encouraged to opt out of local education authority control. However, given the limited success of the grant-maintained schools policy – only 1,188 schools (some 5 per cent of the 24,500 state secondary and primary schools) had opted out of local education authority control by the time of the 1997 election –potentially the most far-reaching aspect of Conservative plans for the delivery of local education was the proposal to create 'locally maintained schools'. Legislation was promised which would convert all state schools into legal entities, with charitable status and the ability to borrow against their assets. It was intended that such schools would take over a range of services controlled by local education authorities, including responsibility for the employment of staff and the allocation of school places. Local education authorities would be left with responsibility for administering budgets, monitoring standards and co-ordinating admissions.

The Labour Party's original intention, as outlined in its 1992 manifesto, had been to re-absorb grant maintained schools into local education authorities. In the event, in a policy document published in 1995 (Labour Party 1995b), Labour stated that it would convert grant maintained schools into 'foundation' schools, with no financial privileges and with local education authority representatives on their governing bodies. The work of the Funding Agency for Schools – the quasi-governmental body established to superintend the payment and monitoring of central government grants to grant maintained schools – would be devolved to local education authorities, who would also be responsible for determining agreed admissions policies for their areas. Local education authorities were seen as playing a new role as 'champions of their parents and communities [and] creating a framework which increases the chances of schools succeeding' (Labour Party 1995b: 14). In contrast to the Conservatives – whose long-term aim was seen by some as the eventual withering away of local education authorities – Labour's plans were seen by defenders of the grant maintained school system as a way of restoring control of education to local education authorities (see, for example, Balchin 1997).

The Conservatives also planned to further reduce the role of local housing authorities, announcing that up to two million council properties would be transferred to the private sector over the next decade. Conservative policy also encouraged the development of public–private partnerships in the field of social housing. Labour also proposed to make use of the private sector in its attempts to develop social housing, and the Party's housing spokesman talked of encouraging the creation of new partnerships through local housing companies, in which local authorities have a holding. As one commentator observed, although the presentation of Conservative and Labour policies on council housing had a different emphasis, the thrust was the same (Rowlatt 1997).

The two main parties also emphasised the use of the private and voluntary sectors in the personal social services. In line with its 'marketisation' approach, the Major Government's plans included the requirement that local authorities contract out residential and domiciliary care services to private and voluntary sector organisations if they could show that they could deliver services more efficiently. Labour, on the other hand, promised to allow local authorities to make their own decisions about whether or not to use the private and voluntary sectors.

The two main parties were divided on the role of local government in the welfare state. The Conservative Party promised to develop 'a new vision' for local government, continuing its attempts to transform local authorities from their traditional role as direct deliverers of services to that of purchasers – the enabling authority. A wider interpretation of the enabling concept emphasises the role of a local authority in using all the powers at its disposal to meet the needs of the local community (see Clarke and Stewart 1988: 1). The Labour Party also had a wider view of the role of local government. In a policy paper on local government published in 1995, Labour argued that local authorities should be given greater freedom to respond to local needs through a new power of 'community initiative' (Labour Party 1995a: 12). The Labour manifesto promised that a Labour government would place on local authorities a new duty to promote the economic and social well-being of their areas.

Labour was also concerned about the need to enhance the accountability of the local welfare state, being very critical of the development of non-elected bodies as delivery agencies of social services at the local level. The growth of such appointed bodies as the governing bodies of grant maintained schools, further education corporations, Housing Action Trusts, housing associations and NHS trusts had given rise to concern among defenders of local democracy about the creation of a 'new magistracy' (see, for example, Stewart 1992). Labour's position on non-elected bodies was that public money should normally be spent by elected individuals, and it had been examining how to restore an elected element to such bodies (see, for example, the oral evidence of Jack Straw, shadow Home Secretary, to the Nolan Committee, Prime Minister 1995: 342).

IMPROVING MANAGEMENT AND EFFICIENCY

As we saw earlier, a key feature of Conservative government policy towards the public sector during the 1980s and 1990s was the emphasis on improved management and efficiency, including the introduction of the 'contract culture'. The need to improve the efficiency and management of the delivery agencies of the welfare state is now a key feature of Labour policies. Thus the 1997 Labour manifesto promised that the Audit Commission – a major instrument of Conservative attempts to encourage efficiency and value for money in local government and the NHS – would be given additional powers to monitor performance and encourage efficiency. On the Commission's advice, a Labour government would, where necessary, send in 'a management team' with powers to remedy failure (Labour Party 1997: 34). As we shall see in the next section, performance indicators are also an important feature of both parties' approaches to public services.

Another manifestation of the search for efficiency and value for money under Conservative governments – Next Steps agencies – is now an established part of the landscape of public administration, particularly in the delivery of social security benefits. The initiative has all-party support and in 1995 the then Labour shadow minister for public services, Derek Foster, stated that a future Labour government would want to maintain Next Steps agencies – 'most are working reasonably well' (Foster 1996: 261). The Major Government's previously announced long-term plans for enhancing efficiency in the civil service had included the continuation of the market testing process and other management techniques.

The Conservatives also reaffirmed the importance of competition as a means of achieving value for money and improving the quality of local authority services. Their manifesto stated that, if re-elected, they would maintain the pressure for higher standards and better value for money by insisting on CCT. Labour, on the other hand, argued in their manifesto that local authorities should not be required to put their services out to tender. CCT would be abolished and local authorities would be required to obtain 'best value' for services. Rather than having to accept the cheapest bid, local authorities should be able to choose higher quality bids which may turn out to be more cost effective (Labour Party 1995a: 9).

There were also differences in the two main parties' approaches towards improving efficiency in the NHS. The Conservatives claimed that the internal market reforms were a success, while the Labour manifesto referred to an NHS 'strangled by costly red tape'. It promised to abolish the internal market, although it would maintain the division between what it described as the 'necessary and distinct' functions of planning and provision of health care (Labour Party 1997: 20). There was to be no return to a system of top-down management. Labour was also committed to cutting the costs of NHS 'bureaucracy', which had increased by £1.5 billion a year since the introduction of the internal market. On the issue of GP fund-holding, Labour moved from previous promises to abolish fund-holding to a pledge to introduce a system in which local commissioning groups of GPs and nurses would 'take the lead in combining together locally to plan local health services' (Labour Party 1997: 21).

The Major Government's plans for the management of the personal social services involved requiring local authority social services departments to follow the NHS model of the purchaser–provider split. In a white paper published only six weeks before the election (Department of Health 1997), the Government argued that local authority social services departments should no longer be direct providers of residential and home care services for the elderly, but should purchase such services. If elected, a Conservative government would have introduced market testing for much of the delivery of the personal social services. Local authorities would have been required to contract out these services if private or voluntary providers could have demonstrated that they could run them more efficiently. The Labour Party rejected the privatisation of care homes, believing that local authorities should be free to develop a mixture of public and private care.

THE CUSTOMER ORIENTATION

As befits a policy seen by some commentators as Mr Major's 'big idea', the Citizen's Charter was an important element of the Conservative Party's plans to take the public sector into the next century. In a White Paper (Prime Minister 1996) published some seven months before the election, the Major Government made it clear that it intended to develop the Charter programme further. The election manifesto itself promised to build upon previous reforms and deliver even better quality public services, undertaking to require all government agencies to apply for the Charter Mark, the award given to organisations which develop excellence in delivering services. Labour was also committed to many of the ideas underpinning the Citizen's Charter. Indeed, when the Charter had first been announced in 1991, Labour had accused the prime minister of stealing the idea, its 1987 election manifesto having proposed a Quality Commission to ensure efficient, responsive and high quality local authority services. Labour had also pioneered the ideas of the Charter through such developments as customer service contracts in York and other local authorities. Thus 'the spirit of the Charter initiative is one which unites, rather than divides, the major political parties' (Rao 1996: 179).

A central component of the customer orientation, and the Citizen's Charter, is the provision of information and the publication of details of performance. The Conservative Party manifesto re-emphasised the importance of more information for the consumers of social services. Thus the section on education promised 'full information' on the performance of schools. There was also a pledge to publish more information on how successfully NHS hospitals are treating patients (Conservative Party 1997: 21 and 27).

The Conservatives had long been committed to targets and performance measurement and the Labour Party now fully embraced this approach. Thus the Labour manifesto promised that each local authority would be required to publish a local performance plan which would include targets for service improvement. Labour also believed that the Audit Commission should give more emphasis to raising standards, suggesting that it could be refocused to incorporate a Standards Inspectorate (Labour Party 1995a: 11). This emphasis on high standards of performance was also reflected in the requirement that local education authorities draw up education development plans detailing how standards will be raised and setting clear targets (Labour Party 1995b: 14). The Conservative manifesto promised to set national targets for school performance and to require individual schools to set targets which relate to national standards.

Both parties also emphasised the importance of performance in the NHS. The Conservative manifesto's promise to publish more information on hospital treatment was directed at helping to 'stimulate better performance' (Conservative Party 1997: 27). The Labour manifesto stated that hospitals would be required to meet high quality targets, with management held to account for levels of performance. Such indicators would place a greater emphasis on measures of quality, with Labour promising a new Patient's Charter emphasising the quality and success of treatment.

Thus, whichever of the two main parties formed the next government, the ideas of charterism looked set to continue. A major criticism of the Charter approach, however, is that it is essentially concerned with fostering the responsiveness of public services – the customer orientation – and ignores the wider meaning of 'citizenship'. In the words of one commentator, the Charter reflects a 'managerial top-down approach' (Bynoe 1996: iv). Citizenship, on the other hand, is about encouraging participation in decision making (see Butcher 1995: 153; Bynoe 1996). A recent report by the Institute for Public Policy Research – a 'think-tank' with close links with the Labour Party – clearly recognises this distinction, recommending that one way forward for the Charter is to develop such initiatives as citizens' juries (Bynoe 1996: 129). This and other devices for revitalising local democracy were included in a Labour Party policy document published in 1995 (Labour Party 1995a: 13), and the Labour manifesto itself promised greater accountability and the encouragement of 'democratic innovations' in local government.

CONCLUSIONS

The Conservative governments of the 1980s and 1990s transformed the organisation and management of the welfare state. A system underpinned by the assumptions of the public administration model of welfare delivery, and dominated by central government departments, elected local authorities and the institutions of the NHS, was gradually replaced by a new set of assumptions and practices associated with the new public management and its emphasis on managerialism and the consumerist ethos. These developments went far beyond the use of private sector management techniques: they involved 'a new way of thinking about the state' (Ridley 1995: 19).

The Labour Party was initially hostile to such developments and the ideas and assumptions associated with them. Thus, the main focus of Labour's proposals for social policy in the 1987 manifesto was not on managerialism, but on the development of policies to meet welfare needs (Cutler and Waine 1994: 137). However, as Cutler and Waine (1994: 137–8) have pointed out, the 1990s saw a growing consensus between the two main parties on the management of the welfare state. Labour's 1992 election manifesto embraced the vocabulary of targets and performance in its proposal that health authorities have Performance Agreements which set local targets (Labour Party 1992: 16). In what was seen as an attempt to outmanoeuvre the Conservatives, the 1992 manifesto also espoused a consumerist ethos (Cutler and Waine 1994: 138, 45). Thus Labour proposed the appointment of a Health Quality Commission and an Education Standards Commission. It also promised to set up a Quality Commission (incorporating the work of the Audit Commission), develop customer contracts for local authority services and require local authorities to carry out annual surveys of customer satisfaction.

By the time of the 1997 general election, the Labour Party had clearly adopted much of the language, and many of the practices, of the new public management which had been such a feature of Conservative government approaches to public sector reform in the 1980s and 1990s. Although there were concerns about accountability, there was a general acceptance of the break up of central government departments into Next Steps agencies. Targets and performance were key elements in the 1997 manifesto, although Labour placed more emphasis on quality of service indicators in defining performance targets. Although Labour promised to abolish the NHS internal market, the purchaser–provider split – now labelled planning and provision – was to remain. The Audit Commission was to remain a key instrument in the promotion of efficiency in local authorities. Even though CCT was to be replaced by a 'best value' approach, the contracting out of local authority services would continue to be a feature of local service delivery.

The terminology of managerialism and consumerism was also to be found in the early pronouncements of Mr Blair's newly-elected Government. Thus a major item in the programme of legislation set out in the Queen's Speech two weeks after the election victory was an education bill intended to raise the standards of local education and set local education authorities improvement targets. The Government's commitment to a performance-based culture was reinforced by the announcement of new-style NHS performance indicators assessing the quality of treatment. Other early initiatives included the announcement that selected local authorities would pilot the 'best value' regime intended to replace CCT.

Thus, despite the changes in emphasis of the new Labour Government, there is much continuity with the approaches of the previous administration. The clock will not be put back to the old public administration model of welfare delivery. However, the assumptions, practices and consequences of the new public management raise important issues. Developments in the management of the welfare state since the early 1980s have given rise to a number of concerns – the proper role of elected local government, and its relationship with central government, in the delivery of public services; the way in which the fragmentation of public services has reduced accountability; the 'democratic deficit' created by the growth of non-elected bodies; the narrow view of citizenship contained in the charterism approach.

There are welcome signs that the Blair Government recognises these concerns. One of its first actions was to sign the Council of Europe's Charter of Local Self-Government, which commits signatory member states to guarantee 'the right and ability of local authorities, within the limits of the law, to regulate and manage a substantial share of public affairs under their own responsibility and in the interests of the local population'. In the same week, the new government's minister for local government, Hilary Armstrong, promised to begin a new partnership between central and local government and to 'reinvigorate' local government (Calpin 1997). Labour's recognition of the defects of the local 'quango state' was reflected in the early announcement that the membership of the boards of health authorities and NHS trusts would be made more representative of their local communities.

Much more radical changes may follow. In its submission to the Nolan Committee on Standards in Public Life, the Labour Party called for a process of 'democratic renewal' and a Governance of Britain Act. The principles on which this would be based included the greater decentralisation of government to ensure the direct involvement of citizens in local decision-making and the increased responsiveness of public services to people's needs; greater transparency so that governmental processes are more open; and more accountability to enable government and the public services to be subject to proper democratic scrutiny at national and local levels (see Foster

1996: 258). Labour clearly recognised that, by themselves, measures to improve the efficiency and responsiveness of the delivery agencies of the welfare state are insufficient. Managerial changes need to be accompanied by wider political and constitutional reform.

REFERENCES

Balchin, B. (1997) 'Leave our fine schools alone', *The Times*, 4 April.

Butcher, T. (1995) *Delivering Welfare: The Governance of the Social Services in the 1990s*, Buckingham: Open University Press.

Bynoe, I. (1996) *Beyond the Citizen's Charter: New Directions for Social Rights*, London: Institute for Public Policy Research.

Calpin, D. (1997) 'Armstrong's radical reforms set style for central/local relations', *Municipal Journal*, 6 June.

Clarke, M. and Stewart, J. (1988) *The Enabling Council: Developing and Managing A New Style of Local Government*, Luton: Local Government Training Board.

Conservative Party (1997) *You Can Only Be Sure With The Conservatives*, election manifesto, London: Conservative Central Office.

Cutler, T. and Waine, B. (1994) *Managing the Welfare State: The Politics of Public Sector Management*, Oxford: Berg.

Department of Health (1997) *Social Services: Achievement and Challenge*, Cm 3588, London: HMSO.

Farnham, D. and Horton, S. (eds) (1996) *Managing the New Public Services*, 2nd edn, Basingstoke: Macmillan.

Foster, D. (1996) 'Labour and public sector reform', *Parliamentary Affairs*, 49, 2: 256–61.

Greer. P. (1994) *Transforming Central Government: The Next Steps Initiative*, Buckingham: Open University Press.

Griffiths. R. (1988) *Community Care: Agenda for Action*, London: HMSO.

Harden, I. (1992) *The Contracting State*, Buckingham: Open University Press.

Hood, C. (1991) 'A public management for all seasons', *Public Administration*, 69, 1: 3–19.

Labour Party (1992) *It's Time to Get Britain Working Again*, election manifesto, London: Labour Party.

—— (1995a) *Renewing Democracy: Rebuilding Communities*, London: Labour Party.

—— (1995b) *Diversity and Excellence: A New Partnership for Schools*, London: Labour Party.

—— (1997) *New Labour: Because Britain Deserves Better*, election manifesto, London: Labour Party.

Prime Minister (1995) *Standards in Public Life: First Report of the Committee on Standards in Public Life*, Vol.2: Transcripts of Oral Evidence, Cm. 2850-II, London: HMSO.

Prime Minister (1996) *The Citizen's Charter – Five Years On*, Cm. 3370, London: HMSO.

Rao, N. (1996) *Towards Welfare Pluralism: Public Services in an Era of Change*, Aldershot: Dartmouth.

Ridley, F. F. (1995) 'Towards a skeleton state? Changes to public sector management', in J. Wilson (ed.) *Managing Public Services: Dealing With Dogma*, Eastham: Tudor.

Rowlatt, J. (1997) 'Rise of the sell-off solution', *Guardian*, 2 April.

Stewart, J. (1992) 'The rebuilding of public accountability', in J. Stewart, N. Lewis, and D. Longley, *Accountability and the Public*, London: European Policy Forum.

Chapter 3

Taxing and spending the people's money

Susanne MacGregor

SHIFTING IDEOLOGIES OF WELFARE

Public expenditure is at the heart of social policy. The 1976 spending cuts, on conditions imposed on a Labour government by the IMF, marked the end of the great expansion of the welfare state. Since then, although demands and needs have grown, restraining public expenditure has dominated thinking on social policy.

Debate about the appropriate extent of state action was continuous throughout the fifty years that followed the 1940s reforms. Over this same period, living standards in Britain more than doubled (Jacobs 1996: 82). But more recent increases in material wealth were accompanied by increased poverty and inequality (Joseph Rowntree Foundation 1995; McFate *et al.* 1995) and, some argue, a decline in the quality of life (Jacobs 1996: 82). The critical questions on public expenditure now are:

1 How much of their increased income and wealth are people prepared to devote to paying for human services as opposed to other consumption goods?
2 Which, if any, of these should be financed and provided *publicly* (with all sharing on the same terms and conditions and contributing collectively) and which *privately* (by commercial or non-government organisations and paid for individually through cash, personal or occupational insurance)?
3 How much are people willing to forgo of their own current income either to plan for contingencies at different points in the life cycle (or when they or their family may become dependent) or to support those who are less fortunate than themselves?

Few people have a firm grasp on what they pay into and what they gain from public finance (see Figures 3.1 and 3.2). Although 'taxes' as an issue may be a little different from the issue of 'paying for welfare', the fact that such a high proportion of government expenditure goes on 'welfare' or into 'social areas' means that there is a close connection between the two. But the mixed economy of care is complex. The shift from direct to indirect taxation, and shifts between tax allowances and cash benefits, obscure the facts. Mixtures of private and public financing and of private and public provision of services add to the difficulty. Inflation complicates calculations comparing trends over time. With such technical problems, one might expect debate about paying for welfare to be a political no-go area. Yet this is clearly not the case. The tax–spend issue is central to electoral behaviour.

With the move from a 1940s citizenship to a 1960s more egalitarian model of social policy and thence to a 1980s quasi-market approach, the meaning and impact of taxation for the electorate have changed. The social solidarity of the old welfare state rested on a shared awareness of risk (Baldwin 1990: 10–21). Now, increasing social diversity has reduced the range of risks considered to be so general and uniform as to justify collective financing and universalistic provision. 'There but for fortune go you and I' is less often felt to be the case. Debate switched from how to provide optimum standards to all, to how much or how little to provide for emergencies or to meet basic needs, and on what conditions such provision might be made available. The view began to gain ground that a more efficient system would be one where individuals made their own arrangements to suit their own circumstances. The state's role would be to provide a basic minimum floor and to regulate the social market.

But as these ideas gained ground, there grew also increasing concern about social breakdown, indicated especially by rising rates of crime and disorder. Perhaps, some argued, state involvement, public expenditure and taxation were needed to weld things together, to encourage social cohesion and overcome exclusion (Dahrendorf Report 1995). Leaving things to the market left too many gaps in the spaces-in-between, between the corporations, families, associations, and other groups identified as key players in the quasi-market social economy. The reconstruction of the public sphere would require public provision, thus increased taxation and public expenditure, (Hutton 1995).

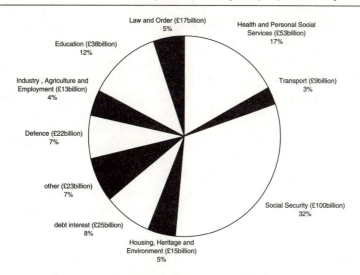

Figure 3.1 Current spending (£billion – 1,000 million)
Source: Government spending plans 1997–98, adapted from 1997 Liberal Democrat manifesto, page 63

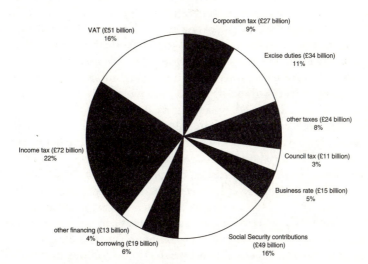

Figure 3.2 Current taxation (£billion – 1,000 million)
Source: Government revenue plans 1997–98 adapted from 1997 Liberal Democrat manifesto, page 63

CONTROLLING PUBLIC EXPENDITURE

The share of the national income which contributed to financing education, housing, health, income maintenance, and social care services grew roughly tenfold over the twentieth century (from about 2.6 per cent to about 25 per cent). Half of this amount covered transfer payments (cash benefits largely through social security). But also, as income increased in post-war years, half of the additional gains went on public services, a rising share on education and social services provided at local government level, which had implications for a Treasury needing to control inflation.

Increases seemed inexorable. The shape of public expenditure changed (with shifts from housing to unemployment provision, for example), there were some changes at the margins, and the culture and conditions of provision altered, but the underlying rise was left untouched by even radical Thatcher governments. The high point of 55.7 per cent of total government spending being welfare expenditure (education, health, housing, personal social services and social security) in 1977/8 was almost equalled in 1987/8 at 55.6 per cent. As a percentage of GDP, welfare spending stayed in a range from 21 to 25 per cent between 1973/4 and 1987/8, just before the third term Thatcher administration put social policy at the top of its agenda. Yet even these ambitions were undermined by boom and bust economic cycles. In the 1990s, the aim to control public expenditure and reduce taxes had to give way to the goal to reduce the burgeoning public sector borrowing requirement (PSBR). The deep recession prior to the 1992 election had 'forced unplanned expenditure on benefits *and* the government [had] needed tax cuts to win the election' (Glennerster 1997: 62). The PSBR rose to nearly 8 per cent of GDP in 1993/4.

Cash limits have had a disciplining effect. And in the 1990s, reforms in Treasury processes aimed to tighten the link between tax and spending decisions and budget announcements. Some very tough expenditure rounds were carried through in 1994 and 1995 (Glennerster 1997: 65). The effect has been further to increase the power of the Treasury *vis-à-vis* spending departments. As ever, the areas most vulnerable to impact are capital expenditures and public sector pay. Capital expenditure on major programmes (in absolute terms) fell from £16bn in 1975 to £8bn in 1995. In 1974, £7bn was spent by the government on house building; in 1995, this sum was £1.9bn.

From the mid-1980s to the mid-1990s, direct income taxation on the highest income groups was reduced while other forms of taxation rose. Central government came to control a very large share of local government expenditure. Public expenditure has been restrained but not radically reduced. The introduction of private sector business disciplines and limiting the influence of professionals and lobby groups (with a move from a paternalistic to a quasi-market welfare state), helped to reverse the upward trend. But public expenditure still accounted for 43 per cent of national income in the mid-1990s. The tax reductions of the 1980s were wiped out by the tax increases of the early 1990s.

Getting budgets under control is now the goal of all OECD economies, actively promoted by the IMF. Tight fiscal control means cuts in public spending, especially if public sector borrowing is too high.

In February 1993, the Conservative government announced it would undertake fundamental reviews of all public spending. The Treasury began to involve itself more directly in social policy – moving from its traditional concern with the total budgets of departments to consideration of the internal details of expenditure – especially in social security, health, education and at the Home Office. The Treasury 'redefined its objectives and its organisation to express an interest in the wider economy and society' (Deakin and Parry 1997).

These 1990s constraints would apply regardless of the party in power. Plans to bring about radical restructuring began to be formulated internally by both Conservatives and Labour. It seemed that only the Liberal Democrats were prepared to talk about taxation: the Dahrendorf Report noted this had become 'almost taboo in British public debate' (Dahrendorf Report 1995: 40).

In mid-1996, a fresh purge on public spending was announced in an attempt to deal with the PSBR, standing then at £27 billion. Sceptics believed this might herald tax cuts prior to the election but, in the event, in his autumn budget, Kenneth Clarke remained true to his commitment to fiscal prudence. After 1997, a crisis of funding in the public sector is predicted (IFS 1997; Millard 1997) exacerbated by the fact that the decay of the infrastructure can hardly be much longer ignored. The Treasury had been making preparations for this. A review in mid-1996 (leaked to the Press and entitled 'Strategic Considerations for the Treasury 2000 to 2005') included a range of options, such as obliging individuals and families to take out private insurance to cover retirement, unemployment or incapacity and drastic cuts in state support for education above the age of 16.

CHANGING LABOUR POLICY

Labour had lost out in 1992 to the accusation that it threatened 'tax bombshells'. In 1996, the Conservatives attempted to relaunch this attack with their 'New Labour, New Danger' campaign. But Labour strategy was well-prepared and had concentrated on burying the old Labour 'tax and spend' image. This had alienated some who were dismayed that the party appeared no longer interested in issues of tax and redistribution of wealth.

It is worth noting that existing systems do involve considerable redistribution of income, with the top 10 per cent of the income distribution paying over 25 per cent of all taxes and receiving less than 5 per cent of all spending, both direct and indirect. The top decile actually includes households with what some might see as quite modest incomes ('to be in the top decile required a joint net income for a two adult, childless household of only £25,000 in 1994–95' (Dilnot 1996). Andrew Dilnot of the independent Institute for Fiscal Studies (IFS) has long argued that there are really only two choices. 'One is a large and continuing increase in taxation, funding a return towards a more universal public welfare state ... [t]he other is explicit recognition that the tax we pay now is insufficient for a broadly "continental" model, and we should therefore target public spending more directly on those most in need, and either leave the better off to make their own decisions or compel them into private provision' (ibid.).

Labour has taken a clear step away from the Croslandite view on social provision (Crosland 1963). The party had embarked on a review of welfare state expenditure, utilising the process of a hundred-strong National Policy Forum, designed to discuss issues in depth. Fundamental to this was the idea that Labour had to be seen to be making a credible effort to control spending. The new soundbite was 'not to tax for tax's sake'. The new approach rejects the idea that the state should be the sole provider, in favour of government acting as the guarantor and regulator of all provision but the administrator of only some (Smith 1996). The centrepiece of Labour's new policy paradigm was that success would be measured by reductions in the size of the social security budget as people were moved from benefit into work. At the same time, Labour and Conservatives were also converging in planning proposals which would involve more use of private insurance.

However, a NOP poll in early 1996 showed that the public was still sceptical about new Labour's claims to want to cut taxes as the economy improves – 41 per cent still believed Labour would put up everyone's taxes. The Labour Left proposal to increase taxes on those earning over £50,000 was a potential weakness for Labour, threatening to repeat the calamity of 1992.

January 20 1997 was a defining moment for Labour when Gordon Brown, as shadow Chancellor, pledged that neither the top nor the basic rate of income tax would be raised over the next five years. In a lecture on public finances (attracting attention through being trailed in the early morning *Today* programme (BBC Radio 4)), he stressed the key word summing up his approach – *prudent*. He emphasised that there were no Labour public expenditure commitments that required raising additional taxes beyond the windfall tax. He also ruled out VAT on food, children's clothes, books, newspapers and public transport. His ambition was, he said, to introduce a new lower starting rate of tax of 10p to encourage people to go back to work and to help all hard-working families. At the same time, he moved to forge new links with business, promising to reward work and leave most Thatcherite industrial reforms in place if, in return, the business community would enter into partnership with Labour to reform education and welfare. Thus was new Labour's constituency marked out – an alliance of hard-working ordinary people and progressive business.

The next month, however, a Guardian/ICM poll showed 60 per cent still believed a Labour government would increase public spending over the next five years. Only 25 per cent believed Labour would keep its promises to hold to existing levels of income tax: 55 per cent believed Labour would increase rates.

THE PARTIES CAMPAIGN

In 1992, led by Neil Kinnock, the Labour Party had campaigned on the slogan 'It's time to get Britain working again'. To carry through their promises on health, education and other services, they would introduce fair taxes. 'Attacking poverty is an essential component of Labour's programme for national recovery and prosperity' the manifesto said (Labour Party 1992: 12). Child benefit would be increased, as would pensions, and low-paid people would be lifted out of taxation. 'To achieve these goals, we will reform the national insurance and income tax system', they pledged (ibid.). The ceiling on national insurance contributions would be abolished. The basic rate of income tax would remain unchanged at 25 per cent as would the 40 per cent rate. A new top rate income tax of 50 per cent would apply to individuals with an income of at least £40,000 a year. Individual employees on earnings up to at least £22,000 a year would be better off, they claimed.

In very direct contrast, the 1997 manifesto, entitled 'New Labour – because Britain deserves better', heralded 'better schools, better hospitals, better ways of tackling crime, of building a modern welfare state, of equipping ourselves for a new world economy' (Labour Party 1997: 1). The test was trust: 'there have been few more gross breaches of faith than when the Conservatives under Mr Major promised, before the election of 1992, that they would not raise taxes, but would cut them every year; and then went on to raise them by the largest amount in peacetime history starting in the first Budget after the election' (ibid.). Labour set out in its manifesto ten commitments, forming their 'bond of trust with the people' (op. cit.: 4). The second of these pledges read 'there will be no increase in the basic or top rates of income tax'. To modernise Britain would involve insisting that all parts of the public sector live within their means (ibid.). A strong and stable economy would be promoted through 'spending wisely and taxing fairly' (op. cit.: 11). They argued that it is a myth that the solution to every problem is increased spending: '[t]he level of public spending is no longer the best measure of the effectiveness of government action in the public interest. It is what money is actually spent on that counts more than how much money is spent' (ibid.). The priority would be to see how public money could be better used.

Labour charged the Conservatives that since 1992 the typical family had paid more than £2,000 in extra taxes. Instead of Mr Major's broken promises, Labour would establish a new trust on tax with the British people. They stressed that Labour is not about high taxes on ordinary families. As well as not raising basic or top rates of income tax, the long-term objective was a lower starting rate of income tax of ten pence in the pound. They would cut VAT on fuel to 5 per cent and review the interaction of the tax and benefit system to promote work incentives, reduce poverty and welfare dependency. There would be adherence to the golden rule of public spending – borrowing only to invest not to fund current expenditure. Qualified by 'over the economic cycle', the aim would be that public debt as a proportion of national income would be at a stable and prudent level.

The accusation was that the Conservatives had mismanaged the public finances. Gordon Brown would be more fiscally and financially prudent than the Conservatives. Under Labour, there would be tax reform to promote saving and investment and a welfare to work budget.

On the contrary, argued the Conservatives, Britain's economy was now the most successful in Europe (Conservative Party 1997). It had the lowest tax burden of any major European economy with the government taxing almost 8 per cent less of national income than the European average. The level of public debt was now one of the lowest in the European Union. They claimed that 'we are the only party that can cut taxes because we are the only party which is serious about controlling public spending' (op. cit.: 7). The goal would be, over the next parliament, for the government to spend less than 40 per cent of national income, virtually eliminating public borrowing by the year 2000. They reminded people that in their election manifesto of 1992 they had promised to make further progress towards a basic income tax rate of 20p. Since then, they said, they had cut the basic rate of income tax from 25p to 23p and extended the 20p band so that over a quarter of all taxpayers now only pay income tax at the 20p rate. The goal would be over the next parliament to achieve the target of a 20p basic rate of income tax while maintaining a maximum tax rate of no more than 40p.

The Liberal Democrats charged the other parties with a 'terrible fatalism'. The solutions they offered 'are all too often puny'. Instead, the LibDems would make education their top priority and invest an additional £2 billion per year in education, funded by an extra 1p in the pound on the basic rate of income tax. In addition to this tax increase, they would introduce a new rate of income tax of 50 per cent payable on taxable income of over £100,000 per year (a proposal which would affect 140,000 out of 26 million taxpayers, IFS calculated). These sums would allow them to take half a million people out of income tax altogether by raising the threshold at which people begin to pay tax. They would also put 5p on a packet of cigarettes and use the money to restore free eye and dental checks for all and freeze prescription charges. Thus like Labour with its windfall tax – but across a wider field – they moved towards hypothecation, justifying specific taxes by showing how the money raised would be spent.

The Liberal Democrats also stressed the issue of trust: a copy of an Annual Tax Contract would be delivered to each UK household following the Budget each year. This Annual Tax Contract would be in keeping with their four Tax Pledges: no taxation without explanation; no promises unless the bill is attached; no more tax without tackling waste; and fair tax for all. Overall, they would spend more on education, health and pensions and decrease government spending on private consultants, publicity and empty properties.

The Conservatives hoped to gain credit for the strong state of the economy – inflation was falling, unemployment was falling and the economy was booming (not the best choice of word). In launching their manifesto on April 2, they stressed their aspiration for a 20p basic rate. They captured attention for a little while by announcing proposals to change the tax allowance for married people – involving an allowance for the married partner who stayed at home to be taken into the account. This would be 'a practical tax measure to help people with caring responsibilities' – but only if they were married. Labour commented that this proposal had not been properly costed and, with the Liberal Democrats, asked how will this tax cut be paid for? Andrew Dilnot of IFS helpfully calculated that 1.9 million families might benefit and the cost would be £1.2bn. What was interesting about this proposal, he added (BBC Radio 4, *World at One*, 2 April) was that it reintroduced notions of social engineering to the tax structure.

On April 24, Labour announced an ingenious way to get more money into the system – to use the mid-week National Lottery to fund innovative local projects in education and health. The Conservatives claimed this proved Labour's plans did not add up. The Liberal Democrats stressed again that the need was extra cash for core services not additional extras, welcome as these might be. The lottery proposal is significant in indicating one possible direction for the future – taxation funding core services and other sources funding 'optional extras'. Once the division between 'core' and 'extra' has been made, such schemes become thinkable.

Throughout the campaign, however, discussions of tax tended to concentrate not on the details of tax proposals but on the question of trust. Labour had a strong message – 'you can't trust the Tories on tax' – whereas all their proposals, they claimed, were fully costed and they would stick to their pledges: they were entering into a 'Contract with Britain'. The Conservatives pointed to possible hidden taxes, for example in the Tartan tax (if Scottish devolution went through) and the real increase in taxation involved in the windfall tax.

The promises being made by both Labour and Conservative were modest and achievable, resonating with the traditional down-to-earth approach of the British people. However, some critics saw the debate as less than honest – Eric Hobsbawm likening it to 'fiscal perjury' on the part of the two main parties (*Analysis*, BBC Radio 4, 3 April 1997). But the Liberal Democrats did try to encourage people to face the public–private choice. Paddy Ashdown argued that people are prepared to pay specific targeted tax increases. They realised, he said, that you can't have tax cuts and better public services.

THE WIDER PUBLIC DEBATE

In spite of the timidity of the main parties, some serious debate did develop during the campaign, especially in radio and television programmes. The issue of how to pay for services began to be discussed and the question of responsibility surfaced.

The Churches in a report on poverty and unemployment (CCBI 1997) focused attention on the poor and attacked the complacency of the contented majority. If redistribution of income through taxation was to be ruled out, the gap between the favoured majority and those left out looked set to widen. The UK, they reminded people, has the widest gap of inequality in western Europe.

As has been indicated, the IFS played a prominent role during the campaign, presenting the facts and raising the key issue of the stark choice that faced the public – if people want better services they will have to pay for them. In their Election Briefing 1997, they stressed the point that '[t]he political debate about the balance between public and private provision in social security, health and education is still undeveloped. Addressing these issues means facing the inescapable trade-off that either the role of private provision must grow, or public spending and taxes must rise, or we cannot have higher consumption' (Dilnot and Johnson 1997: iv). The briefing showed that total general government receipts in the UK in 1997/8 would be around £300 billion, £7,500 for every adult in the UK. Since 1978/79 the tax burden as a share of GDP had risen slightly, from 34.25 per cent to 36.25 per cent. Compared with European competitors, the UK is a strikingly low-tax country, although the tax burden still exceeds that of the US and Japan (whose taxes have been growing however).

The spending plans inherited from the Conservative Chancellor, and to which Gordon Brown was committed for two years, would see overall spending rising in real terms by an average of 0.4 per cent per year, compared with an average of 1.9 per cent per year over the last 18 years. 'None of the major parties seems to have any satis-factory response to the very large gap likely to arise between spending plans and public expectations' (op. cit.: i). 'It is almost certain that over the next five years, either public spending, and therefore tax and/or borrowing, will be higher than planned, or substantial and radical reform of public sector provision will occur, either explicitly or by default' (op. cit.: ii).

Taxes have risen because net incomes have risen. Other pos-sibilities for raising taxes had not been ruled out by the parties, including restrictions in the value of income tax allowances and reductions in the rate of advance corporation tax. IFS regretted that decisions about new taxes were likely to be influenced by a 'trend towards seeking tax increases that can be presented easily, rather than that are economically most desirable', referring here as an example to Labour's proposed windfall tax (op. cit.: iv).

Unlike Blair and Major, Clarke and Brown were willing to debate on television with Malcolm Bruce of the Liberal Democrats. In these exchanges, Bruce performed very well and Brown always played a straight bat. Clarke was his usual rumbustious self, although at times he appeared surprised by the depth of hostility shown by the audiences. Through these and other media discussions, the voters also had a chance to put their views, as in *Voters Can't Be Choosers* (Channel 4 TV, 17 April). Participants here demonstrated dis-satisfaction with the parties' failure to address their concerns, which focused on issues of redistribution, poverty and inequality, deterior-ating public services and the idea that incarceration was the sole solution to crime. Vincent Hanna asked: 'What sort of democracy is this which has closed off these options which people want addressed but are not being addressed?'.

An insight into what might happen if these options were raised was provided in a fascinating programme, chaired by Sheena McDonald (Channel 4 TV, *Power to the People* Sunday 27 April). A representative sample of voters were taken away for a weekend to Manchester Metropolitan University, where they engaged in serious debate on key issues. They were able to question experts and politicians. Support for the Liberal Democrats rose from 11 per cent before the discussions to 33 per cent at the end. The experiment indicated how an informed and attentive electorate, armed with the facts and having debated the issues, would behave – if politics were organised in this way (a real democracy) rather than through contemporary soundbite, media-party arrangements.

AFTER THE ELECTION

On the day the 'long campaign' ended, the City was relaxed at the prospect of a Labour victory. The pound did not fall. Neither the market nor the country could see much difference between the economic policies of the two parties. The Labour Party had successfully turned round its image on spending and inflation. John Major accused Labour of having borrowed Conservative oratory about aspirations but the two parties differed, he said, in how they would try to meet these (Channel Four TV News, 30 April).

An exit poll conducted for BBCTV on 1 May (election day) found 72 per cent would agree to add 1p to income tax to improve schools; 58 per cent would agree to redistribute wealth to the worse off; and 74 per cent agreed there should be no more privatisation. (This of course was a poll of those who actually voted – the turnout at 71 per cent was the lowest since 1935). If Labour had campaigned to raise taxes, would the reluctant Tories who stayed at home have been galvanised to go out to vote? Labour's stance on the tax issue was crucial to winning support among the comfortable classes. The number of Labour MPs in the south east had fallen from 21 in 1966 to 1 in 1987 but it rose at the 1997 election to 36. The London factor, which had played so badly against Labour in the 1980s, appeared to have been buried. In London seats, swings to Labour of up to 18 per cent were recorded.

After the new government was installed in office, in a hot race to capture the headlines each day, the new Chancellor kept well ahead and phrases like 'monster surprise', 'dynamic Brown stuns city' and 'conjuring trick' were used to describe the spate of announcements which followed his appointment. The most dramatic was of a new structure for monetary policy based around an independent Bank of England. In 1946, a new Labour government had nationalised the Bank to prevent a recurrence of the interwar experience. As a symbolic break with the policies of old Labour, this was in a class of its own.

In his first budget, Brown increased taxation. And he found £3 billion for education and health from the contingency reserve. (It was said that Blair and Brown had thought up the idea of committing the contingency well in advance, as early as January, but had kept this secret until Budget day. By doing this, however, they removed their room for manoeuvre around genuine contingencies later.) Leaders in education and health services expressed their delight and even those who had criticised the decision to stick to Conservative spending targets were reduced to silence for a while. Abolition of advance corporation tax refund would remove tax credits paid to pension funds and companies. This was an important innovation raising £2.3 billion in the current financial year, rising to £3.95 billion the following year and £5.4 billion in 1999–2000. 'The tax collected is equivalent to a 5p increase in the basic rate of income tax' (Brummer 1997). This, as Alex Brummer commented, was the true 'tax bomb-shell' in Labour's programme. The changes would impact on middle England through knock on effects on occupational pension schemes. In some compensation to business, the budget included a cut in corporation and small companies taxes.

At the centre of the package was the New Deal, welfare-to-work programme, funded by a £5.2 billion windfall tax on privatised utilities, with water and regional electricity companies bearing the larger share. £1.3 billion of this would be used to refurbish run-down schools, while the rest would go on jobs and training programmes for young and long-term unemployed.

In addition, there were rises in taxes on petrol and tobacco, reduction of VAT on domestic fuel, and release of local authority receipts for house-building, abolition of tax relief on private medical insurance, help to the film industry, suggestions of a move towards the introduction of individual savings accounts, intimations of the introduction of a 10p rate of tax when this was prudent, support for the new University for Industry, a review of tax avoidance, a Comprehensive Spending Review to determine overall priorities for the early decades of the new century, and reinvigoration of the Private Finance Initiative.

The NIESR commented that, as a result, the deficit was likely to fall 'to less than 1 per cent of GDP by fiscal year 1998/9 and [would stay] at a sustainable level for the foreseeable future' (Weale and Young 1997: 4). The immediate increase in direct taxation was £700million; from April 1998, MIRAS would reduce to 10 per cent providing an additional £900million; the ending of tax credits on dividends was a substantial tax change affecting pension funds immediately and would become visible to households in April 1999.

CONCLUSION

For the last one hundred years, government expenditure has grown as demands for education, health and social security (pensions especially) have increased. The choice made, as IFS Director Andrew Dilnot repeatedly and valiantly pointed out during the 1997 election campaign, has been to spend on these areas as countries have got more affluent. The issue is not one of affordability – it is one of choice. But throughout the election campaign, and before that in the years up to 1997, no party was willing to launch a public debate on this issue. The Liberal Democrats to their credit did begin to do so in this election – but perhaps because as a minority party, they were able to take the risk. The message that you cannot win elections by talking about taxation has prevented parties from exercising a leadership role on this critical social question. Rather the issue is presented as one pre-determined – that the economy cannot afford (or risk) higher taxes.

The main slogan of the Conservatives during the election campaign was 'Britain is booming. Don't let Labour ruin it'. While the electorate was not convinced that Labour would ruin it, and while they suspected that boom was not what they wanted – stability would be better – it is the case that Labour inherited a much better economic situation than it would have done if it had won in 1992 and better than at any other of its post-war election victories. Conservative unpopularity was partly to do with having had to raise taxes to prevent a fiscal crisis early in its fourth term. The tax issue is still fundamental to electoral success. While many criticise Labour for its timidity on tax and redistribution, the approach adopted by Gordon Brown made strategic good sense.

The questions dominating discussion at the end of the first 100 days of the new Labour administration focused on how radical could the new Labour government, with its record majority, afford to be – if it did indeed want to be so? In electoral politics, the basic question is 'what do the people want?' Evidence from public opinion polls throughout the 1980s and early 1990s had shown rising willingness to pay more in tax to fund specific services from which all benefit (not however to finance unpopular groups like the unemployed). But the two main parties remained sceptical that these attitudes would influence behaviour once in the privacy of the polling booth.

Those arguing that people would act on their expressed attitudes point to the Liberal Democrats' increased vote in the 1997 election. They argue that voters simply wanted to get the Tories out – Labour could have capitalised on this and proposed increased tax and spend and still won (Brittan 1997).

Experience and evidence indicate that, to be willing to pay more, the public would have to see taxes as in their own interest, not just as a matter of altruism. There is strong evidence that paying for welfare through taxation is the most efficient, effective and fair way (Burchardt and Hills 1997). Decent public provision in health and education benefits the poor as well as those hard-working, ordinary people who are now identified as Labour's core constituency and the poor would gain a lot directly from adequate levels of income support.

While new Labour's approach has been clearly set out, the devil will be in the detail of implementation. The jury remained divided. Are Labour's priorities socially progressive? Will it be possible to shift expenditure within budgets to produce a fairer outcome? What will the tax–benefit review come up with? Will they be successful in shifting resources between budgets, particularly in reducing social security through welfare-to-work thus freeing money for education and health? Will the commitment to the Conservative spending limits prove to be an unnecessary limitation, since bouyant tax revenues may lead to the deficit melting away faster than expected? This raised immediate questions about why the strains on services (like long waiting lists in hospitals, bed shortages and winter health service crises, leaking roofs in schools and collapsing ceilings in universities) needed to be tolerated right through to March 1999.

For the British people, the big question which they will have to face in the next decade is: 'Are you prepared to live with the consequences of being a low-tax country, if these consequences are low benefits, high poverty and inequality, and less efficiency and declining standards in public services?'

REFERENCES

Baldwin, P. (1990) *The Politics of Social Solidarity*, Cambridge: Cambridge University Press.

Brittan, S. (1997) 'Better than you deserve', *Financial Times* May 3/4.

Brummer, A. (1997) 'Radical thrust that tends to conceal itself', *Guardian* 3 July, p.13.

Burchardt, T. and Hills, J. (1997) *Private Welfare Insurance and Social Security: Pushing the Boundaries*, York: Joseph Rowntree Foundation.

CCBI (Council of Churches for Britain and Ireland) (1997) *Unemployment and the Future of Work*, London: CCBI, Inter-Church House.

Conservative Party (1997) *You Can Only be Sure with the Conservatives*, election manifesto, London: Conservative Party.

Crosland, A. (1963) *The Future of Socialism*, revised edition, New York: Schocken Books.

Dahrendorf Report (1995) *Report on Wealth Creation and Social Cohesion in a Free Society*, (Chairman: Lord Dahrendorf) London: Commission on Wealth Creation and Social Cohesion.

Deakin, N. and Parry, R. (1997) 'The Treasury and Social Policy after the 1997 Election', paper presented to the annual conference of the Social Policy Association, Lincoln, July.

Dilnot, A. (1996) 'High taxes or low, bills still have to be paid' *Guardian*, Monday 20 May.

Dilnot, A. and Johnson, P. (eds) (1997) *Election Briefing*, London: Institute for Fiscal Studies.

Glennerster, H. (1997) *Paying for Welfare: towards 2000*, third edition, Hemel Hempstead: Prentice Hall/Harvester Wheatsheaf.

Hutton, W. (1995) *The State We're In*, London: Jonathan Cape.

IFS (Institute for Fiscal Studies) (1997) 'Election briefing', London: IFS.

Jacobs, M. (1996) *The Politics of the Real World*, London: Earthscan.

Joseph Rowntree Foundation (1995) *Inquiry into Income and Wealth*, York: Joseph Rowntree Foundation.

Labour Party (1992) *It's Time to get Britain Working Again*, election manifesto, London: Labour Party.

—— (1997) *New Labour – Because Britain Deserves Better*, election manifesto, London: Labour Party.

Liberal Democrat Party (1997) *Make the Difference*, election manifesto, London: Liberal Democrats.

McFate, K., Lawson, R. and Wilson, W.J. (eds) (1995) *Poverty, Inequality and the Future of Social Policy*, New York: Russell Sage.

Millard, M. (1997) 'The politics of public expenditure control: a problem of politics or language games?', *Political Quarterly* 68, 3, July–Sept pp. 266–75.

Smith, C. (1996) 'Social justice in a modern world', London: Institute Public Policy Research.

Weale, M. and Young, G. (1997) 'Economic prospects for the UK and policy recommendations', *National Institute Economic Review* no. 161, July, pp. 3–5.

Chapter 4

Jobs, unemployment and the European Union

Valerie Symes

INTRODUCTION

One of the most striking changes that has come about in recent years has been the emergence of consensus between the two main political parties in the UK on both the causes of unemployment and the way forward to create new employment. Consensus is not new. It existed more or less for the whole of the post-war period up to the 1970s. At that time the consensus was based around the Beveridge imperative of full employment as the primary objective of economic policy. Fiscal and monetary policy were manipulated to produce, as far as possible, a level of aggregate demand in the economy that ensured that those who wished to work would be able to find employment.

This all changed for several reasons. The massive oil price shock of the mid-1970s resulted in price increases which were exacerbated in Britain by the archaic system of free-for-all wage bargaining. The tripartite system of decision making, common in many other European countries, where the social partners (employers, employees and government) agreed on wages, productivity and working conditions with regard to long-term economic objectives, had never been adopted in Britain. The outcome was that the UK, by the beginning of the 1980s, suffered the highest inflation and unemployment levels of all major industrialised European countries. At the same time a shift in the composition of employment, as a result of structural change, was taking place. Manufacturing industry was hardest hit with a loss of nearly three million jobs between 1971 and 1985, due partly to competition from the newly industrialising countries and partly to technological change. The loss of jobs in manufacturing industry in Britain was overall greater than for the rest of Europe and much higher than for OECD countries as a whole between 1973 and 1990 (Symes 1995). The answer to these problems for the Conservative government, from 1979 onwards, lay in using macro-economic policy exclusively to control inflation and deregulating, or making more 'flexible', the labour market in order to lower the costs of employment, increase competitiveness and encourage the creation of new jobs. This supply-side neoclassical approach to unemployment was in sharp contrast to the protection of employment levels through Keynesian policies, previously supported by both major parties. In the 1983 General Election Labour still strongly supported employment policies based on reflation, the protection of jobs through import controls and the introduction of works' councils, although the first two of these had disappeared by the 1987 General Election campaign.

Deregulation in the 1980s was largely concerned with the erosion of trade union powers, followed in the 1990s by the 1993 Trade Union and Employment Rights Acts, which abolished the power of wages' councils to determine minimum levels of pay, and measures which made redundancy easier and less costly for employers. But as Robinson (1997) has pointed out, the labour market was already fairly lightly regulated prior to 1979, compared to other EU countries where higher levels of social protection prevailed.

In the 1997 General Election campaign the main thrust of Labour Party economic policy was to reflect the Conservatives' policy of keeping public expenditure levels and taxation unchanged, continuing with low inflation as the major economic priority through manipulation of interest rates. Employment problems were also seen as soluble through flexibility in labour markets, and the policy solution for the unemployed lay in education and training. The main bone of contention was over the willingness of Labour to sign up to the European Social Chapter of the Maastricht Treaty, where an opt-out for Britain had been obtained by John Major in 1991, on the grounds that it would destroy British jobs. Before looking at how the various issues and policies were dealt with during the campaign, it would be useful to examine the recent experience in the UK of employment growth and unemployment in order to explain why, perhaps, the policies of the two major parties varied so little.

JOBS AND UNEMPLOYMENT SINCE 1992

During the 1992 General Election, unemployment stood at around 10 per cent. Since then it had fallen, especially during the two years preceding the 1997 election, to 6.2 per cent (February 1997), measured on standardised OECD criteria. The basis for measurement is important because, as we shall see, it became an issue in the election campaign. The number of unemployed fell from around 2.5 million to 1.8 million. For the same period the number in employment rose by 900,000. The fall in unemployment did not match the rise in employment as those not registered as actively seeking work took up around 20 per cent of the new jobs. If the unemployment rate is compared with other countries for the same period, the UK was well below the average EU rate. There was an increase in unemployment in Germany 1996–97 from 10.4 to 11.2 per cent, and in France from 12.1 to 12.8 per cent. Job creation and growth were, however, lower in the UK than in the USA where unemployment was just over 5 per cent.

It was to the USA that the Conservative government looked for recent policy initiatives such as the introduction of the Jobseeker's Allowance and the quasi-workfare scheme, Project Work, piloted in the Medway area and Hull in 1996. The combination of neoclassical free market ideology together with the implication that the taxpayer should no longer fund the 'workshy' had been an attractive electoral formula in the USA. The majority of voters were employed and doing well and there was a low election turn-out among the poor and unemployed in this 'culture of contentment' (Galbraith 1992). So it was clear to the government that what was acceptable in middle America was surely the right path to follow in middle England.

The success of the Conservative Government in creating jobs and reducing unemployment compared to most of the country's European partners, and the fact that a relatively liberal Clinton administration operated on similar lines to the Conservatives, meant two things for Labour. On the one hand, any proposal for radical change in employment policy would appear to be going against the grain of a winning formula, and, on the other hand, this policy direction was to some extent justified by being endorsed by a Democratic presidency with which it had close links. So the Labour Party kept to the basic tenets of a flexible labour market with a re-packaging of the compulsory elements of policy in a 'welfare-to-work' initiative, of which more below.

Europe was to be presented as a cautionary tale by the Conservatives. Other European member states had, it is true, a much higher degree of workers' protection and workers' rights than the UK, and this was to be attacked as the major reason for their very high levels of unemployment and as a justification for dismantling trade union power in the 1980s. (It must be said that high unemployment in Germany, France and Italy was largely due to cuts in public spending enforced to meet the Maastricht criteria for European Monetary Union (EMU), and in Germany's case also to the delayed costs of re-unification. The Netherlands, run on a corporatist tripartite model, managed to achieve a lower level of unemployment than Britain.) The attack on European employment levels was also used by the Conservatives to point up the success of John Major in dealing with Europe to Britain's advantage, through gaining an opt-out to the Social Chapter. This became important as the Eurosceptic wing of the Conservative Party gained impetus during the campaign. The Labour Party confirmed that it would join the Social Chapter as soon as it was elected. This difference of opinion became the most important issue in the battle over unemployment policy. In order to assess the validity of claims made concerning the Social Chapter it would be useful, at this point, to see exactly what it says.

THE SOCIAL CHAPTER AND EUROPE

The Social Chapter was an annex to the Treaty of European Union agreed in Maastricht in 1991. It was an agreement on social policy concluded between all member states of the then European Community with the exception of the UK. Article 1 sets out the general principles and has the objectives of: promotion of employment; improved living and working conditions; proper social protection; dialogue between management and labour; and the development of human resources with a view to lasting high employment and the combating of exclusion. Article 2 is concerned with how these objectives could be achieved. Any directives and minimum requirements were to be implemented gradually, in such a way that would not hold back the creation and development of small and medium-sized enterprises (SMEs), the main creators of new jobs.

The remaining Articles are concerned with the Commission's role in promoting and facilitating consultations between management and labour; encouraging cooperation and coordination of action in all social policy fields; and ensuring that the principle of equal pay for men and women for equal work is actually applied. All proposals from the Commission must be adopted by the Council of Ministers before legislation. The UK objected in 1993 to legislation on maximum working hours but a Maximum Working Time Directive was brought in under health and safety directives, which do not require unanimity, later that year. This undermining of the British veto caused anger among the Conservatives and in the election campaign was interpreted, as we shall see, as a direct threat to British sovereignty. There is no specific mention anywhere in the Social Chapter on the requirement for a minimum wage. To date no European legislation has been adopted on a minimum wage.

The recession in Europe and the recent increase in unemployment made the implementation of more regulations on social policy and employment less likely (Church and Phinnemore 1994).

THE GENERAL ELECTION 1997

The main theme of the campaign for the Conservative Party was to emphasise their success in government in lowering unemployment and generating the economic growth which created new jobs during the eighteen months prior to the General Election. Wherever possible Britain's record was compared favourably with other European countries. This happened increasingly as the campaign progressed and the Euro-sceptic wing of the Conservative Party gained ascendancy.

The Labour Party were keen to highlight their 'welfare-to-work' policy, stressing, in particular, various measures to help the young unemployed back to work, with some references to the long-term unemployed. The catchy phrase 'welfare-to-work' encapsulated the implication that unemployment and the number on welfare would be simultaneously reduced. The policy was first introduced in February, before the official election campaign started. After two weeks of the campaign this policy for the unemployed and the issue generally became less dominant.

Both of the two main parties agreed on the advantages of a flexible labour market but with a less rigorous interpretation by Labour, who had promised to introduce a minimum wage. This was to provide a main line of attack for the Conservatives particularly in the latter half of the campaign, where it was combined with the implication that European unemployment was higher than in the UK because minimum wages caused high unemployment. The major line of attack for Labour was to question the official figures for unemployment, suggesting that they were much underestimated.

All modern election campaigns consist of the publication of a manifesto on policies, both in terms of general aims and specific action to be taken, briefings to the press and media appearances by leading politicians. What reaches the public via newspapers, radio and TV is selected, edited and commentated on by journalists. There is a gap between what the political parties wish to present to the electorate and the information actually received. Party manifestos contain the core of the message the parties wish to convey, so these will be analysed first of all before looking at the development of the campaign in the media.

Manifestos compared

In the Conservative manifesto under the heading of 'The Enterprise Centre of Europe', jobs, unemployment policy and business were treated in the same section and were second only to a section on free markets, low tax and growth. The Labour Party put it fourth after education, prosperity for all and helping create successful and profitable businesses. The preamble to unemployment policy in Labour's manifesto stated that there were a million fewer jobs than in 1990 and one in five families had no-one working. The objective stated was a high and stable level of employment, echoing Beveridge. The unemployed 'have a responsibility to take up the opportunity of training or places of work. . . . Labour's welfare-to-work programme will attack unemployment and break the spiral of escalating spending on social security.' Welfare-to-work was primarily concerned with youth unemployment – 250,000 young unemployed people were to be offered one of four options:

- work with a private sector employer who would be given £60 per week for six months to take on a young unemployed worker;
- work with a voluntary sector employer at benefit plus rate for six months;
- full-time study on an approved course;
- a job with the environmental task force.

There was to be no fifth option of life on full benefit. All those under 18 would be offered part-time or full-time education.

The long-term unemployed, out of work for more than two years, were to be helped by giving employers a £75 tax rebate for six months. Both of these initiatives in welfare-to-work would be funded by a one-off windfall levy on the excess profits of the privatised utilities. Lone parents with children at school were to be offered advice by the Employment Service to develop a package of job search, training and after-school care to help them off benefit and into paid work. The section concluded with the subject of fraud and the promise to crack down on dishonesty in the benefit system.

As the vast majority of young unemployed people on income support have only basic education and come from poorer families in inner city areas, the compulsory element of the welfare-to-work programme for the young affects this group particularly, as opposed to the unemployed young middle class who can rely on their families for support. The measure had within it the idea of idle youth rather than youth as a positive and dynamic force for the future. The message on scrounging was reiterated in the final paragraph on fraud. Both messages were clearly directed at ensuring that the predominantly working (or retired from work) electorate were assured that no costs were incurred (windfall tax to provide), and that fears of the dependency culture were allayed.

The question of Europe in the Labour manifesto was dealt with in a separate section 'Europe' where Labour promised to 'lead from the front in Europe' with a detailed agenda for reform. On the Social Chapter there was the promise to sign and the explanation:

> only two measures have been agreed – consultation with employees of large companies and the entitlement to unpaid parental leave. . . . The Social Chapter cannot be used to force the harmonisation of social security or tax legislation and it does not cost jobs. We will use our participation to promote employability and flexibility . . . not high social costs.
>
> (Labour Party 1997a)

This assurance of not costing jobs was to be challenged fiercely by the Conservatives. The good intention of subscribing to employee consultation, an old Labour virtue, was balanced by the concept of promoting 'flexibility', a New Labour attitude. However, in the section of the manifesto entitled 'Successful and profitable businesses', the concept of 'flexibility plus' included a national minimum wage:

> Introduced sensibly the minimum wage will remove the worst excesses of low pay (and be of particular benefit to women) while cutting some of the massive £4 billion benefits bill by which the taxpayer subsidises companies that pay very low wages.
>
> (Labour Party 1997a)

While clearly, as in the proposals on unemployment, a positive attitude to women was confirmed, the message was also that the minimum wage would save on public expenditure and taxation.

The Conservative manifesto was less concerned with policies towards the unemployed than with policies for creating jobs which was 'not just an economic priority but a social and moral one'. The point was made that the UK unemployment rate was much lower than the rest of Europe and falling. It ascribed the success to the curbing of trade unions, opening up markets and cutting red tape, all giving a low-cost economy. To further this end, cuts in company taxation and capital gains tax were offered for the future, when circumstances allow, while business rates were to be reduced in the next Parliament. A section was devoted to the burden on companies and hence jobs of European 'layers of red tape and regulation'. Here the Conservatives stressed their success in recent years in creating employment through deregulation in contrast to the rest of Europe, and at the same time aimed to occupy the moral high ground. These comments were followed by inveighing against Europe for bringing in the Working Time Directive through the back door, and not allowing the UK to operate its veto in the Council of Ministers. The message conveyed was very clearly anti the European social model.

> No Conservative government will sign up to the Social Chapter or introduce a national minimum wage. We shall insist at the Intergovernmental Conference in Amsterdam that our opt-out is honoured and that Britain is exempted from the Working Time Directive.
>
> (Conservative Party 1997)

On policy for the unemployed, targeted training was to continue to be provided by the Training and Enterprise Councils. The unemployed 'have a responsibility to look for work and accept a reasonable offer. That belief underpins our new Jobseeker's Allowance which ensures that no-one can refuse reasonable work opportunities and remain on benefit' (Conservative Party 1997). For the long-term unemployed Project Work was to be extended to all areas through a job and work experience subsidy to employers or community work experience.

The disciplinarian approach to the unemployed, thought to be electorally popular, was clearly put in the Jobseeker's Allowance, also referred to later in a Press briefing (Conservative Research Department 1997a), but the compulsion to work for benefit under Project Work was not clearly spelt out in the manifesto, only the benefits of work experience.

While the main emphasis of the Conservatives was to promote the benefits of a deregulated labour market in creating employment, the emphasis of Labour was towards a socially oriented policy to bring about lower youth unemployment, albeit with a compulsory proviso. Labour supported deregulation through promoting the less offensive term 'flexibility' in their document, but there is little suggestion anywhere that they would reverse the current status quo, except for the introduction of a minimum wage.

The Liberal Democrats' manifesto was much more general in its approach to unemployment. In only one short paragraph it specified a single policy of enabling the long-term unemployed to use their benefit as a wage subsidy to make them attractive recruits for employers; asserted that they will break open the poverty traps that stop unemployed people from working; and would boost investment in infrastructure, promotion of small businesses and energy conservation projects, all of which would create new jobs. While the other two parties were keen to be seen as low tax, careful spending governments, the Liberal Democrats took on board Keynesian ideas of public investment as the way forward for job creation, with the implication, only specified in the case of education policy, that taxes would rise. The issue of unemployment was rarely dealt with by the Liberal Democrats during the election campaign and so will not be discussed in the following section.

THE ELECTION CAMPAIGN

The election campaign of 1997 was the longest in recent history lasting nearly six weeks. Campaigning, however, started before the official date. The parties wished to get over their main ideas in the month or so preceding the actual campaign. This section will look at statements made by party leaders through the media both in official broadcasts, interviews and reports of speeches made. It is presented chronologically in order to show how the issues of unemployment, employment and Europe were presented, and their relative importance at different periods.

On 9 February, John Major, in a speech in Brussels, said that signing the Social Chapter would put half a million in Britain out of work, that over-regulation does not work and he believed social legislation had bogged down the Continent's ability to compete; 'Britain because of its flexible labour market has escaped the economic trap, creating 900,000 jobs in the past four years'. The same report (*Independent*, 10 February 1997) contained the acceptance by

Tony Blair of the case for flexible labour markets and said he did not intend to impose the European model of 'social protection' on British business. But Blair and Brown argued that the way to compete in global markets was to raise the skills of the national workforce not bid down the cost of labour. The arguments on Europe, its system of social protection for workers and the issues of jobs and competitiveness were seen by both parties as a means to endorse the British labour market model, but less enthusiastically by Labour, as flexibility for them clearly did not mean downward wage flexibility, one of the central tenets of neoclassical free-market theory.

The next Press release taken up by the media was a description of Labour's welfare-to-work policy, financed by a £3 billion windfall tax. Details of the scheme were introduced in the Anthony Crosland memorial lecture on 12 February by Gordon Brown who, when being interviewed on the problems of a windfall tax on the utilities, said ' I think what the utilities will now want to do, instead of defending a privileged position, is to work with us so that we can implement this in a sensible way' (*Today*, BBC Radio 4, 13 February 1997). Increasing taxation on undeserving 'fat cat' industries was thus separated from other kinds of tax increase.

A MORI poll on social issues, carried out in several European countries, showed that unemployment was the biggest worry of the British, with 48 per cent of respondents citing it as their highest concern. The same day that this report was published Gordon Brown talked on radio about the plan for youth unemployment in welfare-to-work (*Today*, BBC Radio 4, 18 March 1997). The following day official figures were published showing a fall in unemployment and an increase in employment in the previous month, confirming the recent trend. The announcement that parliament was to be pro-rogued the following week followed shortly afterwards. This early (and unexpected) date for prorogation was attacked by Labour and the Liberal Democrats as a means of deferring publication of the Downey report, which investigated allegations that some Conservative MPs had taken bribes in return for asking parliamentary questions. This 'sleaze' factor in the election, which was to run for more than two weeks, caused speculation in the media that the opposition parties were trying to distract from falling unemployment figures (*PM*, BBC Radio 4, 20 March 1997).

The real campaign was then underway. Gordon Brown made spending on the young unemployed a public expenditure free lunch: 'savings generated by Labour's programme to get 250,000 unemployed young people back to work would be used to cut the budget deficit' (*On the Record* BBC 1 TV, 23 March 1997). This turned potential attacks on the £3billion of extra public expenditure into the economic virtue of sound public finance management. The attack on the Conservatives' record on unemployment began the next day with David Blunkett who maintained that the UK had the worst record of any major industrialised nation for jobless households and that there were one million fewer men in work than when John Major came to power (*Independent*, 24 March 1997). The attack continued following a report under the headline 'Tories plan huge cuts in spending on young jobless' (*Independent*, 25 March 1997) which analysed Conservative spending programmes to the year 2000 showing a 15 per cent cash cut on measures to help the unemployed into work. At the Conservative Press conference Gillian Shepherd, in reply, said that money spent on unemployed people had been reduced because the number of unemployed people had reduced; she then went on to attack Labour for unnecessary expenditure: 'In November 1995 Gordon Brown said that he would spend £3billion to get 250,000 back to work . . . since then we have put 315,000 back to work without a £3 billion tax'.

The question of Europe and jobs surfaced for the first time in the official campaign at the end of March with tit-for-tat comment by Robin Cook and Malcolm Rifkind on the Social Chapter: 'A Labour government would sign up to the Social Chapter as a way of increasing jobs' – 'The Social Chapter is going to see the same sort of unemployment that they have on the Continent' (*Today*, BBC Radio 4, 25 March 1997). This issue was to run and run throughout the campaign with little or no analysis, as will be seen.

On 7 April Tony Blair gave a speech to business people in the City of London and expanded on the concept of 'flexibility plus', which was to include a better-trained workforce, economic stability, partnership with business, leadership in Europe, backing for small firms and investment in infrastructure. The Labour Party aimed to create the impression that it could do all the Tories would do for business and more besides. It was well received.

Then came a *deus ex machina* which threw both the main political parties off course. The UK's eleven main Christian churches published a report 'Unemployment and the Future of Work' which examined the moral implications of having so many living in poverty and unemployment while priority was given to those who were already well off. It specifically attacked the Conservatives' central claim of the creation of a successful flexible labour market: 'The problem is not just one of creating more jobs but providing enough good work for everyone to do ... with decent pay and conditions'. The recommendations of the report were for additional taxes to be levied in order to generate large-scale expansion of employment supported by public spending in many areas, in other words to improve public services while providing worthwhile stable jobs. Taxation of the well-off was seen as a moral issue. This well-publicised report provided a dilemma for the Conservatives who wished to be seen as upholding Christian values, and for Labour who did not want to agree that the flexible labour market had failed in any way or that old tax-and-spend Labour doctrines would help the poor. They had also specifically promised no change in income taxes and financial rectitude as far as public spending was concerned. The Labour response from Gordon Brown was: 'Tax is a moral issue ... but a tax system built on work and fairness is a moral tax', with the implication that the current system was just that (*World at One*, BBC Radio 4, 8 April). The Conservative response from Peter Lilley, some days later, was to question whether tax increases wouldn't negatively affect the dynamic and enterprising economy and job creation, reiterating the party line that the right means to get more jobs was a low tax deregulated economy (*Today*, BBC Radio 4, 14 April).

The main plank of Labour Party policy on unemployment, welfare-to-work, had been more or less buried by this time as far as the media campaign was concerned. On 8 April Gordon Brown had claimed the endorsement of several large companies including 'Hamlyn, BP, Jaguar and businessmen in every region' for the £60 per week rebate scheme for the young unemployed. The chief executive of Jaguar, Nick Sheeley denied this (*World at One*, BBC Radio 4, 8 April 1997), causing embarrassment and confusion in Labour ranks. Apart from an indirect reference in a speech by Tony Blair on investment in education and skilling being the way forward to 'give people the ability to earn an acceptable income and fend for themselves', the scheme did not appear in the forefront of the media campaign from then onwards.

John Major continued to give soundbites on television and radio on the subject of Europe and unemployment. 'We don't want to sign up to the Social Chapter which is a charter for unemployment' (*Today*, BBC Radio 4, 14 April 1997); wanting 'nothing to do with a Europe which had control of jobs in Britain' (*Nine O'Clock News*, BBC 1 TV, 16 April); and did not 'think we should hand decisions about British jobs and employment to Europe' (Conservative Party Election Broadcast, 16 April 1997).

In the meantime Labour were quick to seize on a report that the number of jobless was more than twice as high as the Government claimed, in order to explain why the Conservatives were doing so badly in the opinion polls (*Independent on Sunday*, 13 April 1997). On 16 April a report was published in which it was stated that one in five children were growing up in families where nobody was in work. The National Institute of Economic and Social Research also predicted that Labour's welfare-to-work policies would reduce unemployment to 1.4 million within two years. Both were good news for Labour. The Conservatives combated the first of these claims by saying that the figures were manufactured and included the sick, the severely disabled, people looking after dependants and those studying full time (Conservative Research Department 1997b).

The news, however, of the lowest unemployment figures for six years, announced on 17 April, with a registered unemployment figure of 1.7 million and an unemployment rate of 6.1 per cent caused problems for Labour. Although they repeated the accusation that the headline figure was fiddled, it was clear from statistics provided by the Labour Force Survey (LFS) for the first quarter of 1997, the internationally accepted definition of unemployment, that un-employment had fallen between December and February by some 111,000. This was smaller than the claimant fall of 181,700 but still significant. The LFS figures also showed a rise in employment of 135,000 for the same quarter and a yearly rise of 351,000. Notifica-tions of new vacancies at Job Centres in March were 249,500. Arguing about the figures was not going to be a good strategy for Labour, and from this point onwards, although youth unemploy-ment remained high, Labour more or less withdrew comment to the media on employment and unemployment policy for the rest of the campaign period.

The Conservatives were left with an almost open field and chose to use the triple-purpose tactic of attacking Labour on Europe, jobs and the unions. By the fourth week of the campaign the Euro-sceptic wing of the Conservative Party were becoming more vociferous in the media. Being able to point up the deficiencies of European membership was to John Major's advantage. On 18 April Ian Lang, President of the Board of Trade, maintained that people were increasingly thinking that the Labour Party were in the control of the unions because the Social Chapter included minimum wages and length of working week legislation on which both unions and the Labour Party agreed. 'They want the trade unions to be a social partner. We didn't reduce the power of the trade unions in the 1980s, to great benefit, in order to have this reversed ... it would have a detrimental effect on jobs' (*Today* BBC Radio 4, 18 April 1997).

In the party political broadcasts for the rest of the campaign Labour concentrated on other social policy issues, health, education, the care of the elderly. Nothing was mentioned about jobs or unemployment. The Conservatives continued to push what they saw as the winning formula of Europe and unemployment: 'Labour would sign up to the Social Chapter. This would mean massive job loss' (John Major, party political broadcast, 22 April); 'He [Tony Blair] would agree an employment package with Europe that would give them control over our jobs. We should say no to it and I will' (John Major, party political broadcast, 25 April). Again on 30 April, the night before the election, in the Conservative PPB, unemployment figured as a strong card for John Major: 'Don't give up falling unemployment'.

The campaign over, Labour elected, how would Labour deal with unemployment and the European dimension in the first few weeks in office?

THE NEW LABOUR GOVERNMENT AND UNEMPLOYMENT

Of the six major objectives specified in the Queen's Speech, which set the agenda for the new Government's first year in office, getting young people back to work is one of them (Labour Party 1997c). The policy is dealt with under the manifesto commitment to promote 'prosperity for all' where details of the welfare-to-work scheme for young people are specified. The Finance Bill included the introduction of a windfall levy on the excess profits of the privatised utilities, in order to get young people off benefit and into work. A Bill is also mentioned to establish a low pay commission which will set a national minimum wage. On the subject of Europe the Government promised to implement any agreement which might be reached at the Amsterdam summit.

Tony Blair, the new Prime Minister, went to the Amsterdam summit on 6 and 7 June with the stated intention of making jobs the number one priority for Europe. He wished to encourage other member states to achieve this by means of greater flexibility, a concept accepted in principle in the EU, but not in all the deregulatory aspects which have been the feature of the British labour market under past Conservative governments. The British presidency of the European Union in the first half of 1998 would provide an opportunity to further persuade our European partners of the benefits of the British model, and an opportunity to examine any new ideas on flexibility that the government might develop.

CONCLUSIONS

As Tonge (1997) has pointed out, unemployment does not possess the political importance that it did prior to 1980. The electability of a government presiding over a high level of unemployment was demonstrated in 1983 when a Conservative government was elected despite there being nearly three million unemployed.

In the 1997 election unemployment as an issue did not take centre-stage in either the planning of the campaign, as evinced by the manifestos, or the campaign in the media. One of the reasons for this was that New Labour differed very little from the Conservatives in promoting the general principle that flexible or deregulated labour markets create employment. There is no evidence to suggest that the Labour Government does not believe in this neoclassical approach, in fact quite the reverse, as the flexible labour market theology was stressed as the way forward for Europe at the Amsterdam summit.

The policy prescriptions of Labour for training and work experience were in essence no different in approach to the Conservatives, except that they were extended to cover all young people up to the age of 25, and higher levels of financing for schemes was to be made available. The old Labour strategy of increasing public expenditure to promote growth and jobs was scrupulously avoided, as the economy was to be run by New Labour on the same principles, and under the same public expenditure levels, planned by the Conservatives. The prospect of increased or new taxes, with the exception of the electorally acceptable windfall tax, was to be avoided since they had clearly had such a disastrous effect on Labour in the 1992 election's 'tax bombshell'. The subtext behind running the economy with low inflation and a reduced public deficit through cuts in welfare expenditure, said to be forthcoming from the new employment policies was to emphasise that Labour would run the economy prudently. Cutting the PSBR would also mean that the UK would be likely to meet the criteria for European Monetary Union. One may find a further indication that joining EMU was an aim of the Government when a few weeks after coming to office the Chancellor, Gordon Brown, announced that interest rates were to be set by the Bank of England, free of government control, operating on similar lines to the European Central Bank.

There was a difference in style, however, in the manifesto presentation of policies on unemployment, with Labour being even more disciplinarian in its approach to the unemployed and even more hard on benefit scroungers than the Conservatives. The concepts of Left and Right, or even Centre and Right disappeared from party politics as far as this issue was concerned. Both parties were also concerned to point up their intentions to protect the interests of business in a free market, and ensure that the conditions for competitiveness were met. The ideology of market virtue, confirmed in attitudes to flexible labour markets and the importance of business as the major priority of economic policy-making, the rejection of the welfare state as anything other than a temporary safety net for the unemployed, a dismissal of trade unions and the expressed attitudes towards the unemployed as irresponsible rather than unfortunate, put New Labour into the category where 'markets are assumed to be benevolent and non-market institutions suspect' (Herman and Chomsky 1988).

However, the Conservative record in reducing unemployment and creating jobs in the year prior to the election would have made it difficult to convince the electorate that a change in policy direction was either necessary or desirable. Although Labour made some attempts to dispute the unemployment figures at the start of the campaign, publication of figures showing a further improvement in the situation in the second half of the campaign caused them virtually to abandon employment as an election issue. Surprisingly, the achievements in unemployment and the creation of jobs were not made more of in the Conservative campaign, which focused largely on the Europe issue, attacking Labour as being weak in giving in to Europe against Britain's interests. This issue was probably stressed more in order to prove John Major's credibility to his own party in strong-dealing with Europe than because it was the only real policy difference between the two major parties.

So what of the future for unemployment and employment under the new Labour government? Will the policy of welfare-to-work succeed? Experience in other European countries of subsidised work experience and training shows that it is quite successful in reducing unemployment in the context of general growth in employment opportunities, but otherwise has a tendency to displace existing workers or cause an unsubsidised unemployed worker to remain unemployed through the substitution effect. There is also the possibility that young people on schemes could be recycled with one six-month recruit being replaced with another. Again this is more likely to happen if there is slow growth in the number of new jobs. In the current context of job growth the policy is more likely to show some reduction in youth unemployment. In the longer term the six-month training or work experience is only useful to a limited extent since in the time available no real difference can be made to skill levels. The quality of schemes including length and type of training and the general support given to the unemployed have been shown to make a difference in ensuring longer-term employment and employability (EFILWC 1997). In Britain in the past there has been some difficulty in persuading firms to take on new subsidised recruits, and many of the young may end up in the voluntary task force. If this resembles the Community Programme of the 1980s then results will not be good. As welfare to work schemes develop it will be possible to make a judegment; hopefully at least a short-term respite from unemployment for the young and long-term unemployed will be forthcoming.

REFERENCES

Church, C.H. and Phinnemore, D. (1994) *European Union and the European Community: a Handbook and Commentary on the post-Maastricht Treaties*, Hemel Hempstead: Harvester Wheatsheaf.

Conservative Party (1997) *You Can Only Be Safe with the Conservatives*, election manifesto, London: Conservative Party.

Conservative Research Department (1997a) Press Release, 16 April. London.

—— (1997b) *Questions of Policy*, London.

EFILWC (European Foundation for the Improvement of Living and Working Conditions) (1997) *Job Creation and the Quality of Working Life in Six Member States*, report prepared by V. Symes, Dublin: EFILWC.

Galbraith, J.K., (1992) *The Culture of Contentment*, London: Penguin.

Herman, E. and Chomsky, N. (1988) *Manufacturing Consent: the Political Economy of the Mass Media*, New York: Pantheon Books.

Labour Party (1997a) *Because Britain Deserves Better*, election manifesto, London: Labour Party.

—— (1997b) *Policy Information. Tackling Unemployment*, 10/B, London.

—— (1997c) 'The Queen's Speech. A briefing from the Labour Party Policy Directorate 14 May 1997', London.

Liberal Democrat Party (1997)*Make the Difference*, election manifesto, London: Liberal Democrat Party.

Robinson, P. (1997) *Labour Market Studies*, Luxembourg: Office for Official Publications for the European Community.

Symes, V. (1995) *Unemployment in Europe: Problems and Policies*, London/ New York: Routledge.

Tonge, J. (1997) 'Britain', in H. Compston (ed.) *The New Politics of Unemployment*, London/New York: Routledge.

Chapter 5

'Education, education, education'

Miriam E. David

INTRODUCTION

With the benefit of hindsight it is possible to argue that education was the major issue of the General Election of 1 May 1997, given that the New Labour government was elected with an overwhelming majority and that Tony Blair, the leader of the Labour Party, had consistently argued throughout the election campaign that *'Education, education, education'*, was the top priority. He targeted in particular the need to improve educational standards *'for the many, not the few'* and so committed his government to a reduction in the *class size* of primary schools. Education has been one of the major items on the political agenda over the last two decades but the forms of debate and delivery have changed markedly. This chapter will explore the ways in which education policy had been developed under the Conservative administrations over the previous eighteen years and consider the Labour Party's counter-proposals, first in opposition and during the general election campaign and second during the first hundred days of Blair's New Labour government. The education policies adopted by the Liberal Democrats will be addressed briefly.

Taking a feminist critical policy stance, I want to argue that there are more similarities than differences between Conservatives and New Labour in respect of education policy, from early childhood education through to higher education and adult education. And that, despite there being over a quarter of women MPs in the New Labour government, little attention was paid to gender issues in the first three months of office: nor were such matters addressed in the election campaign, by Labour in opposition nor by the Conservatives in office. The key words to characterise the Tory period of administration regarding education policy are in the notion of *education reform*, which itself is characterised by marketisation, privatisation and deregulation. This has affected all levels of education from nurseries through to adult and higher education. Although there has been a significant shift from the state and government agencies back to families as key in the decisions about education, this has not addressed questions of gender, even though, at the same time, there have been important social and economic changes in families and their structures and processes.

However, gender equity in academic performances and the fact that girls' educational achievements have improved relative to boys', documented especially since the introduction of league tables in 1992 and the publication of examination results in the 1980s, have become topics for media and public concern. This is such that Chris Woodhead, Her Majesty's Chief Inspector (HMI) and Head of the Office for Standards in Education (Ofsted) could write in *The Times* (1996) that the most disturbing problem for education is 'white working class boys' underachievement'. Nevertheless, the central issues during the election were not about gender differences in educational performances but rather whether the performances of all educational institutions – from nurseries through to adult and higher education – were satisfactory and contributing sufficiently to educational and economic opportunities for 'the many and not the few'. How to reprimand and/or redeem 'failing' schools and educational institutions and how to re-assert traditional moral values, particularly about families and family life were at the heart of the political debates. In this respect gender was seen as irrelevant, as to some extent was ethnicity and/or race; equality of educational opportunity once more came to be about access based upon parental socio-economic backgrounds of privilege or poverty (as a proxy for social class issues).

THE INTERNATIONAL CONTEXT OF EDUCATION POLICIES IN THE NEW 'ERA'

Education reforms and social policies have been high on the public agenda in many if not most, advanced industrial societies since education is seen as critical for economic competitiveness (Chubb and Moe 1990; Ball 1994; Whitty *et al.* 1996). In the last two decades the discourse of educational reform has essentially focused on marketisation and privatization to create the conditions for more competition within education in order to improve educational standards – what have sometimes been referred to as either neo-liberal or neo-conservative reforms (Dale 1991; Apple 1997). More-over, parents have been targeted as the main consumers, customers or users of education, best able to decide on the best education for their child(ren) (David 1993; David *et al.* 1993; West 1994). Thus conditions have been created for parents to be able to choose within and between schools at key transitions to and from primary and secondary schools to ensure that their children receive the most appropriate education. By contrast, educational professionals and bureaucrats have been afforded much reduced roles within educa-tional decision-making. Indeed, educational reforms have also re-moved not only educational bureaucracy but also local government decision-making, in favour of decisions at the local school level (Gewirtz *et al.* 1995). The school has indeed been afforded far more autonomy to make decisions and to raise and spend its own resources in the context of wider national guidelines on the curriculum and staffing. The whole panoply of the governance of education has been increasingly privatised and elements marketised. This has given rise to an enormous growth in both strategic and critical research into aspects of education marketisation (Fitz *et al.* 1993, Gewirtz *et al.* 1995; Glatter *et al.* 1995; Whitty *et al.* 1996).

At the same time, moreover, there has been a growing emphasis and expansion of education within the wider market place, including the growth and availability of educational technology and aids to learning, not only in formal educational institutions. Despite this explosion of information technology and educational materials, parents have still been seen as the main arbiters of such goods and services. Indeed, they have increasingly been expected to manage the ever more complex processes of their children's learning. Social democratic discourses have increasingly emphasised home–school relations, including quasi-legal contracts, homework policies and parental participation in school management, especially as parent governors (David 1993; Deem *et al.* 1995). Parental involvement has become increasingly part of a normative discourse about education where once it was largely the domain of professionals and educa-tional bureaucrats. This too has given rise to a tremendous growth in strategic and critical research into aspects of parental participation or involvement in education (David 1993; Hughes *et al.* 1994).

A third emphasis has been the transformation to mass from elite higher education also as part of the impetus to improve economic competitiveness as well as educational opportunities. Again there has also been considerable institutional change, including privatisation and deregulation. Here too the consumer has been empowered at the expense of the educational professionals and bureaucrats. Most recently it appears that the costs of such education may begin to fall more heavily on users than on the state. All of these 'reforms' mark a considerable shift in the ways in which education is viewed and delivered away from the consensual politics of fifty years ago.

FROM CONSENSUS POLITICS ON 'EQUALITY OF EDUCATIONAL OPPORTUNITY'

In Britain there was a coalition government, with a Conservative leadership, in the Second World War which enacted the 1944 Education Act. This piece of legislation became the cornerstone of education policy in England and Wales for the next forty-four years, up to its revisions in the 1988 Education Reform Act (David 1993, 1995). The two major political parties were agreed on its underlying principle of equality of educational opportunity and the partnership between central and local government for the delivery of the education service, such that Mishra (1984) could write that there was a bipartisan political consensus. However, this consensus began to break down in the 1960s over the policy of secondary school reorganisation on comprehensive lines and the particular involvement of families and schools in the processes, such that there were several modifying Acts of Parliament. Nevertheless, the main framework of central–local relations remained intact. Moreover, this was used to expand higher education in the public sector, in the form of polytechnics, creating a binary system, as determined by Anthony Crosland, then Labour Secretary of State for Education and Science, during the late 1960s (David 1980). This new binary policy of higher education contrasted with the abolition of tri- or bipartite secondary education, moving selective education to a later stage. The ostensible commitment remained to expanding equality of educational opportunity particularly on the grounds of social class, as measured by the socioeconomic backgrounds of parents of children. Policies were aimed at reducing parental privilege and increasing children's access to educational opportunities in terms of parental poverty. Gender and ethnicity were slowly entering the policy arena as topics for policy debate and concern in terms of equal opportunities but no legislation was enacted.

The 1970–74 Conservative government continued these policies of educational expansion, especially over nursery and higher education, particularly when Mrs Thatcher was Secretary of State for Education (1970–73). It was aspects of the economy that led to that Conservative administration's demise in early 1974, as Margaret Thatcher has recounted in her autobiography (1993, 1995). The Labour administrations of 1974 to 1979 also continued in a similar vein, most notably with the Prime Minister James Callaghan in 1976 calling for a 'Great Debate on Education' and setting out an agenda for what was then called a common core curriculum for schools and a renewed partnership between parents and local and central government over the delivery of the education service to better fit the needs of the economy (David 1980). At the same time, equality of educational opportunity was redefined to cover not only social class but also issues of gender and ethnicity through general anti-discrimination legislation, in which the educational components were rather limited.

It has been argued, however, that it was partly the Labour government's problems with education's relationship to the economy that led to the demise of the Labour government in 1979 and the ushering in of the first Thatcher administration in which education was scapegoated for Britain's economic problems (David 1980).

THE TRANSFORMATIONS TO 'EDUCATIONAL REFORM'

Although education was a central issue for the new right-wing government in 1979, and two pieces of legislation were enacted very speedily in 1979 and 1980, it took considerably longer for the forms of education policy to be reformed. All the legislation prior to 1988 remained within the framework of the 1944 Education Act (David 1993). The then Secretary of State for Education and Science, Kenneth Baker, announced a major new piece of legislation in his White Paper in 1987 which has been nicknamed Gerbil – the Great Education Reform bill. His explicit intention, at this stage, was to create a new *era* for education in which '*standards, freedom and choice*' would be paramount, thus creating a new framework, giving 'the consumers of education a central part in decision-making' (David 1993: 63) Thus the term *reform* was inserted into the legislation to ensure that the Education Reform Act (ERA) 1988 created a new *era* for education.

This Act did indeed mark a decisive break with the 1944 Act, making it a very different piece of 'conservative' legislation in which freedom, choice and standards were indeed paramount. First, the partnership between central and local government for the delivery of the education service was deliberately broken, and schools, through their governing bodies and a parental ballot, were given the choice to opt out of local control and become grant-maintained (GMS). Second, all schools remaining within local control were given greater autonomy and financial control through local management of schools (LMS). Third, a new central system of national testing, assessment and a National Curriculum (covering ten subjects to be taught throughout the years of compulsory schooling) was devised to enhance educational standards. Thus local authorities' powers were considerably curtailed. Fourth, a parallel system of institutional autonomy was created for higher education institutions, through the same piece of legislation, and all public sector Higher Education Institutions (HEIs) removed from local education authorities (LEAs) and given a new funding body – the Polytechnics and Colleges Funding Council (PCFC) – similar to the traditional universities' funding body – the University Funding Council (UFC) – save that the latter continued financially to support research through what was known as the dual support system. Indeed, new quality assurance mechanisms were also introduced and initially targeted upon research through what were known as the research selectivity exercises.

ERA, 1988 has thus become the new cornerstone for education policy, emphasising educational standards and quality, consumer freedom of choice and institutional autonomy. Subsequent pieces of legislation, particularly under the Major administrations, have enhanced these three elements. Major's most significant move was his Citizen's Charter, first enacted with the parent's charter for education (Tritter 1994). The Education Act 1992 and the Further and Higher Education Act of 1992 have increased consumer choice and deregulation and at the same time created a diversity of new educational institutions, including the new universities, created out of the old polytechnics. They have also introduced new methods of quality control and assurance, particularly through the creation of Ofsted. Equally significant has been the attempt to increase choice for parents of pre-school children with the voucher scheme for nursery education. By the end of the eighteen years of Conservative rule the education landscape had been transformed to institutional variety and diversity, despite the new centralising language of types of institution together with quality assurance mechanisms. However, new central attempts were made to establish minimum standards of quality for educational institutions, and the means developed to close down what were considered to be 'failing' schools or educational institutions.

Interestingly, however, the contradictory moves towards market-isation, privatisation and deregulation, on the one hand, and central-isation and standards on the other had led to evidence of improved educational standards overall, particularly as measured by testing, assessments and end-of-school examinations such as GCSEs and GNVQs. Moreover, these developments have led to greater participation at all levels of education beyond compulsory schooling, in further and higher education. Over this twenty-year period the participation rate of 16- to 18-year-olds in sixth forms and further education has tripled so that about 30 per cent now take A levels. There has been a similar dramatic increase in participation in higher education. The gender gaps in both entry and performance have also been reduced. In some subject areas at GCSE and less so at A level, there is now evidence that girls are outperforming boys (Arnot *et al.* 1996). This has however led to a 'backlash' and consternation among some professionals particularly about boys' underachievements. Thus the policy developments have been extremely complex and with complicated effects on both educational institutions and educational performances. Nevertheless, the Conservative Party continued, during its election campaign, in the run up to May 1997, to argue for institutional autonomy and freedom of choice for consumers of education.

THE LABOUR PARTY IN OPPOSITION

Policies for 'social justice' and education

During its long period in opposition the Labour Party began to reconsider its educational policies and strategies in response or reaction to Conservative policies. Throughout, however, it maintained its commitment to what Anthony Crosland (1956), the Labour ideologue, had called the strong rather than weak definition of equality of educational opportunity; that is, not access but educational outcomes at various levels of education and access to economic opportunities regardless of the social class backgrounds of families. Although gender, race and ethnicity have become issues of concern they have not featured strongly in revised educational policies.

The most far-reaching review of Labour Party policy in opposition was that devised and initiated by the late leader of the Labour

Party, John Smith. In December 1992, after a third disastrous general election and on becoming leader of the opposition he set up an independent Commission on Social Justice (CSJ), chaired by Sir Gordon Borrie, a former Director-General of Fair Trading, and hosted and clerked by the Institute for Public Policy Research (IPPR), an independent left-of-centre think tank, chaired by Baroness Blackstone. Patricia Hewitt, then deputy director of IPPR, was the secretary to CSJ. The Commission was charged with the task of reviewing social policy fifty years on from the Beveridge Report (1942) on *Social Insurance and Allied Services* and setting out a new agenda for social and economic renewal in the context of an 'intelligent' welfare state.

Social Justice: Strategies for National Renewal, published in late 1994, was a wide-ranging review of social policy including education, remaining firmly within the tradition of bipartisan consensual politics on the welfare state. It therefore offered an antidote to Conservative policies with their emphasis on the free market economy and 'business' strategies to deal with current economic and social problems. This excellent and encyclopaedic review set an agenda for the consideration of the recreation of the welfare state at the end of the twentieth century. In this respect, however, the educational agenda was relatively brief, given the overarching commitment to consideration of reviewing and reinstating an agenda for social insurance, income maintenance, welfare and work. However, educational policies were to be far more clearly tied to employment and employment opportunities. Indeed the values of social justice were articulated as: the equal worth of all citizens, their equal right to be able to meet their basic needs, the need to spread opportunities and life chances as widely as possible, and finally the requirement that we reduce and where possible eliminate unjustified inequalities. These values are inextricably linked to promoting economic success, through first turning the welfare state into a springboard for economic success; improving access to education and training and investing in the talent of all our people; third, promoting real choices across the life cycle for men and women in the balance of employment, family, education, leisure, and retirement and finally reconstructing the social wealth.

However, the rhetoric of equal opportunities was not matched by the limited and often contradictory policy proposals or rather 'vision' for an Investors' Britain, in the context of a radically changed labour market. CSJ did assert that men and women alike will need

to maximise their capacity to obtain formal educational qualifications at various stages in their lives and repeatedly update their
vocational skills, interspersing full and part-time paid work with
unpaid work in the home and leisure pursuits. Education and
economic opportunities become, in this review, intertwined in the
dynamics of the market economy and a socially just society.

The CSJ's main educational strategies which set the agenda for the
Labour Party's election manifesto on education are indeed about the
complex links between education and employment opportunities.
Thus it set out an agenda for what has become known as 'lifelong
learning', rather than education being confined to the years of
compulsory schooling from 5 to 16 years old. This has entailed a
revised agenda for lifelong learning starting with early childhood
education in which children would be entitled to opportunities for
nursery education, in line with European policies and developments
(Moss and Penn 1996; Penn 1997). These opportunities would also
be linked with parents', particularly mothers', needs for child care to
enable them to participate in paid employment. Entitlements to
compulsory schooling were to be more closely linked to a programme of improved educational standards and quality assurance
and the continuation of effective partnerships between home and
school to ensure effective learning.

Indeed, a programme of school effectiveness has been central to
Labour party strategies to improve schooling, whatever the socio-
economic circumstances of the children. One of the major findings
of educational research conducted over the last twenty years has been
the evidence that school policies can make a substantial difference to
children's opportunities and development, whatever the context. In
other words, particular school-based strategies are at least as important as are strategies to deal with home circumstances. Nevertheless,
policies to ensure an appropriate relationship between home and
school have also been demonstrated to be critical to improvements
in school effectiveness. Thus strategies to monitor quality and
educational standards through new approaches to school 'inspections' based upon the re-formed inspectorate through the 1992
Education Act have been endorsed by Labour as much as by the
Conservatives.

Where Labour has diverged from the Conservatives has been over
its plans, through the CSJ, for post-school lifelong learning, linked
with entitlements to paid educational leaves through employment
and attempting to develop the concept of a stakeholder society and

expand educational and economic opportunities. However, the commitments to transformations in further education entitlements, linked with adult education, and the creation of new vocational education qualifications, such as NVQs, have continued from Conservatives strategies. The Conservatives did set in train a review of further education, with Labour and Liberal Democrat support, chaired by Helena Kennedy, QC, to consider the relations between vocational training and more academic education and developments, which reported immediately after the general election. Similarly, the Conservatives set up a review of higher education, also with all-party support, chaired by Sir Ron Dearing, to consider the implications of the moves towards mass higher education, in the light of changes in further education, and in particular to consider funding and resource matters. This too reported after the General Election, in July 1997.

THE PARTIES AND THE GENERAL ELECTION CAMPAIGNS

Although the General Election was called early, providing time for an inordinately long campaign, the campaigns of each of the political parties were quite limited and focused. In the case of education, the rubric of all three parties was quite narrow but they all accepted as fact that the two Departments of Education and Employment had been merged and none of them sought to undo this form of central government administration but neither did any of them fully address the links between education and employment. None of them raised the question of either further or higher education, since they had all committed themselves to waiting for the completion of the two reviews, both planned for the immediate aftermath of the General Election. Neither was there much debate about the institutional forms and governance of education, such as the role of local authorities versus that of central government. However, there was a tacit agreement about the developments in quality assurance mechanisms, such as the creation of Ofsted, and the development of forms of testing, assessment and new examinations in the form of GNVQs and GCSEs.

The Conservatives argued for the continuation of their strategies of customer freedom of choice in the context of a variety of educational institutions, regulated only by quality assurance mechanisms, such as Ofsted regular inspections and official league tables of different forms of educational performance, from examination results to truancy counts, etc. They pledged themselves to remain within strict spending limits. The Liberal Democrats argued strongly for improved educational opportunities, to be achieved by means of increased taxation, and particularly an extra penny in the pound on income tax, to pay for improvements in both the fabric and standards of educational institutions.

The Labour Party also focused its election pledges on improving educational opportunities and standards for the many and not the few, and therefore addressed issues of resources rather than the structures of education and forms of governance. However, given the commitment not to raise taxes for at least two years and to stick within the Conservatives' spending limits, there were also limits to how Labour could reorganise and redistribute education. '*Education, education, education*' was more rhetoric than reality about all aspects of educational opportunities for New Labour. Its key pledges were to abolish the nursery education voucher scheme and return funding to LEAs for nursery education, to reduce the class sizes in primary schools, to improve the standards of literacy and numeracy, to create home–school contracts to ensure more effective learning, to establish homework centres for secondary schoolchildren, and to deal firmly with recalcitrant pupils and schools, through developing new management training schemes for headteachers, with mentors drawn from lists of previously successful headteachers. There was little on how to address the issue of local governance of education, and in particular what might happen to the variety of schools, such as grant-maintained and city technology colleges, created by the Conservatives. Lifelong learning was also one of its election pledges, but with little of substance about exactly how either further or higher education would be dealt with.

THE NEW LABOUR GOVERNMENT IN OFFICE

After taking office on 2 May the New Labour government moved swiftly on many of its election manifesto commitments. What is particularly interesting and relevant for the purposes of considering education, is just how important the social and economic changes have been over the last thirty to forty years, creating a 'new class' of professionals and politicians. Thus the New Labour government and its 418 MPs consist of a majority of highly educated people up to and including university education, and including a large number of education professionals, both schoolteachers and academics, and educational activists, especially from the National Union of Students (NUS). In particular, the almost a quarter of Labour MPs who are women are well educated and significantly more likely to be involved in the profession of education than the male Labour MPs.

The Prime Minister Tony Blair created a formidable team for education and employment under the Secretary of State for Education and Employment, David Blunkett. These include several former academics and teachers such as Estelle Morris, Minister for Standards and David Howells, Minister for Lifelong Learning, and the appointment of Baroness Tessa Blackstone, former University teacher of social policy and Master of Birkbeck College, University of London, from the House of Lords, as Minister for Higher Education. In addition, David Blunkett appointed Professor Michael Barber, from the Institute of Education, London University, as his special adviser for Standards and Effectiveness and as chair of one of the two task forces, in his case, literacy. Professor David Reynolds, of the School of Education at the University of Newcastle is chair of the other task force on numeracy. A panel of expert advisors has also been appointed on educational standards, including academics, such as Dr Heidi Mirza of South Bank University.

In the first hundred days the pledge to abolish nursery vouchers was honoured, first in Wales, followed swiftly by England, with relatively immediate effect and ensuring that LEAs were able to continue to develop schemes of nursery education targeted on children in need. Second, David Blunkett committed himself to the reduction of infant school class sizes within the next two academic years. However, this scheme became relatively problematic since the majority of oversize primary classes are not to be found, as originally believed, in the inner city areas, with inadequate school buildings and resources but in the suburban areas. Thus this commitment to improve educational opportunities may not initially benefit children from poor and socially disadvantaged home backgrounds but may benefit children from middle income and middle class families more readily. Moreover, given resource constraints there may initially be problems with recruitment of primary school teachers for these reduced classes as there are reductions through the Teacher Training Agency (TTA) in the numbers of teachers being trained.

In July 1997 David Blunkett published his first white paper entitled *Excellence in Schools* which brought together all of his initial plans for early childhood and compulsory schooling to the year 2002. In the foreword, he asserted:

Education matters. It matters to you and to the children you care about. It matters to the country. Tony Blair and I have made clear that *education is our top priority.*[my emphasis added] We are now reinforcing that by publishing the first policy document of the new Government ... *Excellence in Schools* and that is what I am determined to achieve. Without excellence in all our schools many of our children are not given a fair start in life. That damages them. It also holds back this country as we prepare to compete in the next century. Excellence can be achieved only on the basis of partnership. We all need to be involved: schools, teachers and parents are at the heart of it. We also need the help of all of you: families and the wider community.

(HMSO, Cm 3681: 3)

He then laid out his six policy principles:

- Education will be at the heart of government.
- Policies will benefit the many, not just the few.
- The focus will be on standards in schools, not the structure of the system.
- We will intervene in underperforming schools and celebrate the successful.
- There will be zero tolerance of underperformance.
- Government will work in partnership with all those committed to raising standards.

Each one of these principles has been translated into particular policy proposals covering early years' childcare and education up to the end of primary schooling and ensuring the reduction in infant school class sizes to thirty; plans for raising standards in primary and secondary schools through LEA Education Development Plans and Ofsted inspections; modernising the comprehensive principle for secondary education, with Education Action Zones and a National Grid for Learning; improved teaching and training especially for headteachers and a General Teaching Council; helping pupils achieve through family learning schemes, home–school contracts, national guidelines for homework and work-related learning and finally a new partnership of schools, LEAs, the Department for Education and Employment (DfEE) and other partners to help raise standards.

Similarly in July 1997 both Kennedy and Dearing reported, first on further education and second on higher education. However, the Kennedy report received relatively little publicity and as yet has not been officially responded to by the New Labour government. The Dearing Report, produced five days later than originally planned, in part because the new government had asked the committee to revise its spending proposals, had an immediate and instant official response which made it difficult for any further or effective consultation to take place. Entitled *Higher Education in the Learning Society* the report is encyclopaedic and comprehensive and considers issues from quality and standards through to statistics on all aspects of academic life, running to well over 1,000 pages and with fifteen appended research reports. The issues that have caused most public discussion are not to do with these broad matters but concentrate solely on finances and resources for higher education through tuition fees and maintenance grants for students. The Dearing Committee had responded to the request to reconsider its proposals and came up with a complex mix of charging some element of tuition fees, of £1,000, to economically advantaged undergraduate students, while retaining free tuition fees and some maintenance grants, on a means tested basis, for disadvantaged undergraduate students together with a public loans scheme for all students repayable over twenty years.

The government, in an attempt to pre-empt the Dearing committee's proposals instantly announced the abolition of all forms of maintenance grants for undergraduates and the charging of £1,000 tuition fee to all students annually, along with the development of a student loans scheme for the repayment of the loan for these charges. The government then intimated that it planned to develop these proposals into a draft bill scheduled for the Autumn so that the new scheme of charging fees and abolishing grants could take effect from the summer of 1998, or the beginning of the academic session 1998/9. This then created a further furore over the summer, especially over whether young people leaving school in July 1997 and being encouraged to take a GAP year before starting university in September 1998 would be caught by the charges. The Minister for Higher Education was forced to retract and say that such students who could not possibly have anticipated such a change in their circumstances and had already been accepted for a course starting in 1998, would be entitled to start their higher education in September 1998, on the same conditions as their fellow students who had opted to continue through into higher education and start in September 1997. However, this may be another instance of the probability of more economically advantaged students being further advantaged relative to poorer potential students, since it is more likely that those who choose a GAP year are the relatively privileged rather than the economically disadvantaged.

CONCLUSIONS

Education, education, education has indeed been a major part of the work of the New Labour government as its election manifesto pledged. There have been a plethora of policy proposals and the first white paper to be published has come from the Department for Education and Employment, with swift plans for a second on higher education, and possibly a third on further education. Thus the three levels of education have all been addressed. However, the ways in which they have been addressed are not as different from the Conservative government as the politicians might like to have us believe. Indeed, the white paper is more a continuation of Conservative policies than a divergence from them, laced with more moralism about families and family roles than the Conservatives dared to offer. In this respect, it seems that there may be a return to traditional family roles and values, rather than an opening up of possibilities for women in education and in employment. This is also signalled by the proposals on *Welfare to Work*, on single parent families, also emanating from the DfEE. In addition, some of the key proposals may not achieve the limited redistributions planned, such as the reduction in class sizes. Similarly, the proposals to charge for higher education, in response to Dearing, may advantage the already advantaged rather than produce opportunities for the many not the few. Thus the election pledges have not yet translated into policies that clearly will produce a more socially just society, and one in which there is more racial and sexual equality. Opportunities for all in a market economy may be more difficult to create than the New Labour government anticipated, given the diverse and unequal society that was inherited from the previous Conservative government.

REFERENCES

Apple, M. (1997) 'The politics of education in a conservative age', Charles Degarmo Lecture, at the American Educational Research Association meeting, Chicago, March.
Arnot. M., David, M.E. and Weiner, G. (1996) *Educational Reforms and*

Gender Equality in Schools, (Research discussion series no 10). Manchester: Equal Opportunities Commission.

Ball, S.J. (1994) *Educational Reform: A Critical and Post-Structural Approach*, Milton Keynes: Open University Press.

Beveridge Report (1942) *Social Insurance and Allied Services*, London: HMSO.

Chubb, J. and Moe, T. (1990). *Politics Markets and America's Schools*, Washington, DC: Brookings Institution.

Commission on Social Justice (1994) *Social Justice: Strategies for National Renewal*, London: Institute for Public Policy Research.

Crosland, A. (1956) *The Future of Socialism*, London: Allen and Unwin.

Dale, R. (1991) *The State and Education Policy*, London: Open University Press.

David, M.E. (1980) *The State, The Family and Education*, London: Routledge and Kegan Paul.

—— (1993) *Parents, Gender and Education Reform*, Cambridge: Polity Press.

—— (1995) 'Parental wishes versus parental choice: the 1944 Education Act 50 years on', *History of Education*, 24, 3: pp. 267–76.

David, M.E., West, A. and Ribbens, J. (1994) *Mother's Intuition? Choosing Secondary Schools*, London: Falmer Press.

Dearing Report (1997) *Higher Education in the Learning Society*, London: HMSO.

Deem, R., Brehony, K. and Heath, S. (1995) *Active Citizenship and the Governing of Schools*, London: Open University Press.

Department for Education and Employment (1997) *Excellence in Schools*, HMSO Cm 3681.

Fitz, J., Halpin, D. and Power, S. (1993) *Grant Maintained Schools: Education in the Marketplace*, London: Kogan Page.

Gewirtz, S., Ball, S.J. and Bowe, R. (1995) *Markets, Choice and Equity in Education*, Milton Keynes: Open University Press.

Glatter, R., Woods, P. and Bagley, C. (1995). *Parents and School Choice*, (Impact Studies), Milton Keynes: Open University Press.

Hughes, M. (1996) 'Parents, teachers and schools', in B. Bernstein and J. Brannen (eds) *Children, Research and Policy: Essays for Barbara Tizard*, London: Taylor and Francis.

Hughes, M., Wikley, F. and Nash, T. (1994) *Parents and their Schools*, Oxford: Blackwell.

Kennedy Report (1997) *Learning Works: Widening Participation in Further Education*, Coventry: Further Education Funding Council and HMSO.

Mishra, R. (1984) *The Welfare State in Crisis*, Brighton: Wheatsheaf.

Moss, P. and Penn, H. (1996) *Transforming Nursery Education*, London: Paul Chapman.

Penn, H. (1997) *Comparing Nurseries*, London: Paul Chapman.

Thatcher, M. (1993) *The Downing Street Years*, vol. 1, London: HarperCollins.

—— (1995) *The Road to Power*, London: HarperCollins.

Tritter, J. (1994) 'The Citizen's Charter: opportunities for users' perspectives', *Political Quarterly* 65, 4: 397–414.

West, A. (1994) 'Choosing schools: the consumers' perspective', in J.M. Halstead (ed.) *Parental Choice and Education: Principles, Policy and Practice*, London: Kogan Page.

Whitty, G., Halpin, D. and Power, S. (1996) 'Self managing schools in the market place: the experience of England, the USA and New Zealand, paper presented at Fourth Quasi Markets seminar, March, University of Bristol.

Woodhead, C. (1996) 'Boys who learn to be losers: on the white male culture of failure', *Times*: 6 March: 6.

Chapter 6

The people's health

Helen Jones

INTRODUCTION

During the 1997 General Election campaign, public opinion polls and in-depth interviews consistently identified the future of the National Health Service (NHS) as one of the most important issues for voters, and yet none of the parties prioritised it in their campaigns and the media gave it scant coverage (*Daily Telegraph*, 25 March 1997; *Guardian*, 29 March, 21 April 1997). The explanation for this apparent indifference to a popular issue lies in the party political history of the NHS, and in Tony Blair's overall strategy for moving into Number 10. In its efforts to prove itself 'fit to govern' the Labour Party employed the concept of modernisation and focused on issues of trust, competence, stability, efficiency and anti-bureaucracy, and on switching government resources but not increasing government spending, all of which helped the Party to regain the moral high ground and win power. Policies achieved significance in the Labour campaign when they could be used to illustrate the above issues.

BREAKING THE OLD CONSENSUS

From the early 1950s to the early 1980s, the NHS sheltered under the protection of a party political consensus, built on the 1945–51 Labour Governments' legislative edifice. For thirty years the parties assumed that it would be electorally foolhardy to undermine the foundations of the NHS. Mrs Thatcher proved them wrong when her Government encouraged private health care and from 1983 insisted that local health authorities contract out domestic, catering and laundry services. The post-war consensus over the NHS had come tumbling down and the Labour Party bitterly attacked what it saw as a crumbling service. Even so, the Conservatives actually trod warily. In 1987 Mrs Thatcher felt it necessary to assuage fears when she promised 'The NHS is safe with us'. While opinion polls consistently identified the NHS as a key issue and the Labour Party as better able to run it than the Conservatives, in the 1987 General Election campaign Labour failed to switch its popularity on the NHS into votes and its efforts to exploit its lead on this issue backfired (Butler and Kavanagh 1988: 112).

It was not until Mrs Thatcher had put the keys of Number 10 safely back in her handbag after a third successive General Election victory in 1987 that she felt secure enough to propose a major redesign of the NHS. She was the prime mover in reform, and the Labour Party heaped criticism on her, not only for her Government's policy but also for the way in which her own preference for private treatment personified the Government's approach to health.

Early in 1988, Mrs Thatcher set up a ministerial health review group which she herself chaired. When she feared that the Secretary of State for Health, John Moore, was not up to the task she replaced him with Kenneth Clarke who out-raced Mrs Thatcher in his charge towards change. His headlong rush to introduce changes, his refusal to take advice and experiment with pilot projects, the nature of the reforms he introduced and his bruising style combined to earn him the almost united hostility of the medical profession. Doctors mounted a highly personalised campaign against the reforms proposed by the ministerial health reform group. Even so, a 1989 White Paper proposed changes which were incorporated into the 1990 National Health Service and Community Care Act, and from 1991, put into practice.

An internal market would now operate within the NHS, creating a clear distinction between 'purchasers' and 'providers' of health care. The reforms meant competition between NHS hospitals, and between the NHS and the private sector, which Mrs Thatcher claimed would increase efficiency and so benefit patients. Hospitals were free to opt out of district health authority control and become self-governing Trusts, selling their services in the public and private sectors. If general practitioners (GPs) chose to opt-out they too could control their own budgets and shop around before buying services for their patients (Thatcher 1995: 571, 606–17). Social service departments also became purchasers of care packages for the elderly and disabled, who came under the Government's 'care in the community' policy, roundly criticised for allegedly abandoning the vulnerable to the whims of the market and placing an intolerable burden on families, particularly women, as part of a governmental agenda of cutting back on state provision and assuming that women should and could play a more active, informal caring role.

The Labour Opposition was unremitting in its condemnation of Government health policy. During the 1992 General Election campaign, opinion polls showed that health was again the most important issue to voters and Labour's ability to handle it easily outstripped the Conservatives. Yet, when Labour tried to exploit the issue in an election broadcast, neither Labour nor Conservatives gained from the ensuing spat, known as 'the war of Jennifer's ear', and it remained, along with the 1987 General Election campaign, a warning to politicians of all colours that health was a slippery subject (Newton 1993: 147). John Major's appointment of Virginia Bottomley as Secretary of State for Health, a deeply unpopular appointment in the country as it turned out, served to increase post-election tensions over health policy. In 1994 John Maples (whom William Hague appointed his first shadow spokesman on health) wrote in a Conservative Central Office document, leaked to the press, that it would be best for the Party if the NHS received zero press coverage for a year (Sopel 1995: 252). Neither the unpopularity of the Government's health policies nor the Opposition's remorseless barrage of criticism could budge the Conservatives on their health policy. Instead, it was the Labour Party which moved its position.

REBUILDING A NEW NHS CONSENSUS

Over the course of the last Conservative Government, 1992–97, the Labour Party moved piecemeal towards an acceptance of the new principles of the NHS, as originally conceived by Mrs Thatcher, with a grudging willingness to modify the internal market and a quiet but symbolic dropping of an old Labour pledge to reintroduce free eye and dental check-ups. The new consensus involves the parties focusing on a very narrow range of NHS issues and avoiding public engagement with the unresolved and key issues of funding and rationing.

Signposts along the road to a new Labour Party health policy were erected in 1994 with the publication of the report of the Commission on Social Justice; in 1996 with the Labour Party's *Renewing the NHS*, its main health policy document; and in 1997 with the Party's manifesto. The Commission on Social Justice raised a number of important issues which the Party has not subsequently addressed or incorporated into policy, despite their pressing urgency. The Commission called for charges for the long-term care of the elderly and the need for a social insurance or pension-linked insurance to cover the costs of care in old age, for support for those taking career breaks to care for someone; and for greater involvement by families in residential care. Ignoring this politically and emotionally touchy issue is typical of the way the Labour Party proceeded, that is, by avoiding new policies which have significant financial implications for individuals and the state. The Commission raised other important issues, nevertheless, which did continue to play an important part in Labour Party thinking: the need to tackle inequalities, subsequently given flesh with a commitment from 1996 to create a Minister of Public Health; shifting resources to primary care and prevention; and banning tobacco advertising (Commission on Social Justice 1994).

Much of the content and principle of Conservative health policy has been incorporated into New Labour, but the style of rushed implementation and major upheaval has been rejected, so reinforcing a cautious Labour policy. In health policy, as in so many other areas of policy, Blair is often perceived by commentators as the true heir of Thatcher: while he has ditched her style, he has kept many of her fundamental reforms (*Newsweek*, 28 April 1997; *Guardian*, 16 April 1997). In fact, although there is an element of truth in this observation, the reality is far more complex. The growing consensus over health issues can be detected in the debates within the Fabian Society (to which academics made a lively contribution) and in a broader shift in opinion towards an acceptance of many of the health reforms introduced by the Conservatives. Calls came from across the political spectrum for more private financing of state services.

Private finance will play a larger role in the NHS, so blurring further the lines between state and private health care. Under the Private Finance Initiative (PFI) health care trusts are required to seek private finance for development schemes before bidding for government money. Private consortia will build and run new hospitals, leasing them to trusts. The Labour Party sidestepped the question of whether this growing consensus actually involved a shift in principle by employing the language of 'modernisation'.

'Modernisation' of the Party's organisation and policies has been a constant theme of Tony Blair since 1994 when he became Party leader, and indeed Blair and Gordon Brown personify the modernised party (the subtitle of one of Blair's biographies is '*The Modern-*

iser') (Sopel 1995). Their aim, to make the Party electable, permeated all aspects and levels of the Party. *Renewing the NHS* took 'modernisation' as a key theme and used it to bring Party health policy into line with a shift in public and expert opinion in favour of the mixed economy of welfare. From 1995 footprints indicating halting steps towards an acceptance of the internal market appeared. An article by Hugh Bayley, an academic expert on the NHS (and now Parliamentary Private Secretary to Secretary of State for Health, Frank Dobson), *Renewing the NHS*, and then the manifesto all adopted the idea of local health commissioning, that is, groups of GPs, rather than individual practices, 'purchasing' treatment for their patients. The proposal had a number of advantages. It meant that the Labour Party could save face, for although it acknowledged that the internal market was here to stay, the Party offered an improvement on the Conservatives' version by minimising the unfair advantage one GP's patients might have over another's; by cutting the paperwork; and by avoiding further upheaval which health professionals had all had too much of under the Conservatives. All three documents (borrowing an idea from the Conservatives' education policy) called on institutions to make public their statistics on treatment outcomes, thus offering GPs and their patients the opportunity to make more informed choices. *Renewing the NHS* and the manifesto both indicated that Labour would end annual contracts, a further improvement in the working of the internal market, and indeed a move already underway under the Conservatives; and get PFI, a Conservative policy, off the ground (Bayley 1995; Labour Party 1996, 1997).

THE REDISCOVERY OF HEALTH INEQUALITIES

The consensus does not involve broader health issues, such as socio-economic influences on standards of health and the resultant inequalities. For the Conservatives, lifestyle influences on standards of health are determined by individual choice and are not really a political issue. For the Labour Party, lifestyles are affected by the socio-economic context, and they do not necessarily involve real choices at all.

The 1992 White Paper *The Health of the Nation: A strategy for health in England* set targets for reducing coronary heart disease and stroke, cancer, mental illness, HIV/AIDs and sexual ill-health, and accidents. The strategy adopted for meeting the targets involved creating 'healthy alliances' between various organisations and individuals. *The Health of the Nation* saw improvements in these areas of health coming through changes in the behaviour of individuals and groups; it made no reference to the structure or organisation of society (Department of Health 1992). Yet, many attempts have been made over the years to draw attention to class (and later, gender and ethnic) inequalities in standards of health, most notably in the 1979 Black Report, commissioned by a Labour Government which fell before the Report appeared, and in a 1988 report by the Health Education Council (Inequalities in Health 1988). *Renewing the NHS* drew on the work of Richard Wilkinson who has argued that standards of health in affluent societies are influenced less by people's absolute standards of living than by people's standard of living relative to that of others in the society. Inequalities and hierarchies create psycho-social factors which undermine rather than improve standards of health. Improvements in health will not therefore come from tinkering with the health care system, but from reducing relative deprivation and promoting a more equitable distribution of resources (Wilkinson 1994).

THE MANIFESTOS

The publication of the Conservative and Liberal Democrat manifestos confirmed the agreement which existed over the future of the NHS. The concepts deployed by the Conservative Party in its manifesto and the policies it highlighted could easily be endorsed by the other two parties, with its emphasis on 'progress', 'investment' and a 'modern' health service. It emphasised that the Conservatives were the 'guardians' of the NHS and that under them standards of health and health care had risen. It saw the future of the NHS as anti-bureaucratic and developing in partnerships. It pledged greater public information and devolved power. The manifesto singled out mental health and primary care for special mention (Conservative Party 1997).

Conservative policies were mirrored in the other manifestos. The language, tone and concepts in the Liberal Democrats' manifesto were familiar, for like the other two parties they emphasised anti-bureaucracy, a commitment to a comprehensive and free NHS, accountability, prevention, investment, improving health and health care, rights, and a better internal market. Like Labour they were committed to a ban on tobacco advertising and increasing local influence on health care; like the Conservatives they emphasised choice in health care and the importance of lifestyle on standards of health. Unlike the other parties the Liberal Democrats opposed bed and hospital closures, mentioned their commitment to dentistry and the importance of all government departments taking account of the impact of their policies on people's health (Liberal Democrats 1997).

In its manifesto, the Labour Party recognised poverty, poor housing and unemployment as contributing to poor health and health inequalities. The most radical claim in the manifesto was that 'Labour will set new goals for improving the overall health of the nation which recognise the impact that poverty, poor housing, unemployment and a polluted environment have on health' (Labour Party 1997: 21). How this problem is to be tackled is not clear, but Labour's resolve to assess the impact of all its policies on health was recognised in the commitment to create a new Minister of Public Health, one rare aspect of Labour policy which has picked up where the last Labour Government left off. It was not out of step with Labour's overall strategy, however, for it was part of the Party's attempt to gain the moral high ground and fitted well with its commitments to ban tobacco advertising, anti-personnel land mines and the sale of arms to countries that might use them for internal repression or international aggression; to change immigration and asylum procedures so that they are firm and fair; and to clean up politics. These gestures which helped to create the impression of economic realism married to morality permeated all aspects of Labour's campaign. They were, in fact, two aspects of the one strategy of proving that Labour was 'fit to govern'. The similarity of the parties' policies on the NHS was scarcely relevant. None of the parties used the campaign as a platform for exposition of their policies. Instead policies were used as illustrative weapons in a campaign which circled around questions of trust, competence, and of being 'fit to govern'.

THE ELECTION CAMPAIGN

While it is generally accepted that the British have a passionate attachment to the NHS, the parties' experience of the two previous General Election campaigns taught them that it is not a vote switcher; so, it was not worth the Labour Party's while taking up precious air time with it (Walsh 1997). The Labour Party had to tread warily because with so many interest groups there will always be one which will pop up and denounce a party's health policies. So, while one headline in the *Daily Telegraph* warned that the BMA chief called Blair's health plans 'pathetic', another headline in the *Guardian* announced that 'top doctors' urge Labour voters 'to save the NHS' (*Daily Telegraph*, 18 April 1997; *Guardian*, 28 April 1997). It was important for Labour to avoid the impression that it was still a loose cannon, making policy on the hoof and for this reason no surprises appeared in the manifesto, or during the campaign. Diverting lottery money and promising to honour the Conservatives' year-on-year increases in NHS spending were cautious moves and part of Labour's strategy of proving itself 'fit to govern'; it was, too, part of a new overall consensus on the principles if not the details of the NHS.

Like the Labour Party, the Conservatives had their own good reasons for not prioritising the NHS: the Conservatives have never scored well with voters over the NHS and it was unlikely therefore to be an issue which could steady the Conservative vote. Indeed, Stephen Dorrell, Secretary of State for Health, inflamed hostility to the Conservatives' health policy when he told a woman who had said that she had been waiting for a heart by-pass operation to 'go and register with a fundholding GP'. Labour quickly announced that within five months of taking office they would ban this two-tier and unfair system which gave faster treatment to patients of fundholding GPs. They did not explain how this was to be executed (*Daily Telegraph*, 21 April 1997).

Those with expert knowledge of the NHS's problems would have welcomed a wide-ranging discussion of the NHS's fundamental problems, but one reason for the parties largely ignoring the NHS was that the problems are so extensive that the parties do not have the answers, not an admission any party wishes to make. So, for instance, none of the parties has a solution to the problem of the population living longer in sickness but not in health, although a report underlining this trend appeared during the campaign (*Daily Telegraph*, 15 April 1997). Resourcing the NHS is a major, complex issue to which there are no easy answers. The parties all ignored the issue of how the NHS can be funded in the long-term and yet this is an issue which NHS staff and health service experts all argue is the key problem which politicians need to address. None of the parties offered any solution to funding for long-term care although this is another of the crucial decisions required (*Guardian*, 27 March 1997).

The Labour Party had postponed a decision by suggesting in *Renewing the NHS* that a Royal Commission should be established to report 'quickly' on the problem.

Instead of offering radical solutions, or indeed any solution at all, to the funding crisis, Labour applied to health funding a strategy which it adopted for other areas, that of concentrating on switching resources from one aspect of health care to another: PFI will be reinvigorated; money saved on bureaucracy will go direct to patient care; and more lottery money will be diverted to the NHS.

The spotlight landed on a narrow range of issues, which related to easy soundbites, such as cutting waiting lists, especially for breast cancer patients (*Independent, Daily Telegraph* and *Guardian*, 18 April 1997): at one point Blair's warning that a 'Tory vote will kill the NHS' resounded around the country (*Guardian*, 18 May 1997). Fat cat managers and bureaucracy were easy targets and made good copy. The underlying problems with which governments need to deal were, as predicted, ignored (Brindle 1997).

The question of which party could best be trusted with the NHS has repeatedly emerged as a matter of concern to electors. The Labour Party has always scored better than the Conservatives on the NHS, for even when their health policies are similar, the electorate never quite trust the Conservatives to honour their promises. Labour's historic links with the NHS reinforced the way in which the electorate could 'trust' Labour with the NHS, in contrast to the Conservatives. *Renewing the NHS* had taken 'trust' as one of its central themes. Lack of trust in private health care has lurked in the background for a number of years, and came to the fore in the campaign when a report revealed that old people do not trust private health care (*Guardian*, 14 April 1997).

The longstanding lack of trust in the Conservatives' commitment to the NHS had, from the autumn of 1992, spread to virtually every area of Conservative activity, but the voters' lack of trust was especially acute over the NHS. Gallup Polls found that 85 per cent of those questioned feared that if the Conservatives won the election the NHS might no longer be a good service, freely available to all; 87 per cent feared that old people might not be able to rely on the state to look after them if they became unable to look after themselves; 86 per cent believed that even with tax cuts people might have to pay more towards things such as health care, pensions and education (*Daily Telegraph*, 24 April 1997).

Tony Blair exploited people's lack of trust in the Conservatives' handling of the NHS in a speech to the party faithful in Edinburgh on 17 April which received wide publicity. He warned that every pensioner, every parent, every child, should ask whether the NHS would still be there when they or their relatives needed it. He claimed that nobody believed the Conservatives when they said that the NHS was safe in their hands: 'Ask yourself this question: if the NHS didn't exist, would they ever have invented it? And if they get back, will it ever be there as we know it? They didn't want it. They don't believe in it. They don't use it. And the British people don't trust them to run it.' He did not offer any solution to the problem of funding and running the NHS but exploited the emotive aspects of the NHS, warning that a fifth Tory term would give them 'A licence to kill the NHS as we know it' (*Independent*, 18 April 1997).

People's lack of trust in the Conservatives was linked with the perception that Conservatives were no longer competent. One of the Government's justifications for its health policies in the early 1990s was that they would increase efficiency and choice; but now Labour were believed when they claimed that the Conservatives' policies had actually increased bureaucracy. (That the figures were too complicated for anyone to fathom did not matter; Labour's figures were believed.) Excessive bureaucracy was linked to managers who were linked with fat cats, and thus incompetence, immorality and sleaze circled together nicely. Labour's claim to cut bureaucracy also helped to distance it from the old Labour image of defending vested interests in an overblown state. Labour's criticism of Conservative bureaucracy and its promise to give more control to local people also undermined Conservatives' claims to have pursued policies of openness, accountability and choice: community care policies did not seem to have increased choice and there were suggestions that one NHS trust gagged nurses from speaking out during the campaign (*Independent*, 19 April 1997). The fact that the Labour and Conservative party policies were not so different on the NHS hardly mattered; what mattered was that voters perceived the Conservatives to have pursued policies in a cack-handed fashion. Labour set itself apart by its style as much as the substance of its policies. The Conservatives' long-standing strategy of presenting themselves as the more competent party with the experience of government now counted for nothing. By 1997 they were widely perceived as experienced incompetents.

AFTER THE LANDSLIDE: THE NEW LABOUR GOVERNMENT

Tony Blair's choice of Frank Dobson as Secretary of State for Health promoted more surprise than the Department of Health's policies. The appointment was a gesture to old Labour, and a comfort to those needing reassurance that the NHS would be safe under new Labour. It might, too, be easier for changes to be accepted in the Party if they came from someone identified with old Labour, even if not with the NHS. Hugh Bayley became Dobson's Parliamentary Private Secretary, and Jo McCrae, who had already worked for Dobson for four years, became his special advisor. The Prime Minister honoured a manifesto pledge by appointing a Minister for Public Health, Tessa Jowell, with responsibility for health promotion and public health; Blair appointed Alan Milburn, Minister of State, responsible for NHS structure and resources; and Paul Boateng, Parliamentary Under-Secretary, responsible for social care and mental health.

With the new team installed, the Department of Health sent out signals for the country to expect continuity in the short and medium term, with the promise of change in the long term. The Queen's Speech signalled continuity in health care with its announcement that a short Bill would be introduced to activate the Conservatives' PFI plan. The Bill, to be introduced in the House of Lords, would clarify the power of trusts to sign contracts under the PFI (banks had not approved PFI deals for building new hospitals because of their doubts over this power). That this should be Labour's first public gesture towards the NHS is indicative of the modernisation of its principles. Labour ministers now appear at ease with the principle of putting private capital into a public service. The need for extra money is the burning NHS issue of the day, and a Bill was required to introduce the desired changes to the PFI. (Steps could also be taken in other areas of health policy, as the health ministers were quick to point out, without introducing legislation.) The PFI for all projects, not just health service ones, is to be strengthened by having fewer projects, fewer tenders, more concentrated expertise and more standard documentation (*Financial Times*, 24 June 1997). The Government presented the new building programme as part of Labour's long-standing commitment to the NHS.

In his first policy speech in office, Dobson confirmed that the structure of the NHS would remain intact for the 'foreseeable future'; ideas would be tested and while he reiterated the manifesto pledge to scrap the internal market, the new system for commissioning health care instead of GP fundholding would undergo pilot projects before the Government introduced a new system. The testing and evaluation of projects means that changes are unlikely this side of the next General Election (*Guardian*, 20 May 1997). Alan Milburn outlined the principles on which new purchasing models must be based: 'Equal access for all, based on clinical need; high quality outcomes; and a service that is delivered efficiently' (*Financial Times*, 21 May 1997).

Policies more closely associated with the Labour Party emerged more gradually. So, Dobson announced that changes to the internal market would await a White Paper and a review would be undertaken of the distribution of NHS cash according to local need. While not ending GP fundholding, no more practices were to be allowed to become fundholders, and there were moves to prevent patients of fundholders being advantaged. New schemes are to be tested, so it is unlikely that the current system will be dismantled or significantly altered before the new century. Bureaucracy is to be cut by reducing invoicing and switching from annual to longer-term contracts (already planned by the Conservatives).

During the Election, the parties managed to avoid confronting awkward questions of funding, but within six weeks of the Election, Labour's media management failed when Dobson admitted that the health service review underway would consider all options, which included paying to see GPs. The story rapidly flooded the media, competing for space with Tony Blair's PR coup when he was filmed at his first semi-public meeting. Ministers quickly issued assurances that the Government would not pursue any policies incompatible with the manifesto commitments. Dobson's slip highlighted the appalling spending dilemma of the Government, but it was disingenuous of him to claim that the Labour Party could not have foreseen the state of the NHS's finances: in March 1996 widely reported figures showed trusts and health authorities £200 million in debt; in Opposition Alan Milburn had drawn attention to the parlous state of the NHS finances, and during the election campaign the Institute for Fiscal Studies released figures which underlined the problems (*Observer*, 15 June 1997).

In office, the health team quickly turned its mind to what will be the overwhelming problem for the NHS, that of funding. They devised projects to make savings: fraud had been exposed as rampant in the NHS, with GPs, pharmacists, dentists and opticians making fraudulent claims, and the Government announced plans to clamp down on fraud, and thereby save tens of millions of pounds (*Guardian*, 24 June 1997). They announced 'Health Action Zones' for inner-cities to bring together NHS bodies, local authorities, community and voluntary groups and local businesses. The stated aim was to bring health care closer to home with more basic services delivered in local health centres and complex treatments in regional hospitals, but the Department of Health must also have been attracted by the possibility of tapping into Department of Environment money (*Guardian*, 26 June 1997).

As the budget drew closer, public warnings and media exposure to the financial crisis facing the NHS intensified. At the annual NHS Confederation Conference, pleas were made to the Government to stem the debts running at £1 million a day (*Guardian*, 23 June 1997). Just before the budget Dobson gave a public warning to Gordon Brown, 'We cannot succeed unless the NHS succeeds' (*Financial Times*, 1 July 1997).

Gordon Brown did pull a financial rabbit out of the budget hat for the NHS with an extra £1.2 billion for the NHS to be taken from the 1998–99 Treasury Contingency Reserve. (This is equivalent to 2.25 per cent real increase, less than the average 3.0 per cent annual increases under the Conservatives, and less than the NHS Confederation's demand for a 3 per cent real increase, and the BMA's call for £1 billion for five years.) It harmonised with the Government's anti-bureaucracy commitment by being dependent on administrative reforms to cut red tape. The announcement that the Government would claw back costs of treating road accident victims from insurance companies also fitted with the mood of ensuring that the Government did not lose money, either through red tape, fraud, or inefficiency. It was, too, part of a strategy of mollifying traditional Labour supporters, preventing a back-bench revolt, and making clear that while not all the gestures were towards business, the Chancellor would, nevertheless, maintain a tough line on public spending. Ministers presented the capital investment in hospitals plus the extra money found in the budget as 'a £2.5 billion modernisation package', so underlining a key aspect of Labour's presentation strategy (*Guardian*, 4 July 1997).

Money from the reserves of income is a short-term strategy, it does nothing to solve long-term funding problems. Raiding the reserves, imposing a windfall tax or dipping into lottery money is no way to ensure that the Government's overall management of the economy addresses social needs. It does not alter the need for hard choices to be made over the rationing and distribution of resources. The key areas which still need to be addressed are: funding of long-term care for the elderly; the need for all departments to consider the implications of their policies for health (a Liberal Democrat policy); and how the demands of increased medical technology and rising expectations are to be met.

While Labour's first move was to revive a Conservative policy, and the focus of media attention was on the various ploys for cutting costs and attracting extra money to the NHS, less publicity was attached to the moves already underway to promote policies which fit with Labour's commitment to reduce inequalities and promote fairness. The new Government immediately moved to redeem a manifesto pledge to ban tobacco advertising (but it lost some credit by proposing to exempt Formula 1 from a ban on tobacco sponsorship); in the budget Gordon Brown brought to an end tax relief on private health insurance for the over-60s (much to the disgust of the *Daily Telegraph*), and over its first summer it set out a strategy for reducing inequalities in standards of health. Cross-departmental action, involving the departments of health, environment, transport, education, trade and agriculture, will take account of poverty, poor housing, ethnic minority status, pollution and poor education. The new proposals, to follow from a Green Paper and then a White Paper, will partly replace the 'health of the nation' strategy with its emphasis on lifestyle changes rather than structural ones. Tessa Jowell explained that, 'We want to attack the underlying causes of ill health and break the cycle of social and economic deprivation and social exclusion' (*Guardian*, 8 July 1997).

That policies to reduce health inequalities receive less attention than dramatic and hospital-related ones is partly due to the way in which the media filters health news; it also reflects the softly-softly approach of the new Government towards those policies which are identified with Old Labour. It is hoped that as the Government grows in confidence it will feel freer to highlight not only its policies for the NHS but also its wider health promotion strategy. Unless the climate of opinion and voters' attitudes are assured, and this requires public debate and exposition of the strategy, the Government's media managers will continue to shun it. Yet, the Government could let health take the lead in asserting its values and in pursuing distinctive policies because Labour's opinion poll lead on health is massive, and the public has repeatedly identified health as a key political issue. The means and ends of government cannot be separated: the way in which government operates – trustworthy and competent ministers providing stable government – is important, as are its policies. The latter were often hidden during the election campaign; next time Labour will be judged on both aspects of its record in government.

REFERENCES

Bayley, H. (1995) *The Nation's Health*, London: Fabian Society.

Brindle, D. (1997) 'Health', in Martin Linton (ed.) *The Election A Voters' Guide. A Guardian Book*, London: Fourth Estate.

Butler, D. and Kavanagh, D. (1988) *The British General Election of 1987*, London: Macmillan.

Commission on Social Justice/Institute for Public Policy Research (1994) *Social Justice: Strategies for National Renewal*, London: Vintage.

Conservative Party (1997) *You Can Only Be Sure With The Conservatives*, election manifesto, London: Conservative Party.

Department of Health (1992) *On the State of the Public Health*, London: HMSO.

Inequalities in Health (1988) *The Black Report The Health Divide*, London: Penguin.

Labour Party (1996) *Renewing the NHS: Labour's Agenda For A Healthier Britain*, London: Labour Party.

—— (1997) *New Labour Because Britain Deserves Better*, election manifesto, London: Labour Party.

Liberal Democrats (1997) *Make the Difference*, election manifesto, London: Liberal Democrats.

Newton, K. (1993) 'Caring and competence: the long long campaign', in A. King, I. Crewe, D. Denver, K. Newton, P. Norton, D. Sanders, and P. Seyd *Britain at the Polls 1992*, Chatham, NJ: Chatham House.

Sopel, J. (1995) *Tony Blair: The Moderniser*, Michael Joseph, London.

Thatcher, M. (1995) *The Downing Street Years*, London: HarperCollins, first published 1993).

Walsh, F. (1997) 'Safe in their hands – the health service', in R. Bailey (ed.) *The BBC News General Election Guide*, Glasgow: Harper Collins.

Wilkinson, R. (1994) 'Health, redistribution and growth', in A. Glyn and D. Miliband (eds.) *Paying for Inequality: The Economic Cost of Social Injustice*, London: IPPR/River Orams Press.

Chapter 7

New partnerships for social services

Susan Balloch

INTRODUCTION

During the years of Conservative government, the statutory social services escaped the wholesale reorganisation imposed on health services. Nevertheless, privatisation substantially reduced the role of local government social services as providers of care while enhancing them as purchasers. Since the Residential Homes Act (1984), private residential homes have more than doubled in number and voluntary homes increased by a quarter, while local authority homes have decreased by a third (Department of Health 1996a). In comparison, the domiciliary market has remained relatively underdeveloped, with traditional, local authority home help/home care provision still the most common form and four major providers, BNA, Care Alternatives, Goldsborough and Allied Medicare, dominating the private sector. Here too there are now signs of change – by 1995, 29 per cent of home help/care contact hours were being provided by private organisations, compared with just 2 per cent in 1992 – though the private sector's growth is thought to conceal a large number of market exits (Young and Wistow 1996). The resulting shift in relationships between statutory, voluntary and private social services has raised crucial issues about value for money and the quality of care which received extensive coverage before the 1997 Election.

The election debate on the future of the personal social services can be traced back to the summer of 1996, to a parliamentary debate on the future of social work, timed to coincide with the twenty-fifth anniversary of the Seebohm Report (1968) and to a seminar in which Stephen Dorrell, then Secretary of State for Health, espoused a cost-effective, right-wing model of residual public social services, with a majority of services either contracted out to the private sector or paid for by individuals themselves (Politeia 1996). This was in spite of overwhelming evidence that, as a result of unemployment, low wages and inadequate benefits, many households could not possibly provide their own means of social support (Hills 1996; Kempson 1996). That these views were modified, at least for services for children, before the election, was more the result of recurrent scandals surrounding child protection rather than an acknowledgement of the prevalence of social and economic deprivation among the majority of users of social services.

The debate generated by the right-wing Politeia group placed a heavy emphasis on individual responsibilities and revealed a lack of understanding of social exclusion. This was in contrast to Labour policies for the personal social services outlined by Alan Milburn, Shadow Health Minister, speaking in the parliamentary debate. These had previously been outlined to the Association of Directors of Social Services at their silver jubilee seminar in February 1996 and were based on:

- A nationally led anti-poverty strategy which would seek to tackle the 'unemployment, deprivation and sheer lack of hope' dominating many local communities;
- Social Services Departments joining in partnership with Labour to develop services based on agreed and enforced national standards, eliminating the unfair 'lottery' of community care, and backed by a General Social Services Council to safeguard standards of conduct and practice for individual workers;
- Recognising the local interface between health and social services and assessing the impact of health policies on other caring services;
- Strong local partnerships to co-ordinate the delivery of community care with new, nationally agreed and enforced mechanisms developed to speed up co-operation between health, housing and social services.

At a later date, the core of Labour's anti-poverty strategy became the proposal for a welfare-to-work programme for the long-term unemployed funded by a £3.5 billion windfall tax on the utilities.

The contrast between Conservative and Labour approaches was striking. The first emphasised individual responsibility and the importance of reducing state provision, while the second addressed the impact of economic and social change on social services users and their localities. However, during the election campaign itself these issues received little attention because the personal social services were marginalised by both main parties, hardly featuring in news-paper headlines or broadcasts. The reasons for this will be considered shortly. The omission was surprising given the flurry of welfare initiatives with which the Conservatives had anticipated the election. These had included new plans for a state pension, 'Partnership Insurance Plans' for long term care (Chancellor of the Exchequer 1997), and a White Paper on social services (Department of Health 1997b). These shared a common objective, to cut the cost of welfare to the state and contain escalating welfare bills, and in this respect their proposals seemed likely to be taken forward in some form by whoever won the election. The following discussion will omit further reference to the pensions proposals as these are analysed in Chapter 10.

The White Paper on Social Services: Achievement and Challenge

The Conservative Government's White Paper stated unequivocally that 'the principal responsibility for social care rests on individual members of society and society's own networks of mutual support'. Responsible individuals were to plan to meet their own needs, with every encouragement given to family and friends who were willing to act as carers of those who were unable to provide for themselves. The Paper saw the statutory social services as supporting those meeting care needs in these ways and as commissioners of care only for those whose networks failed. The Paper did not note that supportive networks mainly existed in middle-class and more afflu-ent families and communities and were often absent among poorer groups, particularly those on large housing estates (Finch 1989; Utting 1995).

In its discussion of adult services, both residential and domiciliary provision was firmly located in the private and voluntary sectors, with local authorities only permitted to act as providers of services after a rigorous review showed no better alternative. The main reason for this was to reduce costs which, it was argued, were too high in the statutory sector. The basis for this was a piece of research which purported to show that social services had become less cost effective in the 1980s: between 1978–79 and 1988–89 there had been a 41 per cent increase in real spending but a 10 per cent fall in the volume of services delivered (Bebbington and Kelly 1995). An Audit Com-mission report on Stockport had also shown the cost of a place in a local authority residential home to be over £100 per week more than in an independent residential home. These findings were strongly contested by local authorities, who rightly pointed out that measuring the 'quantity' of services delivered told you nothing about their quality or the severity of the needs being met. Though the annual report of the review teams being jointly run by the Audit Commission and the Social Services Inspectorate has recorded very good practice in a majority of authorities (Audit Commission 1997), the pressure to keep costs down and obtain maximum value for money remains.

The White Paper did not require local authorities to privatise their children's services in the same way as adult services, though planning and commissioning were to be broadened. Widening the framework for Children's Services Plans to give local authorities a strategic planning role and draw in other council departments and health and probation services was recommended. Amendments to the Children Act (1989) were proposed to reassert a proper balance between the rights of the child and the responsibilities of parents and other adults. A specialist child care qualification on the lines of that for Approved Social Workers was also suggested. While these proposals were generally welcomed, the logic of retaining specialist, local authority services for children, but not for older people was unclear. It appeared to be based on an ageist view of need, which did not differentiate between the needs of older people, including the rising number with dementia. It also, however, demonstrated awareness of the costs that specialist public services for older people would involve.

The importance of regulation and inspection of care homes and services was recognised by the White Paper with a plan for these functions to be assigned to new statutory bodies separate from Health and Social Services, although including their representatives. This took into account the concerns of the private sector about the independence of an inspection process based in a local authority. The distinction between residential and nursing homes was also to be ended, with new bench marks developed for care standards.

'A new partnership for care in old age'

The Conservatives' pre-election policy statement followed an earlier Green Paper with the same title (Department of Health 1996b). It set out a scheme for 'partnership insurance plans' for insuring against the costs of care in old age. The need for support rises sharply for those aged over 85. Although the percentage of the population over 80 will only increase by 1 per cent in the next twenty years, in the twenty years after that, with the ageing of those born in the baby boom years of the mid-1960s, a substantial increase will take place (Central Statistical Office 1996). With the number of people over 85 expected to more than double between 2001 and 2041, it was clear to all politicians that more resources would have to be found for both residential and domiciliary services.

The Conservatives' proposals were intended to safeguard home owners from the loss of their homes. Under their government, the problem of long-term care had been made much worse by the withdrawal of free NHS beds for long-term dependent patients, forcing up to 40,000 people a year to sell their houses to cover the costs of residential nursing care. The scheme offered £1.50 of extra protection from the state for every £1 insured privately. Thus to insure a £60,000 house would mean taking out £30,000 of private insurance, receiving a £15,000 top up from the state and drawing on the £16,000 disregard for savings below which individuals would not be charged.

The proposals were widely criticised for their limited applicability. It was estimated that only 5 per cent of the population was likely to be able to afford the high premiums required and that there would be a danger of creating a two-tier system which would do little to reduce the overall costs of care to the state for the majority. Labour claimed that the £200 million which the scheme would cost would be better spent on free residential nursing care. As an alternative, it promised to introduce a long-term care charter, improve care provision through the NHS by getting rid of the internal market and establish a royal commission to look into the broad issues of caring for older people.

No party, however, showed itself ready to grasp the solution reached earlier by the Joseph Rowntree Foundation's Inquiry, a compulsory national care insurance scheme, costing about 1.5 per cent of earnings. The implications of introducing a new tax were simply not acceptable. Yet the experts on Rowntree's committee, who included representatives from the Confederation of British Industries and the Trades Union Congress, were in no doubt that this was the only way to achieve their objective (Joseph Rowntree Foundation 1996). In this sense, the election outcome for long-term care was bound to be disappointing. A royal commission will find the Rowntree evidence a rich source on which to draw. It will need to take into account issues around the social care of younger disabled people and supporting them to lead independent lives, as well as the needs of older people.

ELECTION MANIFESTOS

Apart from concentrating on the lottery of community care, and pledging a royal commission and community care charter, Labour urged a review of mental health services to identify gaps and find better ways of using resources, and focused on developing partnership between health, housing and social services to deliver integrated mental health and community care services.

The Conservatives pursued 'Choice and security for families', echoing two popular election themes. They endorsed the White Paper with a proposed Social Services Reform Bill to create a new statutory framework for social services. Choice for social services users had already been extended through the Community Care (Direct Payments) Act, 1996 and new ways of reinforcing individual choice would be sought. Extra support was pledged for carers through a new respite care programme. Comments about social workers unnecessary 'meddling' in family life provoked an angry reaction from social workers and contradicted a number of positive statements by the Secretary of State about their work.

The Liberal Democrats promised to create a society in which people, whatever their needs, could live their lives with dignity. To this end they too emphasised giving people choice in the services they used and support for carers through a new Carers' Benefit. They proposed an Inspectorate of Health and Social Care to publish codes of practice for residential and nursing homes with the power to close any home that fell short of national standards. They also emphasised protecting people from the excessive cost of care. The threshold for payment for long-term care would be raised and national agreement sought on a system for funding care services that would not penalise thrift.

Thus the three parties all shared a concern for improving the care of older people. Astonishingly, none of them had anything to say on children's services, though various proposals for older teenagers were made in the context of care and control. Neither did any of the manifestos have a specific focus on social services. (In the case of the Labour Party manifesto, this may have reflected the lack of emphasis on social services in the report of the Commission on Social Justice

(IPPR 1994).) As in the Hansard daily reports, and in the last two Budgets (November 1996 and July 1997), discussion of social services was subsumed under either community care or health. Yet the personal social services employ nearly a million workers, cost upwards of £10 billion and provide services to a wide range of users of all ages (Balloch 1997). It would seem, therefore, that the main political parties were in tacit agreement that social services would not provide them with good headlines nor elicit public sympathy.

To explain this major omission we need to realise that the social services were, and still are, seen as providing a marginal service used by people who are 'not like us', even though increasing numbers of people need their help. In addition, the Conservative Government had characterised people on benefits, many of whom would be social services users, as 'scroungers'. The bad press endured by social workers since the 1970s was also partly to blame. But perhaps most importantly, as explained by David Hinchcliffe in the 1996 parliamentary debate mentioned earlier, 'One of the major problems faced by social work throughout its long history is that its existence is a permanent reminder to politicians of their failure to deal with social and political issues' (Strong 1996: 23).

Concerned at the lack of interest in social services, some voluntary organisations lobbied Members of Parliament and local councillors with election manifestos of their own, seeking support for improved funding for social services. Voluntary organisations were particularly concerned about the ways in which they found themselves compensating for under-funded services, as well as becoming bound by contracts which restricted their flexibility and choice. The Community Care Alliance, an umbrella group of voluntary and community organisations committed to improving the quality of community care, called on all the political parties to recognise the significance of the voluntary sector in the provision of community care services and in the support it was providing to individuals, families, groups and communities. MIND, the mental health charity, used its manifesto to call for national minimum standards for community services and for the full involvement of service users in decisions about their care and support. It emphasised national minimum standards for community care and an injection of new resources to improve provision. This was something which none of the parties had promised and Gordon Brown, as the Shadow Chancellor, had made it clear that there could be no extra funding for local government.

SINCE THE ELECTION

Within the new ministerial team at the Department of Health, the appointment of Paul Boateng, a practising barrister and previously Labour's legal affairs spokesperson, as Junior Minister with responsibility for social services, children's mental health services and family issues, came as a surprise. Some feared that it might mean a downgrading of social services as a political priority, particularly in the competition for funding, but others saw the appointment of a Black barrister, who had actively supported the voluntary sector in the change of family law, as a sign of a fresh approach.

Social services funding

Boateng quickly made it clear that local authorities should expect no injection of new resources. In response to a question on increasing community care funding he described social services funding for 1997 to 1998, part of the local government settlement, as a closed issue, with plans for local government expenditure for 1998–99, including those for personal social services, to be announced in the Autumn (Hansard Written Answers, 9 July 1997: col. 505).

In anticipation of this, the Local Government Association with the Association of Directors of Social Services released a budget survey based on reports from eighty-nine authorities in England and Wales. These authorities had cut their social services budgets by an average of 3.88 per cent, or £2.5 million per authority. While variations between authorities are substantial, reductions had been achieved through increased charges for services (83 per cent), introduction of new charges (38 per cent), the closure of establishments, with over 2,280 places lost, stricter criteria for access to services and changes to conditions of service. While children's services have mostly been protected, the brunt of the budget cuts affected adults and particularly older people. Of particular concern is the pressure felt by a few authorities to place people in residential care rather than support them in the community when this was more costly (unpublished report, LGA/ADSS 1997).

The extent of under-funding of community care had been highlighted before the election by rulings from the High Court and the Law Lords on community care provision. In the first instance, a case was brought by two care home residents in Sefton after their council had refused to subsidise their placements to the full amount required under government rules: the High Court ruled that local authorities could take the personal finances of an elderly person into account when deciding if to provide a placement subsidy, even if those finances fell below the £16,000 threshold at which local authorities were normally required to meet part of the costs. The Court of Appeal then overturned the High Court ruling on 31 July, and reaffirmed the principle that local authority funding should be triggered once personal assets fell below £16,000. Sefton Council said that this new ruling would cost them an immediate £2 million.

The Law Lords' decision to support Gloucester Council's withdrawal of home care services because it could not afford them (House of Lords 20 March 1997) aroused widespread public anger. The action had been originated by the Royal Association for Disability and Rehabilitation (RADAR), taking Gloucester Council to court after it had withdrawn or cut back home care services and revised its eligibility criteria. RADAR contended that the Council could not make such moves simply to compensate for its £2.5 million overspend in 1994–95. A letter from the President of the National Pensioner's Convention claimed that 'At a stroke, the Law Lords have threatened the vital home-care service which millions of older and disabled people rely on' (*Guardian*, 26 March 1997).

After taking office, Paul Boateng commented 'Sefton was totally unacceptable, but I don't see the same thing about Gloucestershire. I mean a local authority's resources are a factor. We have got to be realistic, it is just one factor.' (Downey 1997: 11). On this basis the government refused to back a private bill introduced into the Lords to prevent local authorities withholding or withdrawing care services on grounds of lack of financial resources. Lord Ashley, who had introduced the bill, said he was shocked at the inadequacy of the government's response. Similar sentiments were echoed by the major charities for disabled and older people, fearing continued uncertainty over the services people might reasonably expect to receive.

In the delivery of services, value for money has remained a firm objective. However, the political platform has changed. In a discussion of Wiltshire social services in the House of Commons, it was noted that it was 'for each local authority to decide how best to arrange their community care services to meet the needs of their population. We have made it clear that it is not important whether services are provided by the public, private or voluntary sector. What is important, and what the Government are committed to, is that people will receive services which are of high quality, are responsive to their needs and wishes, and which deliver value for money' (Hansard Written Answers 22, July 1997: col. 564). The belief that privatisation does not necessarily mean more flexibility and efficiency, and that public services may still prove a good option, has the backing of recent research. This found in one authority that greater flexibility and choice of home care had resulted from changes in in-house services promoted by an SSI report and the *threat* of competition; in contrast, in a London borough with a block contract for home care with the independent sector, problems of service delivery similar to those typical of in-house services were encountered (Lewis *et al.* 1996).

The responsibility of local authorities for their own financial arrangements was also emphasised in response to a question on respite care. Boateng commented 'No sums are specifically earmarked for respite care within the total community care funding which local authorities receive. Support for carers is an integral part of community care and authorities are expected to provide an appropriate range of respite and other support services. However, the precise level and type of services locally are a matter for individual authorities to determine in the light of local needs and priorities' (Hansard Written Answers, 21 July 1997: col. 417).

As there are as yet no grounds for thinking that the new Labour government will increase funding for the statutory social services, local authorities' scope for improving service delivery will remain limited.

The General Social Services Council

The need for a regulatory body for social services staff has been under discussion for some years. Although Labour's commitment to the principle of a General Social Services Council (GSSC) had been clearly expressed before the Election, and the Conservative's White Paper criticised for its exclusion, no reference to the GSSC was made in either Labour's election manifesto or the Queen's speech. A short period of uncertainty was dispelled when the new government's support for the GSSC was confirmed at a meeting of a parliamentary panel in May. The purpose of the GSSC will be to protect the public by providing a register of social work and social care practitioners, set standards of conduct and practice, and act as a regulatory body by dealing with complaints from users and others about serious breaches of those standards. The GSSC's membership will not be exclusive to professional social workers, but exactly how its boundaries will be drawn has yet to be decided. Groups to be registered early on will require a political decision but are expected to include field social workers and team leaders, residential child care staff and senior staff in residential homes for adults (Brand 1997).

The GSSC should provide a new measure of protection for the public and a means of restoring public confidence in social work, while new powers will be available to social services users who are to be involved in decisions about standard setting and enforcement procedures. Supported by their own, relatively recent networks, by some of the voluntary organisations and by a handful of social services departments, users have begun to make clear what standards they think they have a right to expect in both health and social care (Beresford and Harding 1996). Their 'empowerment', recognised for example in the Community Care (Direct Payments) Act, 1996, is slowly beginning to change ideas about how services should be delivered and about the roles and training of the staff responsible. In the long run, these developments could have major implications for both social services organisations and personnel .

Education and training for social work

The Council's establishment will have an effect on other central bodies in social work, such as the National Institute for Social Work, the professional associations and the government's inspectorates. A quinquennial review of CCETSW took place during the autumn of 1997. This was to 'assess the extent to which the functions of the council are necessary for the achievement of the Government's policies and whether there is scope for rationalisation, market testing, privatising, contracting out or transferring all, or part of its functions to another body' (Hansard, 23 July 1997: col. 599). CCETSW will be disbanded.

The strategic context in which the review takes place reflects growing concern about unqualified social services staff working in both statutory and private and voluntary services. A Sainsbury study of the mental health workforce highlighted the lack of knowledge and qualifications of non-medical staff (Onyett et al. 1995). In a study of the statutory social services workforce recently completed at the National Institute for Social Work, the low level of educational and professional qualifications among residential and home care workers in the statutory sector, who together make up nearly three-quarters of social services staff, was thought to be a particular issue for concern (Balloch *et al.* 1995). Most of these are low-paid women, a majority of whom work part-time. The low take-up of National Vocational Qualifications (NVQs) in social care by these staff has meant that plans to raise their level of qualification have not as yet been successful. The LGA/ADSS report mentioned earlier noted that a number of authorities are seeking to change conditions of service and replace workers with less qualified and cheaper staff. It also recorded that a small number of authorities were planning reductions in training.

It is possible that, within Labour's welfare-to-work programme, some of the long-term unemployed 18–25 year olds will be encouraged to join the social care workforce. If their willing commitment to such work is matched by relevant training, all will benefit, but a caveat must be issued of the danger of pushing unemployed young people into low-paid work with no clear career structure. In the long run both they and users of social services will suffer.

In addition, a survey of staff who work in voluntary and private residential and nursing homes, estimated at 553,200 individuals, revealed that less than a third of these held qualifications; among 4,424 residential child care staff, excluding managers, 82 per cent had no relevant qualifications (LGMB 1997). These staff often have poorer terms and conditions of work than those in the statutory sector and no continuum of training. Many are young and, without the attraction of training and a proper career structure, only stay in post for short periods, denying residents any continuity of care. For managers and those interested in a career in residential and nursing homes there may also be a need for a new health/social care qualification and training, attached to a clearer career structure. Many staff are qualified nurses with no previous social care or management training.

Partnership for a seamless service

It is not only in residential and nursing homes that health and social services need to unite to provide a 'seamless service'. Partnership between social services, health services and housing is also being given prominence in the new parliament in the debate on public health (Chapter 6). The vigour injected into this by refocusing on the relationship between poverty, poor health and mortality is likely to strengthen the demand for an integration of services for social care, health and housing. Determination to attack the root causes of deprivation and disadvantage is already beginning to bring about radical changes in the organisation of social services departments and in the joint delivery of services.

Nowhere is this more important than in the mental health field where the reduction in residential and hospital beds has left the minority in need of intensive care heavily dependent on community services. A Green Paper brought out by the Conservatives in February 1997 acknowledged the difficulties that had arisen in providing people with severe and enduring mental illness with 'a safe, effective and seamless service' (Department of Health 1997a, para. 1.7). The Paper laid out four options for change to improve partnership arrangements between health services, social services and housing. However, a consensus has emerged that exposing public mental health services to any further reorganisation would be unwise. Problems are being experienced, not because of a lack of organisational structures for partnership, but because of non-compliance and deficits in areas where partnership arrangements have not been developed. There was concern during the election, for example on the part of MIND, that mental health issues were ignored. It remains to be seen if Labour will assign to these the priority it gave them in its election manifesto.

Equal opportunities

Policies to support equal opportunities are of special importance in the personal social services as Black and other ethnic minorities, people with disabilities and women are disproportionately represented among service users. A strong emphasis was placed on equality in both the Commission for Social Justice (ibid.) and the Labour election manifesto. Since the election, however, it is only women in need of child care or as single parents who have clearly benefited from new policies. There have been several parliamentary statements about the need to give greater support to people with severe disabilities, but no action as yet. The disappointment of Black and other ethnic minorities at the lack of a clear strategy has been expressed by Sir Herman Ouseley, Chair of the Commission for Racial Equality. It is too early in the life of this Parliament to pass any judgements, but it will be interesting to reflect on developments in another year's time.

CONCLUSION

Both continuity and change are reflected in this chapter. Continuity of financial stringency is clear – there has been no increase in resources for the personal social services and the emphasis on obtaining value for money is as strong as it was under the Conservatives. Even though mandatory privatisation has been halted, there is still widespread support for a mixed economy of welfare and the rapid growth of private residential care is continuing unabated. No longer, however, does an emphasis on individual responsibility mask the social and economic deprivation of unemployed people and others on low incomes and their communities. New strategies promoting welfare-to-work, community development, public health, community safety and user empowerment, have the potential to change the whole context within which the personal social services operate. The implications for the personal social services and service users could, in the long run, be extensive.

REFERENCES

Audit Commission (1997) *Joint Reviews of Local Authorities' Social Services: Stockport*, London: HMSO.

Audit Commission/Social Services Inspectorate (1997) *Reviewing Social Services*, London: HMSO.

Balloch, S. 'Issues facing the social services workforce' in M. May, E. Brunsdon, and G. Craig, (1997) *Social Policy Review 9*, London: Social Policy Association.

Balloch, S., Andrew, T., Ginn, J., McLean, J., Pahl, J. and Williams, J. (1995) *Working in the Social Services*, London: National Institute for Social Work.

Bebbington, A. C. and Kelly, A. (1995) 'Expenditure planning in the personal social services: unit costs in the 1980s' *Journal of Social Policy*, 24, 3: 385–411.

Beresford, P. and Harding, T. (1996) *The Standards We Expect*, London: NISW.

Brand, D. (1997) 'Right register' *Community Care*, 10–16 July: 23.

Central Statistical Office, (1996) *Social Trends*, London: HMSO.

Chancellor of the Exchequer *et al.* (1997) *A New Partnership for Care in Old Age*, CM 3563, London: HMSO.

Department of Health (1996a) *Statistical Bulletin: Community Care Statistics*, 1995, London: Government Statistical Service.

—— (1996b) *Developing Partnerships in Mental Health*, CM 3242, London: HMSO.

—— (1997a) *Developing Partnerships in Mental Health* CM 3555, London: HMSO.

—— (1997b) *Social Services: Achievement and Challenge* CM3588, London: HMSO.

Downey, R. (1997) 'Minister's Counsel for Care', in *Community Care*, 12–18 June: 10–11.

Finch, J. (1989) *Family Obligations and Social Change*, Cambridge: Polity Press.

Hills, J. (ed.) (1996) *New Inequalities*, Cambridge: Cambridge University Press.

House of Lords, *Opinions of the Lords of Appeal for Judgement in the Case: Regina v. Gloucestershire County Council and the Secretary of State for Health(Appellants) ex parte Barry (A.P.) (Respondent)*, 20 March, 1997.

IPPR (Institute of Public Policy Research) (1994) *Social Justice: Strategies for National Renewal*, London: Vintage.

Joseph Rowntree Foundation (1996) *Meeting the Costs of Continuing Care: Report and Recommendations*, York: Joseph Rowntree Foundation.

Kempson, E. (1996) *Life on a Low Income*, York: Joseph Rowntree Foundation.

Lewis, J. with P. Bernstock, V. Bovell and F. Wookey (1996) 'The purchaser/provider split in social care: is it working?' *Social Policy and Administration*, 30, 1, March: 1–19.

Local Government Association and Association of Directors of Social Services (unpublished) 1997 Budget survey.

LGMB (Local Government Management Board) (1997) *Independent Sector Workforce Survey 1996: Residential Homes and Nursing Homes in Great Britain*, London: LGMB.

Onyett, S., Pillinger, T. and Muijen, M. (1995) *Making Community Health Teams Work: CMHTs and the People who Work in Them*, London: Sainsbury Centre for Mental Health.

Politeia (1996) *What Future for Local Authority Social Services?*, London: Politeia.

Strong, S. (1996) 'Food for thought' *Community Care*, 1–7 August: 23.

Utting, D. (1995) *Supporting Families, Preventing Breakdown*, York: Joseph Rowntree Foundation.

Young, R. and Wistow, G. (1996) *Domiciliary Care Markets: Growth and Stability? Report of the 1996 Survey of UKHCA Members*, May, Leeds: Nuffield Institute for Health.

Chapter 8

Home truths

Mark Liddiard

In most post-war elections, housing has been high on the political agenda. Housing, particularly in the immediate post-war decades, was an issue of the utmost political significance. Central to a Conservative campaign of the 1950s, for instance, was their pledge to build 300,000 homes, and more than Labour. But where was housing in the 1997 General Election? Does it still carry the same weight, or is housing little more than a peripheral issue? Despite recent skirmishes over residualised housing estates and begging, housing and homelessness are low political priorities. Despite the fact that the British housing market in 1997 is very different to that inherited by the Conservative administration in 1979, housing is now one of the UK's least contested areas of social policy. In many areas of housing, the policy differences between the main political parties are negligible.

The low political profile of housing, and the apparent consensus surrounding many policy issues, seems incomprehensible given the real problems facing housing in the UK. As we enter the new millennium, one and half million homes are unfit for human habitation and three and half million are in urgent need of repair, while there is a widely accepted need for some 100–120,000 new social homes a year. This chapter is therefore split into several sections. It begins by examining the housing market and housing policy in the UK in 1997, and how they differ from those inherited by the Thatcher government in 1979. It then focuses upon several key changes, in particular, the rise and expansion of owner occupation; the related decline of public rented housing; the deregulation of the private rented sector and problems with housing finance. The second part of the chapter then considers how the main political parties in 1997 have sought to respond – or indeed not respond – to these developments. The paucity of debate about housing in the 1997 General Election reflects the unwillingness of the main political parties to engage with housing – for a variety of different reasons – and a wider shift in public attitudes towards housing in general.

THE HOUSING MARKET AND HOUSING POLICY IN 1997

The UK housing market of 1997 is very different to that of 1979. One can justifiably argue that housing has been the area of social policy upon which the Thatcher revolution had the greatest impact. Undoubtedly, housing in the UK underwent a transformation after 1979. The most obvious change was the dramatic expansion of home ownership – a development which came to haunt the Conservative government in the early 1990s. Integrally linked to this development was the widespread sale of council housing under the Right to Buy legislation introduced in 1980. Both these developments left the new Labour government with a myriad of problems. More insidiously, Conservative administrations also shifted the manner in which the state is financially involved in housing and the housing market. In particular, there has been an identifiable shift away from 'bricks-and-mortar' subsidies, whereby the Government directly gave money to local authorities and others to build more housing, towards a situation of consumption subsidies, whereby the state covers a proportion of people's actual housing costs. This has been most obviously reflected in the rising cost of housing benefit to the Treasury. However, let us begin at the beginning, with a consideration of how home ownership came to dominate housing policy in the way that it currently does.

The rise in home ownership

We have, to use the words of Saunders (1990), become a nation of home-owners. There was a dramatic rise in home ownership between the early 1980s and the late 1990s. In 1981, for instance, the rate of owner occupation in Great Britain was some 54 per cent. Within fifteen years, it rose to some 68 per cent and seems set to rise to 70 per cent or more.

However, this expansion of owner occupation was not equally spread across social classes. While the rate of home ownership has remained fairly constant for professional groups, at 87 per cent in both 1981 and 1996, over the same period, the rate of home ownership for semi-skilled manual households rose from 35 per cent to 55 per cent. Central to understanding this increase were two features – the first and most significant was the 1980 Housing Act, which gave tenants in local authority housing the right to purchase their property after a short period of time – often at a very substantial discount on the market price. A second and related point was the overwhelming belief, even certainty – explicitly encouraged by the Government at the time – that real house prices would continue to rise, equating owner occupation with the accumulation of wealth. Both of these features were central to the Thatcher governments' expansion of home ownership. Yet both issues also came to create real problems for many owner occupiers when the home ownership dream became the home ownership nightmare in the early 1990s. In fact, the problems encountered by so many home owners in the early 1990s, and which were important political issues in the General Election of 1992 – namely, high rates of repossessions and negative equity – stem from the Government's mismanagement of the housing market.

Central to Conservative housing policy from 1979 was owner occupation. However, the Government saw the main obstacle to an expansion of home ownership as one of access – ensuring that the groups traditionally excluded from home ownership were given greater access to this tenure. The Right to Buy legislation certainly sought to remedy this, as did the Government's deregulation of the financial sector and building societies. The 1986 Building Societies Act, for instance, changed the manner in which home ownership was organised. From a system of mortgage rationing, lenders began to compete for customers by their willingness to lend, and moved to a system of lending on demand. Lenders became willing to offer far higher multiples of income than they had traditionally done, and loans were increasingly calculated on the basis of more than one person's income. Consequently, many households were encouraged to purchase their homes, promoted by easier access to the tenure and the pervasive belief that house prices would continue to rise indefinitely. Indeed, this was the implicit view of the Government and even some academic commentators who should have known better: 'far from falling in the future the real price of owner occupied housing is likely to continue to rise just as it has in the past' (Saunders 1990).

The result of these changes, however, was a very different owner-occupied sector to that previously seen in the UK. In particular, and

largely as a direct consequence of the Right to Buy, owner occupation was no longer an exclusive tenure in the way that it had
previously been. On the contrary, home ownership became a mass
tenure, as far higher numbers of semi-skilled households entered
owner occupation.

Fatally for the future of home ownership, this expansion of
demand, coupled with greater ease of access to owner occupation
through both the Right to Buy and financial deregulation, sparked
an inflationary house price spiral. These rising house prices were
exacerbated by changes to the system of tax relief in respect of the
first £30,000 of each loan, whereby two people could each qualify
for tax relief on the same loan. In 1988, the Chancellor, Nigel
Lawson, moved to replace the system and the limit was applied to
the property rather than the loan. However, because three months'
notice was given of the impending change, this made the rush to enter
home ownership at a time of rising house prices and interest rates
even more pronounced. The result was a flood of new property
purchases, often on the part of borrowers who had based their loans
on multiple incomes.

It was ironic that Nigel Lawson's so-called 'economic miracle' was
soon to have a serious and dramatic impact upon the UK housing
market. Following the recession of the early 1980s, employment and
real incomes began to rise – as did poverty and inequality – with the
result that, when coupled with Government taxation programmes,
there was an explosion of consumption, credit and house prices in
the late 1980s. The Government then began to raise base interest rates
to try and stem the surge in borrowing and consumption, and in turn
control the rise in inflation. The result of this economic policy,
however, was to lead the country into recession, as high interest rates
began to cripple industry and led to rising levels of unemployment.

The implications for the housing market were stark – as base
interest rates rose, so did mortgage interest rates. While mortgage
interest rates had been 9.5 per cent in May 1988, within just two years
they had risen to 15.4 per cent. Of course, there had been recessions
before in the UK and slumps in the housing market. However, what
was so significant about the recession of the early 1990s was the fact
that, as a direct result of the Government's housing policies, rising
unemployment was taking place against the background of a very
different housing market. In particular, there were now far more
home owners than had previously been the case, who in turn were
now vulnerable to the vagaries of shifting interest rates. Crucially,

many of these new home owners had borrowed heavily in the 1980s – often on the basis of high multiples of income – safe in the belief, actively promoted by the Government, that house prices could only go upwards. Such a situation meant that as unemployment began to take hold, home owners who had borrowed on the basis of multiple incomes were put seriously at risk by the loss of an income. As a result, repossessions rose dramatically. In 1989, for instance, some 15,810 properties had been repossessed in the UK. By 1991, this had risen to 75,540 properties. In addition, by the end of 1991, a quarter of a million households were six months or more in arrears, and more than 90,000 households were in arrears of twelve months or more.

As demand fell out of the housing market, so the owner-occupied sector began to stagnate, as falling prices and difficulty selling property became endemic. There was also a high level of repossessed property for sale – in 1991, for instance, one in four property transactions were repossessions – which in turn further depressed the housing market. As a result, house building was drastically cut with the result that thousands of new dwellings remained unsold. However, the cut in house building became an important component in the economic recession, affecting in turn the construction industry, and allied industries producing consumer goods, such as home furnishings, purchased when moving house.

The problems with the housing market were further compounded by the Conservative government's mismanagement of the situation, fuelled as it was by ideological dogma. For instance, while the collapse of house building further compounded the stagnancy of the housing market, this was not a new phenomenon. The owner-occupied market had experienced slumps before. However, in the past, local authorities had been empowered to take up slack in a depressed housing market by purchasing unsold private dwellings, which had previously helped to avoid the collapse of the market. However, for ideological reasons, the Thatcher government was committed to reducing the role of local authorities as providers of housing. Indeed, this was part of the rationale behind the Right to Buy legislation. The purchase of newly-built property by local authorities, which would have helped to ease the problems of owner occupation, was therefore seen to be inconsistent with Government policy. Only belatedly, in 1992–93, did the Chancellor seek to take surplus supply out of the housing market by providing £570 million to allow housing associations to acquire unsold property. It represented far too little, far too late.

Similarly, when the Government could have eased some of the problems with owner occupation by various forms of intervention, their response was one of almost complete inaction. Only in 1991–92, when forecasts for repossessions were rising –and, crucially, when a General Election was just months away – did the Government encourage lenders to establish various rescue packages. Despite the high degree of publicity devoted to these packages, in the longer term, they were largely ineffectual. In short, the Government's response to these problems was one of almost crippling inaction, while John Major later went on to effectively lay the blame for these problems on purchasers themselves.

In the face of such inaction, it is not surprising that by the mid-1990s, and despite the partial recovery of the home ownership market, there were still some 1,000 repossessions every week. In fact, the Government's response was to restrict further the limited assistance available to home owners. Throughout the 1980s and 1990s, for instance, home-owning households had discovered that on experiencing unemployment, the system of assistance available for meeting housing costs was incomplete and often inadequate. Yet far from exploring the viability of a mortgage benefit scheme, for instance, the response of the Conservative government was actually further to restrict assistance for home owners – cutting Mortgage Interest Relief at Source (MIRAS) from 25 per cent to 15 per cent, and withdrawing assistance for the first six months of unemployment. In the words of Larry Elliott: 'the Government is committed to a trio of objectives – deregulated labour markets; increasing home ownership and diminished help for the unemployed – that are quite simply incompatible. Something has to give' (*Guardian*, 16 April 1996: 18).

More recently, the fortunes of home ownership have been more positive than for some time. There has been a significant but geographically patchy improvement in the fortunes of some parts of the owner-occupied market – linked to general economic improvement (Pannell 1996). There has also been a gradual diminution of the mass problem of negative equity seen in the early 1990s, although the rate of repossessions is still high (Ford 1996). Nonetheless, despite recent very low interest rates, which should promote house purchase, confidence in home ownership as an investment has been seriously damaged, resulting in a far more cautious approach towards house purchasing.

The complacency of the previous Conservative Government when

faced with housing problems they had largely created was undoubtedly an issue in their loss of electoral credibility in May 1997.
However, the long-term legacy of these Conservative administrations was to shift the focus of housing policy fundamentally
towards owner occupation. Whatever the virtues of home ownership
– and there are undoubtedly several – the exclusive focus upon this
tenure and the consequent neglect of other housing tenures has
created severe problems for the UK's housing market. Nowhere is
this lack of balance more starkly highlighted than in the contrasting
treatment of public rented housing.

The decline of local authority housing

While owner occupation was enjoying active encouragement and
promotion by the Government, public rented housing was specifically targeted as a focus for 'rolling back the state'. The Thatcher
government was ideologically opposed to the notion of local authorities as housing providers. We have already seen that the Government's ideologically-led refusal to allow local authorities to purchase
surplus property exacerbated the stagnation of the housing market.
Of course, the Right to Buy legislation meant that the fortunes of
both owner occupation and public rented housing have been inextricably linked. If the moves to develop home ownership were the
first revolution in housing policy, the decline of local authority
housing was the second.

The 1980 Housing Act gave council tenants the opportunity to
purchase their home at a very substantial discount on the market
value, depending upon the length of occupation. In 1984, the
qualification period was dropped to just two years and the maximum
discount on the market price rose from 50 per cent to 60 per cent
while, from 1987, the maximum discount available on flats was raised
to 70 per cent of the market value. With such generous incentives,
the Right to Buy proved a great success. By 1986, for instance, more
than a million council houses had been sold into the owner occupied
sector. To date, over 1.7 million local authority homes have been sold
– a crucial component in the expansion of owner occupation.
However, while the Government hailed the Right to Buy as a
successful social revolution, it is important to acknowledge that this
legislation has left a long and difficult legacy for policy-makers to
address.

The first point to note is that the Right to Buy was not so successful simply because of the generous financial incentives offered by the Government to encourage council tenants to purchase their property. On the contrary, the Thatcher government operated a clear carrot and stick approach. If the carrot was a chance to access the home ownership dream at knockdown prices, the stick was sharply rising council rents, particularly between 1981 and 1983. Indeed, in the first six years of the Thatcher government, subsidies to council tenants were cut by 31 per cent while, at the same time, subsidies to owner occupiers rose by some 212 per cent.

It is also important to recognise that council house sales were not distributed evenly either between estates or across the housing stock. On the contrary, Forrest and Murie (1990) present evidence of a very marked spatial variation in sales. Unsurprisingly, the properties which were sold first were the most desirable properties in the most desirable areas. As a result, good local authority housing stock was increasingly eroded, while the stock that remained, and which was still available for rent, was invariably of much poorer quality. Given these differential rates of sale, and the lack of new building, so new tenants of local authority housing have been faced with a more limited choice of less desirable property. In the words of Forrest and Murie: 'These parts of the council sector are exhibiting less social mix and a greater concentration of social malaise. They are nearer to the ghettoised estate than they have ever been' (1990: 168).

Deregulated private rented housing

If recent housing policies, such as the emphasis upon owner occupation and the corresponding neglect of public rented housing, have created a myriad of problems, the Conservative government's approach towards the private rented sector was similarly ill-considered. The private rented sector in the UK has experienced a very long-term decline, from some 90 per cent of all housing stock in 1914, to just 8 per cent in the 1990s. Given the decline in the public rented sector, and the financial barriers to owner occupation, the Conservative government was keen to expand the private rented sector, to help meet housing demand. They believed that the regulation of the private rented sector had effectively hampered its development with many potential landlords discouraged by the regulations, rent control and tenancy agreements in force in this tenure. The Conservatives therefore introduced the 1988 Housing Act, which effectively deregulated the private rented sector. As a result, there was certainly some expansion in the amount of private rented stock, although it seems likely that this increase had more to do with the problems being experienced by owner occupiers, who were increasingly willing to rent their homes to avoid arrears and repossession. However, a consequence of the 1988 Housing Act which is more widely accepted is that private rent levels increased dramatically as a result of deregulation and, with mass unemployment and many tenants on benefits, these rent increases were reflected in rising housing benefit costs.

Housing benefit

Housing benefit is a means-tested support aimed at assisting the very poorest tenants with their housing costs. Housing benefit, however, has become a high-profile issue in many political debates because of sharply rising costs to the Exchequer. There have been several reasons for the growth in housing benefit costs, not least the impact of mass unemployment. However, much of this increased cost directly arises from the Government's deregulation of the private rented sector and the cutting of housing subsidies to both local authorities and housing associations, all of which have led to rising rent levels. In other words, there has been a transformation in the way in which housing has been financed in the UK – a shift away from subsidising the production of housing towards a situation of subsidising the consumption of housing. Rather than assisting with finance to build new permanent properties which would then be available for rent, the Government sought instead to help people directly with their housing costs, often paying large amounts of money to dubious landlords with ultimately nothing of permanence to show for their money.

This scenario is highlighted by considering the cost of bed and breakfast accommodation for homeless families, still widely used by some local authorities. In addition to the obvious benefits of permanent good quality accommodation, as opposed to poor quality temporary accommodation, the Government estimated in 1987 that the first-year cost of building a family home to rent in London was £8,200 compared with the then average £15,540 bed and breakfast hotel bill. Yet, fuelled by crude ideology rather than financial common sense, the Government was still willing to see thousands of homeless families housed in bed and breakfast accommodation, rather than subsidise the production of new housing. In other words, there has been a transfer of resources from public expenditure on housing (through capital investment) towards other forms of expenditure (such as housing benefit). Nowhere is this disastrous housing policy of the last Government more aptly illustrated than in the context of housing associations.

Housing associations only account for some 4 per cent of the UK housing market and so their contribution to housing stock is relatively small, but nonetheless important and very welcome. Indeed, the Thatcher government hoped that housing associations would come to replace local authorities as mainstream providers of housing. Since 1974, the expansion of housing associations was based upon grants – Housing Association Grants – paid on new developments to ensure that the housing association charged affordable rents. This enabled housing associations to develop in a financially generous and relatively risk-free environment, while in return housing associations provided a range of quality accommodation at affordable rents, often to tenants with special needs.

In 1987, however, the Department of the Environment proposed a change to introduce more market discipline into housing associations, and raise rents to market levels. The objective was to increase the volume of rented housing that housing associations could produce for the same level of public expenditure. As a result, Housing Association Grants, as a proportion of costs, have been dropping in value. In 1989/90, for instance, the grant covered some 75 per cent of development costs, while in 1995/96, it was just 55 per cent.

Housing associations have responded to this shortfall of income in an obvious way – by raising rent levels. Indeed, the 1988 Housing Act meant that housing associations were increasingly responsible for setting their own rent levels. In light of the financial uncertainty that faced many housing associations, it is not surprising that the rent levels of new stock increased fast. Between 1988 and 1991, for instance, rents for new housing association dwellings rose by 104 per cent, at a time when prices generally rose by just 26 per cent. Yet housing associations have traditionally catered to tenants on incomes below the national average, and often have a very high proportion of tenants reliant on benefits. These rent increases therefore led to dramatic increases in the costs of housing benefit. Indeed, the Government even acknowledged that housing benefit would 'take the strain' of rising rent levels. Yet any financial savings made by the Government through cutting subsidies to housing associations, were therefore lost through increased housing benefit costs. In the process, the Government also created a dependency trap, whereby rent levels are often so high that many tenants could not hope to find employment paying wages sufficient to cover their housing costs.

The rise in housing benefit costs, however, has become a big political issue in itself. In 1994, for instance, Jonathan Aitken, then Chief Secretary to the Treasury, predicted that the cost of housing benefit would rise, in 1996/97, to some £11.5 billion a year – three times the amount for 1988/89. Even the Department of Social Security acknowledged that much of this increase was a consequence of rising rent levels. Yet the response of the Government – far from making incisive moves to control rent levels – was instead to tighten eligibility and cap housing benefit levels in a number of ways. Arguably, these changes did not succeed because they failed to address the root cause of rising housing benefit costs – escalating rent levels. Instead, these changes seemed only to further marginalise some of the most vulnerable tenants. Young people under 25 have been particularly affected by restrictions in their eligibility for housing benefit. I have argued elsewhere that the last Government's housing policies, coupled with quite punitive attacks upon the benefit eligibility of unemployed young people, helped to create and sustain the youth homelessness problem of the 1990s (Hutson and Liddiard 1994).

Paradoxically, the rent increases in all tenures that have directly resulted from Government housing policies actually conflicted with Government economic policy. A low grant and high rent policy only serves to increase inflation, which in consequence can lead to job losses and high public expenditure on index-linked benefits and pensions. Such rent increases also have wider impacts upon the economy. Even in the context of low inflation rates, employees will be more unwilling to exercise restraint when rent levels – a significant part of the weekly budget – are rising dramatically. Between 1990 and 1994, for instance, average earnings rose by some 24 per cent. Yet over the same period, rent levels in local authority and housing association properties rose by some 60 per cent and 80 per cent respectively.

In short, housing policy in this country was literally turned upside down during eighteen years of Conservative administration. Owner occupation was expanded to the point of collapse; vast amounts of good quality local authority stock was sold off at a discount and despite huge housing demand; the poor quality and rising costs of the remaining stock have left new tenants in local authority properties both marginalised and residualised; both the private rented sector and housing associations have experienced dramatic rent increases – albeit for different reasons – and the cost of housing benefit has exploded, as has the problem of youth homelessness. In other words, the new Government faces a housing market in crisis. How did the different political parties address these issues in the context of the 1997 General Election?

THE 1997 GENERAL ELECTION AND HOUSING

The 1997 General Election was a very interesting election, not least because of an almost complete absence of debate about housing. Even a cursory study of the party manifestos show that housing was politically sidelined. In the fifty-page Conservative manifesto, for instance, housing warranted just half a page – and the dominance of home ownership was tangible. While the Conservative manifesto had few surprises, with its emphasis upon helping 'local authority and housing association tenants to buy their homes, or move to houses which they buy' (p. 19) and 'encouraging a thriving private rental market' (p. 19), the Labour manifesto was more intriguing. The commitment to the phased release of capital receipts from council home sales, and increased protection for tenants in private rented accommodation, were anticipated. However, what was more notable was the emphasis given to owner occupation. Given the relative lack of attention given to housing in the manifesto, and the very real problems facing housing in the UK, the significance attached to the problem of 'gazumping' in Labour's manifesto was surprising: 'The problems of gazumping have reappeared. Those who break their bargains should be liable to pay the costs inflicted on others, in particular legal and survey costs. We are consulting on the best way of tackling the problems of gazumping in the interests of responsible home buyers and sellers' (p. 26).

While other political parties, such as the Liberal Democrats, did show a more rounded approach towards housing policy, it must be remembered that the political agendas of the Election were largely framed by the two main political parties. In fact, the paucity of debate about housing and the dominance of home ownership in debate are very interesting, and reflect a number of themes. Both main political parties were certainly reliant upon the electoral support of home owners. Yet both the Conservatives and Labour also had good – albeit different – reasons to down-play housing as a political issue.

There are certainly a number of reasons why the Conservatives were hesitant to move housing to the top of the political agenda. The main reason, of course, is the fact that so many people were affected by the collapse of the home ownership market, either directly, through negative equity and repossessions, or indirectly, through a loss of confidence in home ownership as the tenure of choice and wealth accumulation. At the 1992 General Election, the Conservatives enjoyed a twenty-point lead among home owners. This was not unduly surprising, given that the Conservatives have long been seen to be the party of home ownership, particularly in the face of initial Labour opposition to the Right to Buy legislation. Indeed, because of the traditional association between home ownership and voting Conservative, many commentators claimed that the 1980 Right to Buy was a political masterstroke, transforming Labour-voting council tenants into Conservative-voting home owners. Of course, the impact of this legislation was not quite so straight-forward, but nonetheless the expansion of home ownership did not do Conservative electoral prospects any harm, at least, not initially.

In contrast to the 1992 Election, when much was being made of building society rescue packages, and belated assistance for beleaguered home owners, the 1997 Election took place in a very different context and against a very different public perception of the Conservatives. Far from being the supportive party of home ownership which they had presented themselves as in 1992, events in the years leading to May 1997 witnessed a real disregard for the interests of home owners – reducing MIRAS from 25 to 15 per cent; withdrawing assistance for unemployed home owners and then even blaming home owners themselves for the problems of negative equity and repossessions. In this context, it is not surprising that many home owners felt betrayed by the Conservatives, and voted accordingly. In contrast to 1992, for instance, in the run-up to the 1997 election, Labour's lead among home owners was more than 13 per cent. Given their record of inaction in the face of the collapse of the home ownership market, it is not surprising that many Conservative strategists were keen to underplay housing as an election issue.

While there was good evidence by 1997 that owner occupation was in recovery – neutralising negative equity and soothing the nerves of many owner occupiers – even this recovery was not necessarily good news for the Conservatives. Not only has this upturn in the market been heavily determined by geographical location and property type, but the upsurge in some sectors of the market had raised again the problem of gazumping, and the Government's failure to take action (Bar-Hillel 1997).

It is ironic that the very success of the Conservative's promotion of home ownership led to a far larger proportion of the population being affected by the fortunes of home ownership than would previously have been the case, with all the attendant political implications. Indeed, no political party could hope to win the election without the support of millions of home owners.

In light of the political significance of home owners, it seems surprising that the Labour Party did not make more of the Conservative's disastrous record on home ownership. However, Labour was hesitant to raise the political profile of housing, for reasons outlined by Kellner (1997). Despite the higher level of support for Labour among home owners, when asked which party had the best policies for home ownership, the results were more worrying for Labour. The results of a Gallup survey, for instance, found that among home owners, 44 per cent thought that the Conservatives had the best policies for home ownership, as opposed to just 25 per cent for Labour. In other words, while Labour was some way ahead of the Conservatives in terms of support among home owners, the poll still showed that some 20 per cent of Labour supporters – or three million votes – thought that the Conservatives nonetheless had the best policies for home ownership. Of course, this reflects the fact that for most voters, housing is not the sole or even main issue determining electoral preferences. However, these figures may also reflect the fact that the traditional notion of the Conservatives as the natural party of the home owner remains, encouraged as it has been by a period of rising house prices and low interest rates. By implication, it also implies a lingering suspicion of Labour's economic competence, at least in the context of home ownership. For this reason alone, many Labour strategists were hesitant to move housing and home ownership onto the main political stage, despite the Conservatives apparent vulnerability. Indeed, Peter Kellner (1997) forcefully made this point: 'the Tories could turn the housing issue to their advantage in the coming election – if they can scare voters rigid about what would happen if Labour won' (p. 9).

Some Tory strategists did take this point further – with their 'New Labour, New Mortgage Risk' campaign, for instance. Indeed, the number of rises in interest rates since the Election has been one of the few areas in which Labour have seemed politically vulnerable during their initial honeymoon period. Nonetheless, in retrospect, it seems clear that neither of the main parties were keen to place housing, even home ownership, high on the political agenda, albeit for different reasons.

If home ownership did not really find itself at the centre of the political stage, then it is not surprising that other housing issues failed to gain the political coverage that they deserved – there were simply too few votes in them. Home owners, after all, now represent almost three-quarters of the electorate. The fact that owner occupiers outnumber council tenants by some four-to-one means that whatever the serious problems with other housing tenures, housing finance and homelessness, and the really pressing demand for new housing, these issues do not carry the potential voters to make them politically expedient. The neglect of these themes in the last election was disgraceful, given the state of crisis that housing in the UK now finds itself in. Even when issues such as homelessness or problem estates were raised, they were invariably discussed in quite individualistic terms – with the main political parties competing fiercely for the votes of middle England, often with crude political gesturing, rather than serious and informed debate.

A further issue is the fact that many housing commentators detected a tangible sense of confusion surrounding a number of Labour's housing policies, which in turn may have dissuaded Labour from focusing upon this area. In particular, there has been some long-standing debate about Labour's policy in relation to the release of capital receipts – the proceeds from the sale of council housing that local authorities have been restricted from using. Labour has long claimed that they are committed to the phased release of capital receipts, to provide funds for new housing and renovating old housing stock, while in the process giving a valuable boost to the construction industry. However, at the same time, in their efforts to promote their financial prudence, Labour have pledged to avoid any increase in the Public Sector Borrowing Requirement (PSBR). Yet the two objectives have been technically incompatible. Under current Treasury rules, any release of capital receipts would increase public borrowing, and in turn inflation. It would therefore be impossible under the current financial regime to increase housing investment without either increasing taxes; cutting investment elsewhere, or changing the Treasury rules. Given the fact that Labour pledged to keep public spending within the Conservatives' projected limits for two years, it was initially very unclear just what Labour was going to do. Unclear policies have the potential to become political disasters and this may be another reason for the exclusion of any serious discussion of housing.

In fact, during its first 100 days, the progress of the new Labour government in housing terms was encouraging. Labour immediately published a bill to allow the release of £5 billion of banked capital receipts for housing investment by modifying Treasury rules, and two significant housing policies of the Conservatives – compulsory competitive tendering for housing management and changes to the homelessness legislation – were dropped. Nonetheless, in spite of these welcome developments, it was very unclear just how housing policy would develop under the new Government (Dwelly 1997). After all, despite the inclusion of released capital receipts, total housing investment is set to fall to just £2.1 billion in 1999/2000 – less than half the amount spent by the Conservatives in 1994 (*Roof* 1997).

Probably the most obvious reason for the neglect of housing in the 1997 General Election was the fact that it is no longer seen to be a political priority by the electorate. In 1945, for instance, Gallup asked 'What do you think is the most urgent home-front problem that the Government must solve in the next few months?' Cited by some 54 per cent of the electorate, housing was easily the most important issue, as opposed to just 13 per cent who mentioned the second-placed issue – employment. The political significance of housing was tangible until at least the 1970s. In contrast, regular MORI surveys in 1996 and 1997 showed that just 7–10 per cent of voters cited housing as 'one of the most important issues facing Britain today' (Kellner 1997). In short, in the eyes of many voters, housing is no longer a mainstream issue. In this sense, it is not surprising that housing was largely neglected in the 1997 General Election.

However, public attitudes and opinions towards welfare are contextual, and can reflect a number of themes. I have discussed elsewhere, for instance, the role of the media in promoting a perception of homelessness as a problem of individual pathology, rather than a consequence of structural changes in the housing market. Actively promoted by the Conservative government, who in turn helped to set media agendas, such interpretations of homelessness are now a prominent feature of public attitudes towards homelessness (Liddiard, forthcoming). Similarly, one could argue that the low priority accorded to housing as a political issue by the public, is itself a consequence of Government policy. The British Social Attitudes Survey, for instance, also shows that for most of the population, housing is not a political priority (Taylor-Gooby 1995). The findings from this survey are very interesting, and have attracted considerable comment. What does seem clear, however, is the centrality of self-interest in reflecting public preferences for more state intervention. Universal state services from which most of the electorate benefit, such as education and health, attract high levels of public support. Indeed, these were the two most important issues of the 1997 election. Yet selective services, such as social security, receive considerably less public support, because fewer of the public actually benefit from these services, or at least perceive themselves as benefiting. From once being something of a universal service, the rise in owner occupation and the residualisation of local authority housing stock, has led to housing becoming an increasingly marginal-ised and selective welfare service. In turn, housing has become less of a political priority for most of the population. This public perception is perhaps ironic, given that MIRAS and subsidies to home owners are a very considerable burden upon the Treasury. Nonetheless, the notion that housing provision is somehow beyond the remit of state provision has become pervasive, actively promoted as it was by successive Conservative governments.

In conclusion, it is evident that the 1997 General Election was characterised by a paucity of debate on housing; homogeneous and uncontested housing policies; and public indifference to housing as a political issue. In the context of the 1997 election, history may show that housing policy was Margaret Thatcher's greatest triumph.

REFERENCES

Bar-Hillel, M. (1997) 'It's still in a mess', *Roof*, 22, 2: 10.

Dwelly, T. (1997) 'The council comeback', *Roof*, 22, 4: 20–3.

Ford, J. (1996) 'High-wire recovery', *Roof*, 21, 4: 24–7.

Forrest, R. and Murie, A. (1990) *Selling the Welfare State*, 2nd edn, London: Routledge.

Hutson, S. and Liddiard, M. (1994) *Youth Homelessness: The Construction of a Social Issue*, London: Macmillan.

Kellner, P. (1997) 'Poll bombshell', *Roof*, 22, 2: 9.

Liddiard, M. (forthcoming) 'Homelessness – the media, public attitudes and policy-making', in S. Hutson and D. Clapham (eds) *Homelessness – Private Troubles and Public Policies*, London: Cassells.

Pannell, B. (1996) 'Recent developments in the housing and savings markets', *Housing Finance*, 31: 3–6.

Roof (1997) 'Editorial – homes and rules', *Roof*, 22, 5: 5.

Saunders, P. (1990) *A Nation of Home Owners*, London: Unwin Hyman.

Taylor-Gooby, P. (1995) 'Comfortable, marginal and excluded: Who should pay higher taxes for a better welfare state?' in R. Jowell, J. Curtice, A. Park, L. Brook and D. Ahrendt (eds) *British Social Attitudes: The 12th Report*, Aldershot: Dartmouth.

Chapter 9

Poverty and social security in a changing Britain

Carey Oppenheim

INTRODUCTION

Poverty set the General Election campaign alight only fleetingly when the Churches' Report on *Unemployment and the Future of Work* was published. It threw down the gauntlet to the political parties questioning how far their policies would address disadvantage. This public reticence about poverty sits alongside a dramatic sharpening of inequalities between rich and poor over the last eighteen years. The growth of poverty and inequality has been widely researched (Hills 1995; Kempson 1996; Oppenheim 1997a). The Households Below Average Income (HBAI) statistics produced by the Department of Social Security show that between 1979 and 1993/94 the numbers living in poverty (defined as 50 per cent of average income after housing costs) grew from 5 million (9 per cent of the UK population) to 13.7 million (24 per cent) (DSS 1996). The rise for children was even steeper – from 1.4 million (10 per cent of all children) in 1979 to 4.2 million (32 per cent) in poverty in 1993/94. Inequality, whether measured by income, earnings, health, housing or wealth, has grown since the late 1970s. The HBAI documents the rising disparities in income over the 1980s – real incomes after housing costs of the bottom tenth fell by 13 per cent, compared with a rise of 40 per cent for the average and a steep rise of 65 per cent for those in the top tenth. Inequality measured by expenditure also showed a sharp rise but not as stark as income (Goodman and Webb 1995).

ORIGINS AND INFLUENCES

The context in which governments make social policy has changed markedly from that which shaped the developments of the post-war modern welfare states. Global labour and capital markets have brought higher rates of unemployment and economic inactivity and substantial increases in inequality and poverty. They have also generated strong pressures to deregulate and create flexible labour markets with sharp rises in wage dispersion and part-time, temporary and casual employment, particularly in the UK and USA.

Alongside these economic transformations have come changes to family patterns and the growing social and economic independence of women. The development of more heterogeneous societies, greater individualisation and choice have created new expectations and demands of a welfare state originally shaped by notions of uniformity. These new needs and demands come at a time when the public appears to be reluctant, or at least ambiguous, about support for higher taxes to meet those needs (Oppenheim 1997b). The more restricted capacity of national governments to tackle the major economic and social transformations is one important reason shaping the more tentative approach of all political parties.

A second reason for reticence in discussing poverty and inequality, despite its glaring evidence, is the political reading of public attitudes to these questions. Unpicking public attitudes is an important part of painting the backdrop against which political parties set their priorities. According to Taylor-Gooby's (1995) analysis of the British Social Attitudes Survey, the public view poverty as a serious problem, but are reluctant to finance services and benefits which primarily benefit the poor (see Table 9.1). An important fault line is the varying degrees of support for different parts of the welfare state. The evidence consistently shows much higher levels of support across the political spectrum for spending on *universal services* – health and education – than on other parts of the welfare state. Conservative supporters are less likely than Labour supporters to nominate social security and housing as priorities. In addition, there is some evidence to show that the 'contented majority' – the group who experienced a 40 per cent rise in real incomes since 1979 – are less likely to support spending on the poorest.

The British Social Attitudes Survey undertakes a more detailed look at priorities within social security. Brook and colleagues (1996) found that there are marked differences in support for benefits, which are based not on whether the benefit is universal but on perceptions of the beneficiaries themselves. For example, pensions and benefits for the disabled carry much higher levels of support than

Table 9.1 Perception of the level of poverty, 1994

	Conservative (%)	Lib Dem. (%)	Labour (%)
There is quite a lot of real poverty in Britain today	54	67	79
Poverty in Britain has been increasing over the last ten years	50	75	78
Poverty in Britain will increase over the next ten years	35	57	64

Source: Taylor-Gooby, P. (1995) 'Comfortable, marginal and excluded: Who should pay higher taxes for a better welfare state?', in Jowell, R. *et al.* (eds) *British Social Attitudes, The 12th Report*, Aldershot: Dartmouth.

Note: the British Social Attitudes Survey is an annual randomised survey of approximately 3,600 respondents; 'party' labels reflect whether respondents identify with a particular party, either considering themselves as supporters of it, closer to it than other parties or more likely to vote for it in a general election.

Table 9.2 Social security benefits as priorities for extra public spending, 1995

Benefit	Percentage naming each benefit as first or second priority
State pension	68
Benefits for disabled	58
Child benefit	33
Unemployment benefit	25
Benefits for single parents	12

Source: Brook, L. *et al.* (1996) 'Public Spending and Taxation', in Jowell, R. *et al.* (eds) *British Social Attitudes, The 13th Report*, Aldershot: Dartmouth.

benefits for the unemployed and lone parents, in part drawing on notions of the deserving and undeserving poor (see Table 9.2).

The interpretation of public attitudes is a difficult task. Much of the evidence reveals ambivalence and tension between different views which suggests that there may be more fluidity than politicians suppose. While there is strong cross-party support for universal services, differences emerge, both between parties and according to income group, in relation to services or benefits for the disadvantaged. In the context in which all parties, but in particular the Labour Party, were pitching for the centre-ground and Middle England, it is perhaps not surprising that their reading of public attitudes was cautious. For the Labour Party this is reinforced by the experience of the 1992 General Election when its promise to raise taxes and increase benefits brought damaging Conservative accusations of 'tax bombshells' and the 'double whammy'.

The Conservative legacy to Labour encompassed both an ideological and policy inheritance. The Conservatives redefined the debate on poverty and inequality in three important ways. First, they saw their role as providing a minimum for those in poverty rather than tackling the broader questions of social injustice. Instead, the market was to cater for rising living standards (Hoover and Plant 1989). The 'trickle-down' theory assumed that a growing economy would automatically provide improved living standards for those at the bottom. Second, they attempted to deny the existence of poverty – from John Moore MP's 'End of the Line for Poverty' speech in 1989 to Peter Lilley MP's refusal to comply with the UN Social Summit's requirement to set out a national strategy to tackle poverty. Third, there was a strong emphasis on personal responsibility for poverty, heavily influenced by the work of writers like Charles Murray (Murray 1984; Lister 1996). At its most reductionist, the New Right redefined poverty as 'dependence', which was seen as a behavioural problem caused by the welfare state itself. These ideas have shaped the contours and language of a debate in which individual explanations of poverty have had much greater prominence (Oppenheim 1997a).

Social security policy under the former government was underpinned by a number of themes, some of which have come to be increasingly influential across the political spectrum (Oppenheim and Lister 1996). These embraced targeting, primarily through a substantial increase in means-testing; the promotion of work incentives by reducing some benefit levels, the expansion of wage subsidies and extensions of sanctions; a redrawing of the boundary between the public and private sectors, particularly in relation to pensions; and a shift of support from state to family, embodied most clearly in the Child Support Act. Interwoven with these policy changes was an emphasis on the ideas of both obligation and self-reliance. Underpinning all these themes was the partly economic, partly ideological goal of reducing public spending and thereby the role of the state. Social security, with the largest departmental budget, featured centre stage in the attempts to bring spending down.

Labour's 1997 policies are a response to the economic and social changes of the last two decades, ambivalence in public attitudes to poverty and social security, and Conservative changes in approach and policy. Here we look at three influences on its policy framework: the Commission on Social Justice; the work of Frank Field MP; and Gordon Brown MP's discussion of equality of opportunity.

The Commission on Social Justice (CSJ), was an attempt to take a fresh look, in the face of defeat, at the whole range of Labour's policies on the welfare state and was influential in reshaping key elements of the debate on poverty and social security. First, in contrast to the neo-liberal view that policies which reduce inequality harm economic prosperity, the Commission held that these were central to economic success. Thus the case for reducing inequality was given an economic as well as a moral foundation. This, in turn, led to a second theme, the focus on paid work as the principal solution to poverty: 'Paid work remains the best pathway out of poverty, as well as the only way in which most people can hope to achieve a decent standard of living' (Commission on Social Justice 1994: 151).

Third, the CSJ's support for the 'investors', rather than the 'deregulators' or 'levellers', strategy led to a clear rejection of the 'old' redistributive agenda. The levellers represent:

a strategy for social justice based primarily on redistributing wealth and income, rather than trying to increase opportunities and compete in world markets. The Levellers believe that we should try to achieve social justice through the benefits system, rather than through a new combination of an active welfare state, reformed labour market and strong community.

(Commission on Social Justice 1994: 96)

Finally, education and skills were seen as central elements in both overcoming inequalities of birth and status and promoting economic security and prosperity.

On the policy front the overarching themes were translated into proposals for a modernised social insurance to include new forms of work, part-time unemployment benefits, the broad rejection of means-testing, looking at new ways of improving the transition from benefits into paid work, a minimum wage and family-friendly policies. Benefit levels would be reviewed in the light of research into a minimum income standard and the use of tax allowances and reliefs for improvements in child benefit, childcare and the creation of a mortgage benefit for the low-paid.

Alongside the Commission on Social Justice, Frank Field MP has had a marked influence, shaping Labour's overall approach and policies in this area. As chair of the Social Security Committee, prolific author and now Government Minister, Field has challenged some of the central tenets of the traditional left agenda. In *Stakeholder Welfare* (1996), picking up the 'stakeholder' theme initiated by Tony Blair, Field lays out the principles of his approach. First, he stresses the importance of self-interest rather than altruism in underpinning welfare. One of the tasks of reform is to shape self-interest in line with the public good. It is this view that leads Field to conclude that: 'For the time being, the age of large unspecified redistributive acts [has] ended. Politicians who argue otherwise are a public menace. I do believe however that hypothecated redistribution is possible within carefully defined parameters' (Field 1996: 20).

For Field the central issue is not primarily the redistribution of incomes between rich and poor, but the redistribution of paid work between the 'work rich' and the 'work poor'. A second strand of Field's thought is that social security provision is not neutral but has an important impact on people's behaviour and character. In particular, he documents the ways in which means-tested benefits have a detrimental effect on earning, saving and honesty, creating welfare 'dependency'. Third, Field redraws the relationship between state and individual:

> Increasing numbers of voters no longer see the state as central in achieving the good life. Indeed, self-achievement is part and parcel of the good life. . . . Rather than being the leading player, the state is increasingly cast in the role of active umpire, setting rules and ensuring that fair play operates.
>
> (Field 1996: 28)

Related to this view of the state Field attempts to recast welfare institutions which reflect the demise of trust in the capacity of the state to deliver its promises and to draw on the sense of social autonomy which he argues characterises our society today.

His policy proposals, dealt with only in passing here, embody this overall perspective – the development of a proactive income support agency to tackle 'dependency culture'; promoting active rather than passive benefits through the agreement of individual work plans and the conversion of benefit spending into education and training; the revitalisation of national insurance by creating independent stake-holder corporations at arms-length from the state; and the extension of second-tier compulsory stakeholder pensions owned by individuals. There is much greater focus on single parenthood as the major cause of family poverty, with suggestions for an extension of childcare provision alongside tougher conditions for lone parents about availability for work (Field 1997). The proposals are founded on the view that the rapid growth of social security spending distorts overall decisions about public spending.

A third important part of the debate which has steered the Labour policy agenda is the discussion of equality of opportunity and equality of outcome carried out in the pages of the *Guardian* newspaper between Gordon Brown MP and the now Lord Hattersley. Brown's view of equality of opportunity develops ideas from the Commission on Social Justice and provides the framework for Labour's approach in government. For Brown, the goal of equality is the central dividing line in politics. He argues for a maximalist version of equality of opportunity which is 'recurrent, lifelong and comprehensive' (*Guardian*, 2 August 1996). This view of equality continues to have an important role for the state:

> Equality of opportunity is also an essential duty of government: not just a public good to be desired but a responsibility to actively, relentlessly, pursue equality of opportunity as an objective of policy. Equality of opportunity cannot be achieved by markets alone, however dynamic. . . . It is only government that can make equality of opportunity real.
>
> (Brown, The Second John Smith Memorial Lecture, 19 April 1996: 6)

But it also leads Brown to redefine the strategy for tackling poverty:

> For too long we have relied on the tax and benefit system to compensate people for their poverty rather than doing something more fundamental – tackling the root causes of poverty and inequality – by creating employment, education and economic opportunities that help more people out of poverty.
>
> (*Guardian*, 2 August 1996)

Many of these themes echo through the new government's current policies and its attempt to come to grips with a changed landscape – the importance of paid work as a route out of poverty, the redefinition of redistribution as about primary endowments, the emphasis on education and skills, the focus on rights and duties and the adoption of the language of welfare dependency. There is a rethinking of the boundaries between public and private – the state is seen as an 'enabler', 'umpire', 'regulator', 'resource' rather than necessarily being the provider (Kelly *et al.* 1997). Interestingly, this view of the state is more sophisticated than that proffered by the Conservative manifesto, which appeared caught in a rigid divide between a state seen as inevitably stifling and markets seen as inevitably liberating.

THE PARTY MANIFESTOS

'Our priority is to create jobs. This is not just an economic priority, but also a social and moral one. Jobs and enterprise are the best ways of tackling poverty and deprivation.' (Conservative Party 1997: 9). The 1997 Conservative manifesto built on the themes of its eighteen-year period in government, stressing the need to reduce the social security budget as a share of national income by targeting benefits on those most in need, helping people from welfare to work and tackling benefit fraud. It proposed the extension of existing welfare to work pilot schemes such as Project Work (a compulsory work programme) and Parent Plus (voluntary employment advice for lone parents), maintaining the value of child benefit and family credit, refocusing social security support on the traditional two-parent family by cutting benefits to lone parents and the implementation of a tougher anti-fraud programme. The only new policy was the proposal to introduce a transferable tax allowance for people caring for children or adult 'dependants' at home.

'The best way to tackle poverty is to help people into jobs – real jobs'(Labour Party 1997). The 1997 Labour manifesto was more ambitious in its aims, proposing to streamline and modernise the tax and benefit systems to promote work incentives, reduce poverty and welfare dependency and strengthen family and community life. Its welfare to work programme took centre stage, representing its largest immediate spending pledge of £3.9 billion and encompassing the young and older unemployed as well as lone parents. Other policies included at least maintaining the value of child benefit up to the age of 16 (with a review of its role for young people over 16), tackling tax and benefit abuse, the extension of childcare to all 4-year-olds, a national minimum wage, opting into the Social Chapter, the creation of individual learning accounts and a reduction in the marginal tax rate for lower earners, as well as lowering VAT on fuel.

'Our aim is to provide a more effective safety net for the disadvantaged to encourage work without compulsion and to widen opportunities'(Liberal Democrats 1997). The 1997 Liberal Democrat manifesto had a rather broader approach. While touching on welfare to work, it concentrated on other social security policies, proposing to merge income support and family credit, extend benefits to young people and improve benefits for the disabled and carers. In common with the Labour Party manifesto it put forward a regionally-based minimum wage, opting into the Social Chapter, the extension of childcare to all 3- and 4-year-olds and individual learning accounts. It proposed taking the lowest paid out of taxation altogether through a rise in the tax threshold and, unlike both Conservative and Labour, called for a modest rise in the basic and higher rates of income taxes to fund higher public spending, particularly on education.

What are the differences and similarities between each political party's priorities on poverty and social security? All three parties have embraced welfare to work policies though each with a different emphasis. As illustrated by the quotations above, employment-based strategies are seen as the major solution to poverty across the political spectrum. However, there are important distinctions between the parties – Labour's welfare to work programme is much more all-embracing and it shares with the Liberal Democrats a commitment to the minimum wage and the Social Chapter in contrast to Conservative's adherence to Euro-scepticism. Thus, for the centre-left paid work is underpinned by minimum standards and conditions.

The Labour and the Liberal Democrat programmes share a number of other elements: the emphasis on education and training which pinpoints employability as the key to reducing poverty, the expansion of childcare to enable lone parents to undertake paid work (in contrast to the Conservative tax proposal which supported carers at home) and the reduction of the tax burden for lowest earners (again distinct from the Conservative promise to reduce the basic rate of tax). The Liberal Democrats stand alone in proposing improvements to certain social security benefits and a modest increase in progressive taxation to fund higher public spending, focused on education.

Conservative and Labour programmes also share a number of features, including a reduction in the social security budget. The Conservatives see this as part of an overall reduction in the public sector, while Labour are committed to changing the *composition* of public spending, and in particular diverting funds from social security to education. Both place greater emphasis on duties and obligations as illustrated by the elements of compulsion in their welfare to work proposals (the Liberal Democrats specifically state that they are not in favour of compulsion). Both parties advocate clamping down on benefit fraud.

There are two important features of Labour's approach to poverty and inequality which distinguish it from previous years; firstly, the opposition to real rises in benefit levels – 'Blair plans benefit freeze' stated the *Guardian* (29 April 97) – claiming that there would be no above-inflation rises in benefits during a first term of office and second, the rejection of redistribution through the tax and benefit system. A quick glance at the 1992 manifesto highlights the differences – the earlier manifesto proposed increases in child benefit and pensions (financed by higher personal taxation) as well as reforming a number of means-tested benefits such as abolishing the social fund. Today's approach stems both from the drive to reduce the social security budget as well as a view that reliance on social security benefits is not a long-term solution to reducing poverty:

> We got ourselves into a situation where we no longer seemed to be a party of aspiration. We appeared to be the party that represented those who were poor and unemployed – rightly – but it seemed we did not want to help these people up, but level other people down. . . . I believe in a more equal society. I would not be in the Labour Party otherwise. I want a just society by which I mean extending opportunity, tackling poverty and injustice. But we have moved beyond the idea that the way to achieve that is to pay people a few more quid in benefit.
>
> (Tony Blair, *Observer*, 27 April 97)

THE CAMPAIGN

'Churches Slate All Parties' was the *Guardian* headline which greeted the publication of the Council of Churches' Report released early in the election campaign (Council of Churches for Britain and Ireland 1997). The Report included recommendations to reform the tax system to encourage private sector employment, higher taxation to fund public sector employment, creating jobs for the long-term unemployed, a national minimum wage, better conditions of work and fairer bargaining over pay, reform of social security to reduce means-testing (including the abolition of job seekers allowance), and priority for basic skills for young people. While the Report shared a number of policies with the centre-left parties, it raised particularly difficult questions in relation to redistributive taxation and the limits of education and training:

> in the British election campaign the political parties are competing for votes by promising low taxation. When so many are living in poverty and unemployment, it is wrong to give priority to the claims of those who are already well off. None of the political parties has put forward a programme which offers much real hope of improvement to those in the greatest need.
>
> (Council of Churches for Britain and Ireland 1997: 2)

> we also warn against regarding education and training as the solution to all our problems. There will always be some people more skilled and productive than others. It matters a lot how willing the successful and lucky ones are to share their good fortune with the rest.
>
> (Council of Churches for Britain and Ireland 1997: 9)

The Churches' Report represents a reassertion of the moral case for redistribution. In doing so it follows in the time-honoured tradition of the Church as the voice of the poor. Both *Faith in the City* (Archbishops' Commission 1985), published in the early years of the Thatcher era, and the more recent Church Action on Poverty hearings were examples of the capacity of the church to talk about poverty and disadvantage, unfettered by electoral calculation. Poverty did raise its head again briefly in the campaign, though less dramatically, with the publication of the Catholic Bishops' Report on poverty and educational failure and the Child Poverty Action Group's *Britain Divided*. The limited effectiveness of pressure groups, charities and the poverty lobby in finding openings for debating poverty is a reflection not only of the fact that all the parties were appealing to Middle England but also that such groups have had a decreasing influence on a Labour Party anticipating power. Labour was keen to distance itself from being tied to particular causes and promises, as well as wanting to address 'all' rather than just its natural constituency.

THE FIRST WEEKS OF GOVERNMENT

Labour's initial period in power left the impression of the frenetic activity of a party impatient for power. Frank Field's appointment as Minister of State for Social Security and Welfare Reform under Harriet Harman, Secretary of State for Social Security signalled a radical approach to reform. Charged with 'thinking the unthinkable', social security would be subject to his reforming zeal. Two outsiders from the world of business, Martin Taylor, Chief Executive of Barclays and Sir Peter Davies, Chief Executive of Prudential, were appointed to head major investigations into the future of the welfare state – the interaction of taxes and benefits and welfare to work respectively. Their appointments symbolised the new government's commitment to partnership between public and private sectors and a recognition that the private sector has an increasingly important role in the future shape of the welfare state. Such appointments would have been unusual in an earlier era where Commissions were more likely to have been headed by academics. The Chair of the Social Security Committee, likely at times to be critical of government policy, has been placed at some distance from the government in the hands of Liberal Democrat MP, Archie Kirkwood.

The Budget, as expected, announced further details of its welfare to work programme – New Deals for young unemployed, older unemployed, lone parents and disabled people. The term 'New Deal' is not only reminiscent of Roosevelt's rebuilding of post-depression USA but has picked up the Australian Labour Party's approach to pulling policies together under a headline that encapsulates the intent behind policy, for example the Australian 'Working Nation' reforms (Finn 1997).

The bulk of the spending was to be focused on young people. However, the smaller programmes for lone parents and the disabled – some £200 million each – represent a recognition that welfare to work has to encompass those who are not defined as officially unemployed. The New Deal for Lone Parents includes an increase and extension to £100 a week of the childcare disregard for in-work benefits for lone parents with two children. A further £150 million will be available from the National Lottery to fund after-school places. Alongside the extra money for the lone parent welfare to work programme, Labour accepted the Conservative cuts in lone parent premium and one-parent benefit as part of its adherence to the former government's public spending plans. The New Deal for Lone Parents, despite all the media hype, was voluntary.

The sanctions policy is perhaps the most controversial aspect of the government's programme. It has adopted a rather tougher version of the job seeker's regime where young people who refuse all four options without good cause will have their benefit suspended initially for two weeks, and another four weeks for any further refusal. Sanctions will not be imposed if 'good cause' is proved. Hardship payments at the lower rate of job seekers allowance will continue to be available in specific circumstances. The government justified this approach as not only symbolising a commitment to rights and responsibilities, but that the options would be of high quality. While in principle there is a good case for unemployed claimants participating in a work-related activity, matched by a government obligation to provide an adequate income and to ensure that the activity is of value, the detail of such schemes is crucial. If sanctions are too tough, the withdrawal of support is likely to be counter-productive, forcing some claimants into the twilight world of the shadow economy and crime (Oppenheim 1997b). In the Budget, the Chancellor of the Exchequer signalled a number of reforms that the Taylor committee would look at more closely – the reduction of tapers for in-work benefits and the introduction of an earned income tax credit along the lines of that introduced in the US (Meadows 1997).

The Institute for Fiscal Studies' analysis of the distributional impact of the Budget found that the tax and benefit changes alone (including the reduction in mortgage interest tax relief, the rises in petrol and cigarette duty and the decrease in VAT on fuel) resulted in the poorest faring worst, although by a small margin (*Financial Times*, 3 July 1997). However, this assessment is inevitably limited in that it cannot take into account the impact of the welfare to work programmes. Any progressive element from claimants moving into paid work, gaining new skills or work experience is not captured by this analysis.

Peter Mandelson MP's announcement of a new cross-departmental social exclusion unit, to be chaired by the Prime Minister was an important initiative, particularly in the context of the denial of poverty by the previous administration. Promisingly, Mandelson raised the future possibility of improvements in income for the poorest: 'Not only is Labour committed to protect the poor against inflation, we are also determined to do more for those on the lowest incomes when economic circumstances and the re-ordering of public expenditure make this possible' (*Guardian*, 15 August 1997).

Other policies were jettisoned (or at the very least downgraded) by the Government, notably some of the Commission on Social Justice proposals to improve and extend certain social security benefits financed by changes in tax reliefs and allowances. The language of the debate also changed. The terms 'underclass' and 'welfare dependency' were once only the preserve of Conservative politicians but are now used freely across the political spectrum. While there has been a useful recognition by the centre-left of the impact of long-term reliance on social security on individual and community capacities to regenerate themselves, there are dangers attached to the use of such language. It tends to over-emphasize the individual causes of poverty and disassociate those experiencing poverty from the rest of society.

CONCLUSION

> In each area of policy a new and distinctive approach has been mapped out, one that differs from both the solutions of the old left and those of the Conservative Right, This is why new Labour is new.
>
> (Labour Party 1997)

The political tramlines are indeed less distinct in 1997 than in earlier eras as we have seen in our analysis of the manifesto promises on poverty and social security. The redrawing of the parameters of policy have taken place in a tougher international climate, an ambiguity about paying for increased welfare and a changed policy context. Despite this, much is innovative and potentially radical (Oppenheim 1997b). The yoking together of social inclusion and economic stability has been a powerful tool in the critique of neo-liberalism. However, while the economic case for reducing in-equality is important, it tends to overstate the interdependence of social justice and economic efficiency (White 1997). Hence the force of the Churches' salvo in the Election campaign – the need for a moral foundation for redistribution as well. The new government will need to find strategies which improve the well-being of those people who are beyond the reaches of welfare to work. The government's strategy of life-time equality of opportunity is central to its overall focus. The emphasis on prevention, empowering individuals and encompassing a broader notion of the factors that shape people's life-chances with the potential to offer a more all-embracing vision of redistribution, is radical. However, redistributing endowments does not come cheaply; it is a long-term strategy and there will always be a need to protect those who fail in the market place, however good their education and skills. Finally, reducing income inequality will remain important if we are to achieve equality of opportunity. It is hard to see how we can sustain both a more mobile and a socially tolerant society if there is to be an ever increasing gap between rich and poor.

REFERENCES

Archbishops' Commission (Church of England Archbishops' Commission on Urban Priority Areas) (1985) *Faith in the City*, London: Church House Publications.

Brook, L., Hall, J. and Preston, I. (1996) 'Public spending and taxation', in R. Jowell, J. Curtice, A. Park, L. Brook and K. Thomson (eds) *British Social Attitudes, the 13th Report*, Aldershot: Dartmouth.

Brown, G. (1996) 'New Labour and equality', The Second John Smith Memorial Lecture, Edinburgh University, 19 April 1996.

Commission on Social Justice (1994) *Social Justice, Strategies for National Renewal*, London: Vintage.

Council of Churches for Britain and Ireland (1997) *Unemployment and the Future of Work: An Enquiry for the Churches*, London Council of Churches for Britain and Ireland.

DSS (Department of Social Security) (1996) *Households below Average Income, A Statistical Analysis, 1979–1993/94*, London: HMSO.

Field, F. (1997) 'The dependency debate and new directions in the UK', speech given at the 'Beyond Dependency Conference', Auckland, New Zealand, 18 March 1997.

—— (1996) 'Making welfare work, the underlying principles', in A. Deacon (ed.) *Stakeholder Welfare*, London: Institute of Economic Affairs.

Finn, D. (1997), *Working Nation, Welfare Reform and the Australian Job Compact for the Long-term Unemployed*, London, Unemployment Unit.

Goodman, A. and Webb, S. (1995) *The Distribution of Household UK Expenditure 1979–1992*, London: Institute for Fiscal Studies.

Hills, J. (1995) *Joseph Rowntree Foundation Inquiry into Income and Wealth, Volume 2*, York: Joseph Rowntree Foundation.

Hoover, K. and Plant. R. (1989) *Conservative Capitalism in Britain and the United States*, London: Routledge.

Kelly, G., Kelly, D. and Gamble, A. (eds) (1997) *Stakeholder Capitalism*, Basingstoke: Macmillan.

Kempson, E. (1996) *Life on a Low Income*, York: Joseph Rowntree Foundation.

Meadows, P. (1997) 'The integration of taxes and benefits for working families with children', *Policy Options*, June 1997, York: Joseph Rowntree Foundation.

Murray, C. (1984) *Losing Ground*, New York: Basic Books.

Lister, R. (1996) *Charles Murray and the Underclass, The Developing Debate*, London: Institute of Economic Affairs.

Oppenheim, C. (1997a) 'Poverty and inequality', in A. Walker and C. Walker (eds) *Britain Divided: The Growth of Social Exclusion in the 1980s and 1990s*, London: Child Poverty Action Group.

—— (1997b) *The Post Conservative Welfare State: A Framework for the Decade Ahead*, Policy Paper 9, Sheffield: Political Economy Research Centre, Sheffield University.

Oppenheim, C. and Lister, R. (1996) 'Ten Years after the 1986 Social Security Act', in M. May, E. Brunsdon and G. Craig (eds) *Social Policy Review 8*, London: Social Policy Association.

Taylor-Gooby, P. (1995) 'Comfortable, marginal and excluded', in R. Jowell, J. Curtice, A. Park, L. Brook, and D. Ahrendt (eds) *British Social Attitudes, the 12th Report*, Aldershot: Dartmouth.

White, S. (1997) 'What do egalitarians really want?' in J. Franklin (ed.) *Equality*, London: Institute for Public Policy Research.

Chapter 10

Paying for pensions

Barbara Waine

INTRODUCTION

The aim of this chapter is to discuss how old age/retirement pensions policy figured in the 1997 General Election and its immediate aftermath. Although all the political parties had statements on pensions the key debates were fought out between the Conservatives and Labour and they will be the focus of this chapter. However, the political debate in this area will be easier to follow if some key issues and concerns are elucidated. The British pensions system in the twentieth century has operated with a basic state pension and additional pensions. Originally the latter came in the form of occupational pensions. Since the late 1950s the state has also offered additional pensions for those not covered by an occupational scheme: initially this was in the form of a graduated pension but, since 1975, it has been via the State Earnings Related Pension Scheme (SERPS).

During the 1980s, the Conservatives introduced a number of important changes to the pensions regime which they inherited. The basic pension was indexed not to earnings but to prices and, since earnings generally rise faster than prices, this meant that over time the basic pension has and will become of marginal importance. In the sphere of additional pensions, the 1986 Social Security Act introduced a number of changes. SERPS was modified: from 1999 onwards it will be based on lifetime earnings rather than an individual's best twenty years of earnings and between 2000 and 2009 the pension will be reduced from 25 per cent to 20 per cent of earnings. The established occupational pension schemes, where the pension was a proportion of final salary, were retained but such schemes would also be able to operate on a money purchase basis where the pension is based only on accumulated contributions and returns from investments. The 1986 Act offered an important additional choice, the Appropriate Personal Pension (APP) – an individual money purchase scheme – as an alternative to occupational schemes and a modified SERPS. The 1986 measures were justified in three principal ways: demographic changes were seen as leading to an increased 'burden' of the elderly on the working population; the Conservatives claimed that Britain was becoming an 'enterprise economy' in which frequent job changing would become the norm; and finally part of the attempt to create an 'enterprise culture' stressed the importance of extending individual ownership as part of a new 'popular capitalism'.

The shifts in pensions policy related to these concerns. In particular SERPS is a Pay-As-You-Go (PAYG) scheme where current pensions are funded out of taxation and national insurance contributions. The Conservatives claimed that such schemes carried the threat, in the context of demographic change, of unacceptably high levels of personal taxation. They thus supported funded schemes where entitlements are paid for out of employer and employee contributions into a distinct fund and the investment income of that fund. Tax relief on both the contributions, and until 2 July 1997, on the investment income, is available. (With occupational schemes and the APP, employers and employees pay a lower rate of National Insurance contributions – the 'contracted out' rebate – in recognition that provision for an additional pension is being made outside SERPS). The notion of an enterprise economy was also significant for pensions because occupational pensions were associated with a pattern of employment involving long job tenures; in contrast personal pensions were 'portable', since they were individually owned they could transfer when the individual changed jobs. As personal pensions were individually owned, they also fitted in with a notion of the individual property owner and were seen as part of a more general shift involving the spread of owner-occupied housing and shareholding (Waine 1995).

The themes of Conservative policy on pensions in the 1980s and 1990s – a reduction of direct state expenditure and direct state provision, the extension of choice as a means of securing individual independence through property ownership – were carried through into the 1997 election.

PENSION PROPOSALS AND THE 1997 ELECTION

Radical Conservatives

On March 5 1997, the Prime Minister, John Major, and the Secretary of State for Social Security, Peter Lilley, announced a major pre-election initiative – the Basic Pension Plus (BPP) – which would privatise the provision of the state retirement pension for future generations. With BPP, everyone would receive a rebate of £9 per week from their National Insurance contribution (NIC) to build up a fund to pay for their basic pension. It was estimated that a person on average wages would build up a fund worth £130,000, sufficient to provide for a pension of £175 a week at today's prices. In addition, employees would receive a rebate of 5 per cent of their earnings on which they pay NIC to fund an earnings related pension (Lilley 1997). The state though would continue to be involved in the basic pension in three ways: via the development of an effective regulatory regime for the BPP; through the Basic Pension Guarantee (BPG) which would ensure that if a person's fund was insufficient to pay the BPP, the state would top up the pension; finally, those with low earnings who generated rebates of less than £9 per week would receive a state subsidy, while the unemployed, sick, disabled or carers would receive credits towards their BPG. Income support would continue to be available for those unable to build up pensions (Lilley 1997: 2).

The justification for the proposals was consistent with an increasing number of pensioners and a declining working population: a dismissal of PAYG principles as they were thought to involve a lack of saving for the future and a preference for the apparently more secure funded schemes (Conservative Research Department 1997). In addition, both the Secretary of State (Hansard, 13 March 1997, col. 512) and the Prime Minister (Hansard, 20 March 1997, col. 696 written answer) argued that the BPP proposals represented the biggest extension of personal ownership in the UK.

Although BPP took many by surprise (according to Peter Lilley it had been prepared in secret over the previous year (Hansard, 9 July 1997 col. 964)) it did have immediate antecedents. In 1993, the 'No Turning Back' group of Conservative MPs argued that people should be allowed to 'opt out' of the basic state pension and be given a rebate on their NICs to make their own private provision ('No Turning Back' Group of Conservative MPs 1993). This idea was taken further in a 1995 publication from the Adam Smith Institute, *The Fortune Account* by Eamonn Butler and Madsen Pirie (Butler and Pirie 1995). This advocated an individual savings account which would be financed by relief from NICs and income tax and whose prime purpose would be to provide pensions and purchase insurance against a number of other contingencies. (A more extensive treatment of the Fortune Account can be found in *Beyond Pension Plus* which the authors produced as a response to BPP (Butler *et al.* 1997)). The Conservative MP, Geoffrey Clifton-Brown, in a pamphlet published by the Bow Group, had proposed privatising the state pension with universal funded pensions financed by NICs (G. Clifton-Brown 1996). Of course, in a sense, it could be argued that the true antecedent of the BPP is to be found in the work of Friedrich von Hayek a key influence on Conservative governments in the post-1979 years. Hayek argued that while people should be compelled to ensure against contingencies such as old age, the state should not be the monopoly provider of such security (Hayek 1960: 286).

The response to BPP from the pensions industry and the media was broadly enthusiastic (cf Conservative Research Department 1997, Appendix 1 for a selection of commments). Any reservations were about detail, not principles. Tony Blair used an article in *The Times* to oppose the scheme, pointing out the cost to the taxpayer, especially having to underwrite the BPG, questioning the level of the BPP as a percentage of future earnings and pointing to the need for a stronger regulatory regime of private pensions (*The Times*, 7 March 1997). At the same time, as John Plender pointed out, the plan had caught Labour on difficult territory: not only was its own pensions policy far from developed but there was a wide range of opinion within the Party about what that policy should be (*New Statesman*, 14 March 1997). While it can be argued that the pensions policy of the Conservatives has developed on a clear trajectory from 1986 onwards, this has not been the case for the Labour Party.

Modern Labour

The Labour Party had mounted a vigorous opposition to the 1986 pension reforms (e.g. the Standing Committee on the Social Security Bill, 1986) while at the same time supporting SERPS. Thus during the third reading of the Bill, Margaret Beckett, argued that 'SERPS was the most efficient way of providing a good pension and good value for money' (Hansard, 19 May 1986, col. 79). In the 1987

Manifesto, Labour committed itself both to a restoration of SERPS (entitlements under this scheme had been considerably reduced with the 1986 Act), and an immediate increase in the state pension as a first step in re-establishing the link between earnings or prices, whichever was most favourable to pensioners (Labour Party 1987: 4). This commitment was broadly reaffirmed in the 1992 manifesto (Labour Party 1992: 20).

However by the 1997 election, Labour's proposals on pensions had undergone considerable change. A basic state pension, non-means-tested and based on contributory principles would remain, but with annual increases at least in line with prices. Properly regulated second-tier pensions – occupational schemes and personal pensions – would continue: SERPS would be maintained as an option for those wishing to remain in it and developed to create a 'citizenship pension' for carers. The centre piece of the proposals, though, was to be the stakeholder pension for 'those on low and modest incomes with changing patterns of employment, [who] cannot join good value second pension schemes' (Labour Party 1997: 27).

The key changes then between 1992 and 1997 concerned the formula for inflation-proofing the state basic pension; the marginalisation of SERPS; and the creation of a stakeholder pension. Two questions need to be addressed: how can the changes be accounted for and were they unopposed?

In accounting for the change on pensions policy between 1992 and 1997, the general context – a fourth consecutive election defeat and the election of new leaders (John Smith followed by Tony Blair) with the objective of modernising the Party and distancing it from its reputation as a high tax–high spending party – are all important. This perceived need for change was manifested in the establishment of the Commission on Social Justice at the end of 1992 with its focus on the creation of a strategy for national renewal, namely 'Investors' Britain with its emphasis on innovation, investment in skills, the need to shape and regulate markets (Commission on Social Justice 1994: 99–106) and an active welfare state which provided opportunities and promoted responsibility (op. cit.: 20). A pensions policy which related to these objectives was necessary. The Commission accepted that the basic state pension did not meet the needs of the elderly: yet an across-the-board increase was rejected as expensive and poorly targeted. Thus there would be a Pensions Guarantee, at a higher level than the basic pension or Income Support. Pensioners with an income below this guarantee would have it topped up by the state.

Membership of a second-tier pension scheme would be compulsory: the Commission was not prescriptive on the type of scheme but rather confined itself to discussing the advantages and disadvantages of the two options – namely an improved SERPS and funded schemes (op. cit.: 275–81). What is of interest is that for possibly the first time, in a document associated with the Labour Party, SERPS was seen to have disadvantages, in particular its PAYG formula which, it was claimed, could suffer from the political risk of governments changing the rules and the resistance of future taxpayers to 'the increased contributions that would be needed to finance the increased benefits' (op. cit.: 277). Funded schemes whereby people had the responsibility of saving for their retirement and thus created individual ownership rights were seen as avoiding such problems. Indeed, a funded scheme – the National Savings Pension Plan (NSPP) – could be developed for groups such as the low paid, women, part-timers 'to take the place of SERPS' (op. cit.: 282). These proposals, mediated by the Party's 'Road to the Manifesto' publication – *Security in Retirement* – are to be found in the manifesto. The exception is the 'Pensions Guarantee' which appears in the 'Road to the Manifesto', and in the speech of the Shadow Secretary of State for Social Security in a Parliamentary Debate on pensions just before the election was announced (Hansard, 13 March 1997, col. 530) but had been quietly dropped by the time the manifesto was published. Possibly this was because it could have provided the Conservatives with a useful weapon, namely, that a future Labour goverment would means-test all pensioners.

The attack on SERPS was also to come from elsewhere within the Labour Party. Between 1993 and 1996, Frank Field, Labour MP for Birkenhead and Chair of the House of Commons Social Security Committee, writing in a personal capacity, published a number of newspaper articles, pamphlets and books which developed a scenario on future pension provision for the political Left.

Field advocates compulsory universal additional pensions to run alongside the state retirement schemes. He rejects the rebuilding of SERPS for reasons similar to that of the Commission on Social Justice (Field 1995: 176) and in later work states that proposals to rebuild SERPS 'are simply out of time. There does not exist the widespread trust for such a scheme'(Field 1996: 36). In addition he argues that there is widespread enthusiasm for the ownership of one's own pension. Thus Field would close SERPS and redirect contribu-tions into funded schemes chosen by the contributors, with the state subsidising the contributions of low wage earners and those outside of the labour market (op. cit.: 38) and hence ensuring inclusiveness for the bottom 20 per cent in society. Funded schemes would be operated by a multiplicity of providers – friendly societies, building societies – in addition a National Pension Savings Scheme similar to that proposed by the Commission on Social Justice would be established (Field 1995: 180–1).

Thus, by 1997, a significant strand of Labour's thinking on future pensions was characterised by the commitment to a basic state pension, albeit one which would, because of index linking to prices, form a smaller proportion of future average earnings; a dismissal of SERPS/PAYG provision; and a clear preference for funded 'stakeholder' pensions. This was a pensions platform radically at odds with that of the earlier period, 1975–92, and as such it met resistance. Here the Labour Party Conference, in October 1996, was the key event. The pensions debate represented 'Blair's only serious challenge … at the Conference' (J. Sherman, A. Leathley and P. Webster, *The Times*, 3 October 1996). The challenge was thrown down by Barbara Castle, the Secretary of State responsible for the 1975 SERPS scheme. Earlier in the year she had published a pamphlet with Peter Townsend in which she contested many of the proposals for reform and argued for an improved state basic pension and the restoration, and improvement, of SERPS (Castle and Townsend 1996: 10–18, 26–7). Similar proposals had been developed by Peter Townsend and Alan Walker (1995) and Tony Lynes (1996).

Old Labour

In rejecting the New Labour proposals, Old Labour raised central questions about the arguments for the reform of pensions: the extent of the demographic timebomb; the possibly fallacious nature of claims as to the superiority of funded schemes; and the insecurity of personal pensions.

A feature of the debate on pensions is the notion of the 'demographic timebomb': namely an increase in the number of pensioners, especially between 2020 and 2030, accompanied by a decline in those of working age. Fewer people will be available to support the retired (Labour Party 1996: 2). While 'the burden of the elderly' thesis predates the 1980s and 1990s it has been a critical prop in justifying change in this period (e.g. Department of Health and Social Security 1985: 1.28–1.30). Yet, as all Old Labour authors argue, the thesis is highly problematic. This is nicely illustrated by Lynes. He refers to two reports by the Government Actuary in 1986 and 1994. In the former the Government Actuary showed the number of pensioners rising from 9.84 million in 1993–94 to 13.41 million in 2033–34: in the latter report, he estimated that there would be 16.89 million pensioners by 2030–31, assuming pension ages were retained at 60 for women, 65 for men (Lynes 1996: 6). As Lynes notes, the Government Actuary emphasises that 'the demographic and economic assumptions underlying the estimates are inevitably subject to a considerable degree of uncertainty, particularly for the more distant future' (Ibid.). This potential for uncertainty over the size of the retired population raises the suspicion that such arguments are used to sustain a political position rather than being required by demographic imperatives.

Pensions are financed in one of two ways: PAYG where they are paid for out of taxes of current workers 'the intergenerational contract' of the state basic pension of SERPS, or funding, whereby contributions are invested on behalf of members as in a company scheme, or of individuals as in a personal pension. Current fashonable thinking in pensions policy is that with an ageing population, PAYG principles are unsustainable but funding would lead to an increase in savings, hence investment, thus making it easier to pay for pensions in the future (Crawford 1997: 38). Such thinking embodies a number of questionable assumptions: namely, that funded schemes would raise national savings; and that they are immune to political interference by governments (Crawford op. cit.; Wolf, *Financial Times*, 4 March 1997). Indeed, the questionable nature of the argument that funded schemes are superior was exposed at a meeting of the Treasury Committee on 5 March 1997. In answer to a question from Quentin Davies MP, a member of the Committee, William Waldegrave, Chief Secretary to the Treasury, agreed that any pension scheme, either PAYG or funded, 'simply represents a claim on the economy in the future' (Treasury Committee 1997a: 9). As Castle and Townsend (1996: 18) succinctly note 'the choice between funding and PAYG is a political, not an economic one'.

Finally, money purchase schemes which are implied by the stakeholder concept have an inherent problem: namely they depend upon an investment and the returns on this, and hence the final pension can be uncertain (Townsend and Walker 1995: 9; Lynes 1996: 26–7). The proposals by New Labour for a more effective regulatory regime of money purchase schemes, transparency over commissions and administrative charges (Commission for Social

Justice 1994: 282; Field 1995: 180; Labour Party 1997: 27) cannot, of course, control market trends, and hence, final pension outcomes.

The pensions card

In a House of Commons debate on BPP on 13 March 1997, the Conservative M.P., John MacGregor stated that 'the proposal may not be of major excitement and significance to many people in the forthcoming election' (Hansard, 13 March 1997, col. 543). However, events over the weekend preceding the election (25–27 April 1997) were to prove him wrong. On Friday 25 April, Tony Blair played the 'pensions card'. On the *Today* programme on BBC Radio 4 at 8 a.m., it was reported that Blair had said that the government, if returned to office, would privatise old age pensions and that BPP was a threat to existing pensioners. The issue dominated the press conferences of both parties that morning, which was particularly unfortunate for the Conservatives as Mr Major had intended to highlight 'Britain's economic miracle' (G. Jones and R. Shrimsby, *Daily Telegraph*, 26 April 1997). Despite Mr Major dismissing the allegations as 'absolutely contemptible' (C. Reiss, *Evening Standard*, 25 April 1997) and claiming that he was so committed to basic pension that he 'would not only leave Downing Street ... [but] politics rather than abolish it' (G. Jones and R. Shrimsby, *Daily Telegraph*, 26 April 1997), apparently the allegations were sufficient to raise anxieties among pensioners and those closest to retirement, and as Edwina Currie claimed the way in which the government had handled the pensions issue did suggest that it wanted to privatise them (*Express*, 27 April 1997). The *Daily Telegraph* in its editorial of 26 April accused the Labour Party of cynically distorting the Conservative proposals for electoral advantage. However, it could be argued that Blair had merely played the 'pensions card' as the Tories had played the 'tax card' in the 1992 election. Certainly, over that weekend the pensions row was at the centre of the campaign: and the Conservatives were left with no time in the three days before polling to reverse the damaging publicity.

THE AFTERMATH OF THE ELECTION

After its election, the Labour Government moved swiftly on two pensions issues which it had inherited from its predecessors, the mis-selling of the APP and pension sharing on divorce.

The APP had been hugely popular attracting 5.5 million people by the end of 1994–95 (Department of Social Security 1997: Table 1.0). Problems began to emerge in the 1990s and hinged on the possibility of 'bad sales advice' to groups such as teachers, miners, nurses and policemen who believed that they had been persuaded against their long-term interests to leave the security of their occupational schemes or not join one and take out an APP. Following numerous Press stories, in 1994, under pressure from a few occupational pension scheme managers, the Securities and Investments Board proposed that life companies and independent financial advisers should review all cases where people might have been given poor advice on taking out an APP and where such claims could be substantiated make compensation. Redress, though, had been notoriously slow with only 7,000 out of half a million estimated victims of mis-selling receiving any compensation (Treasury Committee 1997b: 1). Indeed, the numbers of victims of mis-selling who had died awaiting compensation (18,742) far outweighed those who had received it (op. cit.: 18).

Within days of winning the election, Helen Liddell, Economic Secretary to the Treasury summoned the heads of twenty-eight pension companies to her office and threatened serious consequences if they missed the end of the 1998 deadline announced by the City regulators. She also added that the Treasury would be monitoring, on a monthly basis, the progress of the companies in resolving the mis-selling scandal, and 'naming and shaming' the laggards (J. Eaglesham, *Financial Times*, 17/18 May 1997).

It is well established that women's income in retirement is usually lower that that of men; this is due primarily to lower earnings when at work and interrupted working lives (Davies and Ward 1992: Ch. 2). In addition, divorce rarely takes account of pension rights and is likely to exacerbate this situation further (Field and Prior 1996). The last Conservative government was put under cross-party pressure to tackle the latter. The Pensions Act 1995 allows the courts to earmark a proportion of a member's pension for a former spouse but with transfer taking place only on the member's retirement. The Labour Government has announced that it will introduce legislation in this Parliament which will bring forward the transfer of pension right to the point of divorce and hence align the procedure with the 'clean break' approach to divorce.

Prior to Labour's first budget, there was considerable speculation on what the Chancellor might have in store for pension schemes. In the event he removed the tax credits which pension funds can reclaim on their dividend income. The Chancellor justified the change on the grounds of encouraging investment (the system prior to the abolition encouraged companies to pay out dividends rather than reinvest their profits) and that many pension funds were in surplus and enjoying a contribution holiday (Hansard, 2 July 1997, col. 306).

The Opposition, in a debate on the measure claimed that it would 'penalise long-term savers' (Hansard, 9 July 1997: col. 955). The debate though, presented the Government with a vehicle for attacking its predecessor's record on pensions, in particular, the mis-selling of the APP and the removal of billions of pounds from the future entitlement of members of SERPS (e.g. op. cit.: col. 981).

There has been considerable speculation as to the impact of the abolition: for example, that it would reduce the income of the pension funds by £5 billion. per year (while raising the revenue of the government by the same amount) and could mean lower pensions or higher contributions. In addition, it could alter the nature of pension provision, in particular triggering a move away from final salary schemes (likely to become more expensive to run with the Minimum Funding Requirement of the 1995 Pensions Act) to company money purchase schemes or accepting no commitment beyond paying into an employee's APP (J. Guthrie, *Financial Times*, 3 July 1997; K. Campbell, *Financial Times*, 21 July 1997). It was also suggested that, as the contracted-out rebate has not been increased, many of those with an APP could find themselves better off in SERPS.

The Pensions Review, trailed at the 1996 Conference, partly to ameliorate the attack of Old Labour, was announced on 17 July 1997 (Hansard, 17 July 1997, cols 239–41, written answer). This represented the final policy move on pensions by the Labour Government before the summer recess.

CONCLUSION

In the course of the election, Labour played the pensions card: by so doing it suggested that its pensions policy was radically different from that of its opponents. In respect of the basic state pension, this was the case. While the Conservatives would, if returned to office, have privatised provision in this area, Labour have promised to retain it, although at such a level that it would be likely to constitute only a small proportion of pensioners' income. However, on additional pensions the distinction between the parties was not so evident.

The key theme of Labour, in both opposition and Government has been the development of a 'modern' responsive pension system and one which provides security. However this security for many people 'can best be achieved by building up their own funded second pension' (Hansard, 17 July 1997, col. 240, written answer), namely the 'Stakeholders Pension', an individual funded money purchase scheme. Clearly this security was not to be provided by the state within the potentially redistributive PAYG mechanism. Security was to be achieved by distributing opportunities not income.

The 'Stakeholders' Pension' has been closely identified with Frank Field and his appointment as Minister for Welfare Reform would seem to suggest a clean break between New Labour and Old Labour in respect of pensions (as well as other aspects of social security). However, the pensions policy of the Labour Government is less coherent than this might suggest. At issue here is SERPS which Field has strenuously maintained should be abolished. The Government has announced, in line with the manifesto, its intention of retaining SERPS. Further, the abolition of tax credits on dividends of pension funds, by reducing the value of the investment funds of those with an APP, is likely to have a significant effect on the numbers remaining in or taking out an APP. Many will find it preferable, unless the contracted out rebate is increased, to return to SERPS, thus making SERPS, by default, a major player in the field again. This opens up the possible irony that at least part of Old Labour's programme could operate due to the tax policies of New Labour. New Labour's much trumpeted commitments not to raise income tax and the need to find other sources of revenue could thus have the paradoxical effect of shifting its pensions policy in a somewhat more re-distributive direction.

REFERENCES

Butler, E. and Pirie, M. (1995) *The Fortune Account: The Successor to Social Welfare*, London: Adam Smith Institute.

Butler, E. and Young, M. (1997) *Beyond Pensions Plus: Developing the Fortune Account*, London: Adam Smith Institute.

Castle, B. and Townsend, P. (1996) *We CAN Afford the Welfare State*, London: Security in Retirement for Everyone.

Clifton-Brown, G. (1996) *Privatising the State Pension: Secure Funded Provision for All*, London: Bow Group.

Commission on Social Justice (1994) *Social Justice: Strategies for National Renewal*, London: Vintage.

Conservative Research Department (1997) *Basic Pension Plus*: Brief prepared for a debate in the House of Commons, 11 March, London: Conservative Research Department.

Crawford, M. (1997) 'The big pensions lie', *New Economy*, Spring: 38–44.

Davies, B. and Ward, S. (1992) *Women and Personal Pensions*, London: HMSO.

Department of Health and Social Security (1985) *Reform of Social Security*, vol. 1, Cmnd. 9517, London: HMSO.

Department of Social Security (1997) *Pension Scheme Contributions 1986/87 to 1995/96*, London: Government Statistical Service.

Field, F. (1995) *Making Welfare Work: Reconstructing Welfare for the Millenium*, London: Institute of Community Studies.

—— (1996) *Stakeholder Welfare*, London: Institute of Economic Affairs.

Field, J. and Prior, G. (1996) *Pensions and Divorce: A Survey Carried out on Behalf of the Department of Social Security by Social and Community Planning Research*, London: HMSO.

Hayek, F. von (1960) *The Constitution of Liberty*, London: Routledge, and Kegan Paul.

Labour Party (1987) *Britain Will Win*, London: Labour Party.

—— (1992) *It's Time to Get Britain Working Again*, London: Labour Party.

—— (1996) *Security in Retirement: The Road to the Manifesto*, London: Labour Party.

—— (1997) 'New Labour: Because Britain Deserves Better, election manifesto, London: Labour Party.

Lilley, P. (1997) Press conference speech to launch *Basic Pension Plus*, 5 March, London.

Lynes, T. (1996) *Our Pensions: A Policy for a Labour Government*, London: Eunomia.

'No Turning Back' Group of Conservative MPs (1993) *Who Benefits? Reinventing Social Security*, London: Conservative Political Centre.

Townsend, P. and Walker, A. (1995) *The Future of Pensions: Revitalising National Insurance*, London: Fabian Society.

Treasury Committee (1997a) *Public Expenditure Survey and Spending Objectives*, HC 355, London: HMSO.

—— (1997b) *The Personal Investment Authority*, HC 387, London: HMSO.

Waine, B. (1995) 'A disaster foretold: the case of the personal pension', *Social Policy and Administration*, 29, 4: 317–34.

Chapter 11

Criminal justice

Security, social control and the hidden agenda

Frances Heidensohn

INTRODUCTION

Party political debate about law and order has a relatively short history in Britain. Two somewhat contradictory features characterise that history: one that 'criminal justice issues have traditionally been subject to a broadly bipartisan approach in Britain' and second '"Law and Order" has traditionally been a Conservative phrase' (Morgan 1989). One analysis of the postwar politics of law and order suggests that there were two phases, the first lasting from 1945 until 1970 and characterised by 'liberal rehabilitative ideas' while the second showed a marked shift in 1970 when the Conservative Party election manifesto raised the issues of crime, protest and disorders and accused the (then Labour) Government of responsibility. Thereafter, the Conservatives developed the issues more forcefully at each general election, stressing their own strong image as *the* law and order party. Labour, on the other hand, either focused on deprivation and social conditions in relation to crime, or, as in their 1992 election manifesto, confined themselves to a very brief commitment, just half a column in a twenty-page-plus document. Crime rose inexorably as a matter of public concern during the 1970s and 1980s and featured inevitably in political and election debates.

While the Conservative Government (in power from 1979 to 1997) claimed the superior position as the natural party of order, this claim was increasingly challenged by Labour, a challenge which proved partially successful so that the ratings of both parties in opinion polls in the early 1990s were similar on this issue (Downes and Morgan 1994). Indeed, if the test of criminal justice policies is reducing the crime rate then, on actual performance the Conservatives fail 'since periods of Labour government have seen lower rises in the recorded crime rate, both relatively and absolutely, than have Conservative administrations' (Downes and Morgan 1994).

The 1997 General Election proved to be notable in several ways for law and order. These can be headlined:

- Overlapping approaches;
- A low key issue, although sleaze and corruption were major ones;
- The importance of the pre-election period;
- The significance of 'stakeholder' debates among criminal justice professionals, the media and academics.

Taken together, a review of these aspects will show how important the 1997 General Election was and how its significance may be perceived in future analyses.

OVERLAPPING POLICIES

The sections of the manifestos of the three major political parties which set out their proposals on law and order are hard to distinguish from each other. They are headed thus:

Which party will make me feel safe on the streets and secure in my home? (Liberal Democrats)

We will be tough on crime and tough on the causes of crime. (Labour)

Our record – a safe and civil society. (Conservatives)

While the Liberal Democrats include other social policies (on housing and the homeless) in the same chapter, the other two list similar concerns and proposals. Both focus on youth crime, drugs, victims, conviction and sentences and community crime. In some cases, the overlap appears almost paradoxical. While both address the question of local community safety, the Conservatives merely emphasised the use of closed circuit TV and voluntary identity cards while Labour proposed 'zero tolerance' of petty criminality and community safety orders to 'deal with threatening and disruptive criminal neighbours' as well as parental responsibility orders (Labour Party 1997). Not only do these policies resemble each other, those proposed by Labour can be seen both as harder than their traditional approach and compared to some of the Tories.

There were, nevertheless, important philosophical differences between the main parties which are summed up by the slogan produced by Tony Blair when Shadow Home Secretary 'tough on crime, tough on *the causes of crime*'. Labour explicitly focused on structural features of society – the widening divide between rich and poor, the growth of a disaffected underclass – and, albeit briefly, insisted that they intended to 'attack the causes of crime by our measures to relieve social deprivation' (ibid.). Clearly, their welfare-to-work and youth programme were designed to do this, and were therefore more in keeping with liberal approaches. What is interesting is the way in which Labour's crime measures were on the whole 'tough' and close to the Conservatives and were consistently presented in this way and not linked to their wider agenda. For instance, their *Tackling the causes of crime*, released in October 1996 addresses unemployment, homelessness and lack of services for young people as causes of crime. Yet, *Setting the pace* the Party's 'plans for fast track punishment for persistent young offenders' issued on 29 April 1997, focuses solely on that subject matter (which had been prompted by the Audit Commission Report (1996) *Misspent Youth*).

NOT AN ELECTION ISSUE

Most commentators discerned few differences between the main parties on crime with the result that there was relatively little debate on the issues during the campaign. After the first two weeks, *The Guardian* Media Watch (with Loughborough University) showed that the news topics covered were dominated by the election itself (26.1 per cent of items surveyed) and the 'sleaze' factor (17.8 per cent). Only taxation featured in more than 10 per cent and crime was not mentioned (*Guardian*, 14 April 1997). What was notable was the way in which, especially during the first week of electioneering, allegations about sleaze and corruption in parliament dominated, while these events were not linked to criminal charges; nor to criminal justice policies. It was fascinating to see how high a profile moral and ethical questions could gain in a British election and also how the regulation of MPs' behaviour came to the fore. Essentially this debate and indeed much of the election was fought over *politics* and *politicians* rather than *policies* and this had huge potential implications for authority and legitimacy of the state and its leaders. After all, the two most basic functions that any government needs to perform even as a 'nightwatchman' state are the external defence of the realm and the keeping of the peace within its boundaries. To achieve both of these, but especially the latter, it must maintain respect and command loyalty.

Pre-election matters

Much comment on the result of the 1997 vote has suggested that it was determined by events which happened some years before and in particular, Britain's departure from the Exchange Rate Mechanism in September 1992. Whether this is true, it can certainly be shown that developments occuring well before the campaign started were important in determining the salience of this subject. There are two aspects to this: the way in which Labour shaped and presented its policies so that it could end its manifesto section on crime with the claim 'Labour is the party of law and order in Britain today!' The second feature is of course that the Conservatives, having been in power for eighteen years, had to defend and fight on their record.

In an analysis of the politics of law and order, published as recently as 1992, the authors gloomily describe Thatcherism, its 'moral stances' and what they 'have done successfully is to define the Labour Party as progressive, which has become synonymous with ir- responsibility and permissiveness' (Brake and Hale 1992: 169). Even the Commission for Social Justice, an independent body set up by the late John Smith, Leader of the Labour Party, presented a stark picture of crime in its review of the state of the nation (1994: 47, *et seq*.) but advocated liberal, progressive policies: a national education campaign to condemn all forms of violence and promote non-violent discipline in schools (ibid.: 322) and diversion programmes for car thieves 'to teach repair and maintenance and to develop negotiation skills' (p. 333).

However, in the same year that this report was published the birth of New Labour occurred and with it changes to the substance and more significantly, the presentation of their law and order policies. Tony Blair had already used the phrase 'tough on crime, tough on the causes of crime' in a speech in February 1993 after the horrifying murder of a 2-year-old boy, Jamie Bulger, had caused national outrage. The 1995 Party Conference document 'Safer communities, safer Britain' does consider 'links between social conditions and crime' (p. 8) and proposes a number of liberal measures such as preschooling, childcare and youth clubs to support families. It contains rather more 'tough' proposals (often related to research or innovation) on 'robust enforcement measures' against drug dealers, new laws on racial violence, as well as stressing the need for greater accountability for the police and wider use of partnerships and multi-agency approaches to crime prevention.

In March 1992 when ICM/MORI surveyed popular views on the two main parties' policies for crime, and law and order, the Conservatives enjoyed a substantial lead (40 per cent compared with 26 per cent for Labour). A year later respondents had greater faith in Labour's policies (Labour 23 per cent compared with 19 per cent for the Conservatives). From then on Labour were normally ahead of the Conservatives on the issue and, at times, were way in front (Quoted in Young *et al.* 1997: 123). This may have been due to actual shifts in Labour policies, but it is also as likely to have been the result of two other factors: Labour's increasingly successful projection of itself in the media and to the public as a (eventually the) party of government and the Conservatives record of failure and even disasters in this field. Jack Straw's presentation of the 'zero tolerance' approach in which he asserted that 'we have literally to reclaim the streets for the law-abiding citizen from the aggressive begging of winos, addicts, and squeegee merchants; make street life everywhere an innocent pleasure again' (Travis 1997), may have shocked civil libertarians but effectively gained him much publicity and emphasised the 'tough' angle.

CONSERVATIVES AND CRIME

Claiming to be able to control the crime problem is hazardous. The risks are high. One risk which is apparent to criminologists and professional commentators is that crime control is an oxymoron. 'Crime' is complex, hydraheaded, illicit and unreachable. In the 1970s it was even pessimistically fashionable to argue that 'nothing works' – no penal or other sanctions are effective. Certainly, Britain, along with many other nations, has seen a fairly steady increase in recorded crime rates over a very long period and further, several accounts link these trends with other social developments, such as unemployment and the business cycle. Modern developments in research as well as in the mass media have led to much greater public concerns about crime. Criminal victimisation has been especially highlighted in the last twenty years because of both of these factors and a 'new' and somewhat discrete concept of 'fear of crime' has a profound impact on the lives of many, especially older, people. That crime was a politically 'neutral' topic for a long period after the

Second World War was due partly to these aspects of it. As the Conservatives so firmly claimed to be the law and order party and were in office for so long, they were bound to have to confront these matters.

Indeed, apart from a short phase at the end of their period of government they did preside over rising crime rates – they roughly doubled – a growing prison population, and various unwelcome events such as civil disorders, football hooliganism (at home and abroad) and increasing violent crime. However, they were also dogged by other disasters: by several hugely embarrassing prison scandals in their last years, by the outcomes of various very long standing miscarriages of justice, and finally by some particularly horrifying crimes.

British prisons could be described as having been in near-permanent crisis during the 1990s. April 1990 saw the longest, most serious disturbance in British penal history: from 1st to 25th April, Strangeways prison in Manchester was partly controlled by rioting inmates, protesting at their conditions. The Woolf Report, which recommended many changes to the system, following the disturbances was never fully implemented. Instead, a major change in the direction of policy led by Home Secretary Michael Howard was promoted, based on the declaration that 'prison works', with the result being a dramatic increase in the prison population. However, a series of highly publicised scandals hit the system: armed IRA prisoners broke out of Whitemoor Maximum Security Prison and the explosive Semtex was found within the perimeter fence, and three men serving life sentences escaped from Parkhurst Prison (also a maximum security establishment). Eventually, Derek Lewis the Director of the Prison Service was sacked. He was to prove a highly vocal critic of the Government and scathing in his views (*Guardian*, 9 April 1997).

While the scale of the prison riots in the 1990s was unprecedented, the impact of such events on policy is not. In the 1960s, for instance, under a Labour government and a reforming Home Secretary, Roy Jenkins, the successive escapes of two Great Train Robbers, Wilson and Biggs and then that of the spy, George Blake, led to the setting up of the Mountbatten inquiry into prison security and major changes in the direction of penal policy. In short, reform and redirection through 'the unpredictable realm of scandal and concern' (Downes and Morgan, 1994: 216) is a characteristic of this area of social policy as it is of personal social services and health, but much less so of social security or employment.

The long period of office enjoyed by the Conservatives obviously exposed them to such hazards, but their credibility (and hence poll ratings) were affected by their claims to effectiveness and indeed their policy energy and productiveness in this area. The series of high profile exposures of miscarriages of justice during this period are also a feature of the system: in the more distant past the use of capital punishment led to the gravest injustices as when the wrong person was executed (e.g. Timothy Evans) or doubts were later raised about evidence (e.g. Derek Bentley). Names of the more recent cases will be familiar, many of them involved Irish people suspected of terrorist offences – the Birmingham Six, Guildford Four, Judith Ward – while others had racial aspects – Winston Silcott – or featured women in abusive relationships and some were 'merely' conventional crimes. While the release of the first Irish people who had been wrongly convicted led to the setting up of the Royal Commission on Criminal Justice in 1991 (the only use of such a body throughout the Thatcher – Major years) the Commission's report was not fully implemented and such episodes were still occurring up to the time of the election, e.g. the Bridgewater case in February 1997. The reports of faked evidence, incompetence and fundamentally of *injustice* which these episodes revealed clearly helped to tarnish the Government's reputation as the party of law and order, not least with some of the minority communities.

An even profounder impact on public opinion was achieved by a number of notably brutal and horrible crimes committed (or discovered) in the final years of Conservative government. Among these were the murder of toddler Jamie Bulger by two other young boys, the massacre of sixteen school children and their teacher by Thomas Hamilton at Dunblane, the West trial at which Rosemary West was convicted of taking part in a series of killings of young women in Gloucester and the murders of headmaster Philip Lawrence outside his school and of student Stephen Lawrence in a racial attack. All of these attracted enormous, sometimes worldwide, publicity and led to calls for the banning of guns and knives. It can be argued that the media deliberately heightened public concern. The *Daily Mail*, for instance, named alleged suspects in the Stephen Lawrence case and challenged them to sue for libel. Two comments are relevant here in relation to the election. First that the government had exposed itself to criticism and to linkage in the public mind with fears about growing crime waves and second because both main parties were increasingly using the media, especially the tabloid Press themselves (Institute for Study and Treatment of Delinquency 1997: 7).

Further evidence of the problematic nature of criminal justice policies for any government plus the added hazards that the late Conservative Government provided for itself, came as the consequences of policy initiatives they had introduced. Administrative and organisational changes dug what Derek Lewis called 'bear traps' in this field. The separation of policy and implementation responsibilities between the Home Office and the Prison Service Agency led to much confusion and embarrassment, including the inappropriate early release of prisoners. The shackling of pregnant prisoners and even of mothers in labour formed another such example. At a quite different level the application of rigorous audit to social policies has very clearly exposed failures in *effectiveness* and *efficiency* and lack of value for money. An admirable addition to the analysis of social policy, such reports provide ammunition against the government. A prime example of this was the critique of the youth justice system in the Audit Commission's *Misspent Youth* seized on by Jack Straw and highlighted during the election campaign.

The Thatcher and Major governments were characterised by emphasised claims about law and order. In fact, policies varied considerably during these years and can be described as having formed two 'circular tours' from harsh to liberal and back again to 'punitive populism'. Many initiatives were launched, nine Criminal Justice Acts were passed between 1979 and 1996. In their final 1996–97 session, the Conservatives still had legislation prepared (or were supporting private members' bills) on firearms, sentencing, the police, sex offenders, stalking and knives. Yet this was a topic which had ceased to work (just like the economy) for them and was a key one on which Labour had gained public confidence. This is a classic example of a policy domain in which 'activity does not necessarily equate with influence' and where being out of office was of benefit.

STAKEHOLDER DEBATES

As noted earlier, criminal justice matters do not readily fit into a party political framework, although there are many important value and ideology differences between those, for instance, who argue for social crime prevention and hence links between welfare policies and crime control and others for whom law enforcement and due process are more central. Such divisions often cut across party lines and may reflect professional distinctions with the magistracy and the judiciary favouring the latter approach (Stenson and Cowell 1991). The 1997 Election was remarkable in two ways. First that a variety of public discussions did take place between 'stakeholders' in the criminal justice system and secondly that these generally revealed that the government had lost the support of many of the participants. One typical example of public debate was the conference sponsored jointly by the *Guardian* and the London School of Economics and held at the London School of Economics in December 1996 which brought together politicians, professionals, academics and journalists and created a Website to which members of the public could contribute comments. Summarising the event, one account concluded that there was an even 'split on whether a Labour government would make any real difference in the field of criminal justice' (*Guardian*, 18 December 1996). Contributors proposed much wider terms of debate and policy solutions than the politicians present (Jack Straw and Sir Ivan Lawrence, former Chairman of the Home Affairs Select Committee). In an issue of their magazine timed to reflect and influence thinking around the election, the Institute for Study and Treatment of Delinquency drew in a wide variety of contributions, including one from Michael Howard, the (then) Home Secretary, Jack Straw and Alex Carlile. What notably characterised the academic and pressure group articles were pleas to *reduce* public expectations of what can be delivered. Writing of policing, Morgan and Newburn assert 'with the major political parties competitively engaging in policing and penal populism, then we will undermine a policing tradition which despite its problems, still has much to commend it'(ISTD 1997). They insist 'there are no simple solutions to the crime and policing problems that confront us' and they specifically challenge the conclusions of the Audit Commission report *Tackling Crime Effectively* which advocated more surveillance and proactive policing.

In the run-up to the election such debates proliferated and many players used the wide media interest in order to present their views and also the greater freedom accorded to some of them to comment. Senior members of the judiciary were extremely critical of the government's policies. Lord Woolf had already attacked the 'prison works' nostrum as short-sighted; Lord Chief Justice Taylor condemned sentencing proposals as 'a denial of justice'. Perhaps the most surprising (and damaging) loss of support was that of the police. The

Chief Constable of Thames Valley was critical of the approaches to policing disorder of both main parties in an article published by the Institute of Economic Affairs (Pollard 1997). He claimed that they could provoke riots and end up targetting minorities. The *Guardian* crime correspondent felt confident that this would be 'certain to provoke a political debate on law and order which has so far been lacking in the election campaign' (*Guardian*, 23 April 1997), but it did not do so.

CONCLUSIONS

Law and order issues are easily subject to gesture politics, to rhetoric and to simple solutions. But crime and criminal justice are complex, often messy, deeply morally implicated areas of human behaviour. Criminologists have claimed for decades that there are no quick-fix answers. Prohibition in the USA is often cited as the classic example of massively unintended and disastrous consequences – organised crime, protection, corruption – of an unsuitable and unenforceable ban on alcohol, which criminalised its production, sale and consumption. Politicians nevertheless seem drawn to proffer simple analyses and initiatives to respond to problems of crime and disorder.

Among the striking paradoxes which characterised the 1997 election and the run-up to it was that while the main parties began with very different views on the *origins* of criminality, they both proposed similar policies. All political parties reflected public concern about crime and security issues. However, Labour and the Liberal Democrats recognised 'the social causes of crime' and linked their welfare policies to the reduction of disorder. Indeed, the Liberal Democrats set their crime proposals in their manifesto section dealing with other 'security' matters such as homelessness. Conservatives, on the other hand, while emphasising individual moral causes of crime, had produced a range of policies during their time in office and were advocating more when they lost power. Despite these diverse origins, the menus published by the main parties resembled each other in their (somewhat narrow) lists of youth justice, policing, drugs and sentencing policies.

Curiously, when one digs more deeply, the policy histories are more diverse and more complex. The Conservatives, for instance, presided over considerable variations during their long period in power. As late as 1991 they had promoted and legislated for a twin-track approach to penal policy which commanded widespread support. Equally, Labour in its pre-election background papers acknowledged social causes of crime and welfare solutions to them. Yet in its manifesto and pronouncements before and during the campaign, there was a tightly-targeted focus on 'tough' measures *and* approaches.

Law and order did not become a central policy issue *between* the parties in the 1997 campaign as it had in some elections in the recent past. Instead, the parties appeared to have achieved a new consensus, albeit on different ground. The inter-party debate then became a matter of which politicians could be trusted to provide greater security for the public. The Conservatives tried to gain advantage on this quite late in the campaign when, on 22 April, Michael Howard promised to cut crime rates by 10 per cent over the next five years. Not only his political opponents attacked him for this rash promise, Judge Stephen Tumim, the former chief inspector of prisons, and Mike Hough, previously a Home Office researcher and co-author of the British Crime Survey, dismissed this as unrealistic. Labour and the Liberal Democrats had raised crime as an issue in the previous week, but it did not take off on either occasion. As *The Guardian* (23 April 1997) noted: 'there is no serious debate. No issue is subject to such deliberate distortions as crime. Politics is demeaned and the public insulted'. Some of the responsibility for these shifts may lie with the mass media, especially the tabloid Press, which have raised crime, especially violent crime stories to very high profiles and have demanded punitive responses from authority.

Arguably, it may not be inappropriate that the complex themes of law and order were not subjected to the unsubtle debates in election campaigns. In the USA, George Bush's use of a particularly horrific murder case in the 1988 Presidential election was seen as very damaging. Instead, a calmer discussion of some of the difficult and troubling issues which this area raised would contribute to greater public understanding and ultimately, sounder policies.

Law and order remain nevertheless both the most basic and among the most difficult areas of public policy. 'Insecurity' was not one of the Five Giants identified by Beveridge as stalking the land and in need of dispatch. No doubt it might now be included, although there are major contrasts with other social policy areas. While social services, for example, have both a history and contemporary aspects of social control, they are seen as having *primarily* welfare purposes. The criminal justice system, embodying directly the state's power over individuals and their (mis)behaviour as well as affecting the stability of society, is somewhat distinctive. Since coming into power on 1 May, the new Labour government has, while maintaining many of the previous government's policies – for example the prison ship moored off Dorset – initiated reviews of many aspects of the whole system. Crime was not a major election issue, indeed the 1997 election could be described as a non-, or perhaps a one-, issue election and that issue was *politics*, their character, the nature and integrity of politicians. One of the observations made by sociologists today is that we live in a globalised world and by political scientists that the state has been 'hollowed out'. Both these features have vast consequences for law and order – for example, organised crime is a highly mobile international business. Much of the approach to criminal justice issues is simplified down into very basic terms. It is unlikely that solutions can be found in that way. Even though the 1997 General Election campaign may have been conducted with a fairly narrow focus, the problems themselves cannot be simplified nor the complex social and structural links ignored.

ACKNOWLEDGEMENT

I am most grateful for assistance provided by Martin Heidensohn in preparing this chapter.

REFERENCES

Audit Commission (1996) *Misspent Youth . . .*, London: Audit Commission Publications.
Brake, M. and Hale, C. (1992) *Public Order and Private Lives*, London: Routledge.
Commission on Social Justice/Institute for Public Policy Research (1994) *Social Justice*, London: Vintage.
Conservative Party (1997) *You Can Only be Sure with the Conservatives*, election manifesto, London: Conservative Central Office.
Downes, D. and Morgan, R. (1994) '"Hostages to fortune"? The politics of law and order in post-war Britain', in M. Maguire, R. Morgan and R. Reiner (eds) *The Oxford Handbook of Criminology*, Oxford: Oxford University Press.
Conservative Party Press Conference Report 'Tough on the Statistics of Crime'. 'Howard Pledges 10 p.c. Cut in Crime'. Michael Hough 'High Cost of Keeping Peace', *Guardian*, 23 April 1997.
ISTD (Institute for Study and Treatment of Delinquency) (1997) *Law and Order Politics, Criminal Justice Matters*, no. 26, Winter 1997. (Articles by Downes, Morgan and Newburn and Bennetto).
Labour Party (1995) 'Safer communities, safer Britain', conference leaflet.

—— (1997) *New Labour: Because Britain Deserves Better*, election manifesto, London: Labour Party.

Liberal Democrats (1997) *Make the Difference*, election manifesto, London: Liberal Democrats.

Morgan, R. (1989) 'Criminal justice', in M. McCarthy (ed.) *The New Politics of Welfare*, Basingstoke: Macmillan.

Pollard, Charles (1997) *Zero Tolerance: Policing a Free Society*, London: Institute of Economic Affairs.

Stenson, K. and Cowell, D. (eds) (1991) *The Politics of Crime Control*, London: Sage.

Straw, Jack and Michael, A. (1996) 'Tackling the causes of crime', leaflet, London: Labour Party.

Straw, Jack (April 29 1997) 'Setting the Pace Labour's Plans for Fast Track Punishment for Persistent Young Offenders', leaflet, London: Labour Party.

Travis, Alan (1997) Home Affairs: Crime and Prisons in M. Linton (ed.) *The Election: A Voters' Guide. A Guardian Book*, London: Fourth Estate.

Chapter 12

The greenest election ever?

Sue Barber

INTRODUCTION

It would be impossible to deal with all the issues which are on the green agenda in one short chapter. Transport and pollution, energy consumption, food safety, housing, social and environmental welfare, and political organisation are just some of the areas which a green perspective takes into account. Here we shall look briefly at the key environmental issues of transport and pollution and the policy perspectives impacting on these over the last 10 years. The rest of the chapter is concerned with how green issues were taken up in the 1997 election and the first budget. The conclusion speculates on how things may develop during the present term of government.

THE LEGACY OF PRIVATISATION

At the end of the 1980s, the government under Margaret Thatcher continued to stress the role of the market as paramount in environmental as well as other policy areas. This militated against environmental protection via regulation and remained unchanged in 1997 as the Conservatives' Green manifesto revealed (Conservative Party 1997). Yet the fact that a Conservative Green Manifesto was published at all speaks of some influence, albeit indirect, of the Green movement. The Conservatives pointed to the fact that they had published plans for sustainable development, made some moves to integrate pollution inspectorates and created a new Environment Agency, and introduced what they termed the first environmental tax in the form of the landfill levy. However, the Greens would argue that many issues, not least those of transport and the control of pollution, continued to be stymied by the road lobby.

We now have a deeply entrenched car culture. Changing it is agreed to be one of the key ways to develop greener living. The Conservatives, like Labour before them, actively promoted car ownership, and at the same time played their part in supporting the British car industry. Many jobs exist in related industries such as road building, supply of fuel, insurances and so on. Garner (1996: 166–8) makes the point that the road lobby, (within which is the motor industry, motorists' organisations, bus operators, road haulage companies, road construction and oil industries), depends upon the car culture. The lobby's influence totally eclipsed that of the environmentalists throughout the four terms of Conservative office. They successfully argued for more roads, and fiercely opposed moves towards more integrated pollution control. The latter is something which all environmentalists argue is crucial to turning the tide and decreasing environmental degradation and related ill health. In theory, the Environment Agency, set up in 1996, has the power to do this. In practice, the reality is that control is patchy, and prevention virtually non-existent. In 1989, the Conservative government announced that it would be increasing the budget earmarked for road building from five to twelve billion pounds over a ten-year period. This led to increased traffic and pollution.

In recent years, awareness has been growing that more roads may not be the panacea leading to the kind of tomorrow people want to live in. More roads has meant more cars, more traffic congestion and pollution, gridlock and 'road rage', increased ill health and a run-down in public transport, especially that which used to carry freight. 82 per cent of those polled by MORI for the Real World Coalition said they wanted government to promise 'much tougher policies to protect the environment' and 'a transport programme with clear targets for reducing road traffic' (MORI/Real World 1997).

The Conservatives in office privatised much of the public transport system. By handing over the responsibility of maintenance and investment to private companies, some pressure was taken off the public spending borrowing requirement (PSBR). However, privatised companies received massive grants of taxpayers' money (Harper 1997a). Environmentalists argued that the splitting of responsibilities would lead to the very same chaos which provided the rationale for creating a system of co-ordinated public transport in the first place. The Labour Government is committed to developing an integrated transport system. It appears that coordination and regulation as well as partnerships between public and private sectors will be central to its policies. Renationalisation of public transport is not on the agenda. The Labour Party manifesto signalled that local authorities would have greater powers to control local traffic. Protracted recession in which cutting public expenditure has been a hallmark, forms part of the same picture and should not be taken out of the context of decreases in income tax which could otherwise have been used, in part, for such investment. We could also make a connection between the widening gap in wealth between richer and poorer UK citizens, and the run-down of services such as public transport upon which those who are not wealthy depend and which is very much a political issue.

The future of the London Underground became a particular subject of debate. Unless the Treasury put in extra funding, London Transport's grant was set to fall from £918 million in 1996–97 to £150 million in the year 2000 (Harper 1997b). It was estimated that some £2 billion in new investment would be needed over the next five years. Labour appeared to favour some form of semi-privatised underground system.

The legacy of privatisation was also visible with regard to water. The role and powers of Ofwat were the subject of controversy, especially in the months preceding the election. Ideology differentiates new Labour's approach from that of its predecessor. The Conservative policy of 'private finance initiative' or PFI was just that – privatisation. One assumes that Labour's 'public private partnership', or PPP signals that the government will want a greater say than their predecessors in how the system is organised and run. Ofwat, the independent regulator set up under the Conservatives to oversee the privatised companies, has turned out to have too little power to enforce standards and hold privatised companies to their investment and maintenance targets. Efficiency was the watchword of the Conservatives who fiercely defended their decisions to privatise on the basis that the market was the best, indeed the only means of delivering efficient systems run in the public interest. New Labour on the other hand were quick to introduce new regulations compelling water companies to carry out maintenance and investment by agreed deadlines. The record relating to pollution, and therefore to the quality of service provided, shows that some powerful business interests will attempt to resist greater regulation. Formulae for cutting emissions suggested by the European Union (EU) and the United Nations (UN) have been rejected, revised and delayed. There are signs however, that new Labour intend to play a high profile role in gaining agreements internationally to help to combat pollution and climate change, although early signs are that further revisions to EU and UN targets will be to scale down the process in the hope of gaining wide agreement and action as the Earth Summit II and the Kyoto meetings showed.

THE MANIFESTOS AND THE ELECTION CAMPAIGN

The manifestos revealed that the main parties were all concerned with environmental and green issues to varying extents. In comparison with the 1992 election, when environmental issues were notable only by their virtual absence (Carter 1992: 442) the 1997 manifestos were 'greened', but not the campaigns. In the campaigns the traditional concerns of the economy, education and health dominated. The Labour and Liberal parties gave some time to transport policy, yet this remained a secondary issue. Pollution, food safety, energy efficiency, and what may be widely referred to as 'green living choices' such as improvements to housing, changes in production technology and consumption patterns, connections between ill health, poverty and the natural and built environments were absent from the campaigns, despite the fact that many of these issues were hitting the news headlines in the weeks and months preceding the election. It is ironic that the campaign took place at a time in which extraordinary roads protests and other environmentally-oriented social action was very much in the news. For example, there were protests against an additional runway at Manchester airport and against hunting. Also in the news, public outrage about food safety was evident in the light of the BSE scandal. Yet the campaign failed to tackle these head on. 73 per cent of those polled by MORI for Friends of the Earth (FOE) and the Royal Society for the Protection of Birds (RSPB), said that environmental issues should have been given higher priority in the campaign (FOE/RSPB 1997).

The manifestos of the two main parties revealed very little. Manifestos are often written in 'safe' language, indicating only the general direction that policy formulation might follow, rather than giving much away in terms of specific programmes of action. The Liberal Democrats alone claimed to offer a 'menu with prices' (Liberal Democrats 1997: 7). All of the three main parties claimed that whatever they might do in government, it would cost the taxpayer no more overall than they were paying already. All three parties gave commitments to setting environmental policy in the context of reviewing all government policies. All made some mention of raising environmental taxes and relating these to creating new jobs.

The Labour Party manifesto

The Labour Party's document was correctly characterised as cautious yet it did make significant changes to the priorities of government and outlined that there would be several initiatives to come which are relevant to the green agenda. Here is an example of their cautious language which reveals a possible change to their traditional values:

> We will put concern for the environment at the heart of policy making, so that it is not an add on extra, but informs the whole of government, from housing and energy policy through to global warming and international agreements.
>
> (Labour Party 1997: 4)

A new minister for Public Health was promised whose remit would include looking at the impact that poverty, poor housing, unemployment and a polluted environment have on health (op.cit.: 21). Labour also pledged to develop an integrated transport policy; to make cycling and walking safer; to review vehicle excise duty to promote low-emission vehicles; to work with the automotive industry to develop clean cars for the future (op. cit.: 28–9); and to decrease carbon emissions by 22 per cent by 2010 (op. cit.: 39). They pledged to promote energy conservation and renewable energy (op. cit.: 17). They set new targets for the recycling of waste at 25 per cent. They assured us that they would reform the Common Agricultural Policy to enhance the environment (op. cit.: 30) and that they would establish an independent food standards agency. All of these commitments can be seen in the light of the high profile that the issues have had in recent years. In particular, air pollution and lack of food safety are widely thought to pose a high risk to health, and governments have been criticised time and again for their irresponsibility and failure to prevent major crises. The number of children and old people suffering from asthma is at an all-time high and it is thought that one probable cause is carbon emissions from vehicles (Women's Environmental Network 1995). Before the election the scandal of the BSE crisis had brought the lack of governmental integrity into the media headlines while outbreaks of *E coli* highlighted the lack of care in food handling by vendors. An environmental audit committee in Parliament was also pledged.

Home energy-efficiency schemes linked to an environment task-force made up of those unemployed and aged under 25 was another measure announced in Labour's manifesto (Labour Party 1997: 19). This is part of the Welfare-to-Work programme which could result in environmental awareness being raised and examples of good practice developed (see Chapter 15).

The Conservative Party's Green manifesto

What was most striking about the Conservative Party's manifesto was that it was written in the language of sustainable development, as laid out in Agenda 21 (a document agreed to by more than 120 countries, signed at the United Nations Conference on Environment and Development 1992 which outlines an agenda framework for the twenty-first century). Sustainable development is a concept which the Conservative government, and in particular John Gummer, the previous Secretary of State for the Environment, had publicly supported since 1992, especially in the international arena. It is also a concept which is used interchangeably with 'green' by many involved in initiatives related to Agenda 21. One of the success stories over the same period was that of the local Agenda 21 initiatives. Yet the future of these, and their ability to bring real change remains in the balance as most have few or no financial resources and no statutory status. The values of *laissez-faire* and voluntary action remained firmly at the core of the Conservative's record in government, manifesto and campaign.

Leadership was also stressed in the Conservative manifesto – as it was in the Labour one. The Conservatives chose to call their Green manifesto *Leadership Abroad, Responsibility at Home*. The concept of leadership is not revered by the Green movement. Their belief is that leaders, or spokespeople, should not stay in power for too long, as they are likely to become corrupted and out of touch with those they represent. Much of what the previous Conservative government can point to by way of an environmental programme can be traced to international agreements such as Agenda 21. These speak of grand international potential, and they can inspire. Inspirations, particularly those outlined in Agenda 21, are left open-ended for each nation to put specific meaning to. This allowed the Conservatives to use rhetoric, with very little commitment to the kind of major structural and behavioural changes implied.

The role of the individual as a responsible and voluntary citizen was central to the viability of the Conservatives' policy stance. They compared the virtues of this approach with the supposed heavy-handed regulation stamp of any potential Labour government (Conservative Party 1997: 10, 13, 20).

The Liberal Democrats' manifesto

The Liberal Democrats used a passionate language which was redolent of green issues. Their traditional values of local democracy, and social and economic justice maintained through a rigorous market economy and government intervention remained central. Of the three main parties, it is they who have developed policies on environmental issues in the past and can therefore claim some credibility and continuity in terms of their Green values. They stressed greater accountability from government, a strong civil society built 'from the bottom up' (Liberal Democrat Party 1997: 7), a promise to 'redress the balance between the powerful and the weak, between rich and poor and between immediate gains and long-term environmental costs'(op. cit.: 7). It has often been said of the Liberal Democrats, and of other minority parties operating in a system of 'first past the post', that they can afford to be bold, where the main contenders tend to be more pragmatic. The latter, it is argued, need to be able to keep any promises that they make. There may be some truth in this.

The Liberal Democrats committed themselves to greening the economy. Conservative and Labour language was non-committal and indirect compared to the Liberal Democrats, who used clear, direct language. They pledged to develop new economic indicators, designed to measure quality of life, progress and wealth. This is exactly what think tanks such as the New Economics Foundation called for (Mayo *et al.*, 1997: 4 and passim).

LABOUR'S FIRST BUDGET

Although some expected significant environmental tax reforms, the Chancellor's first budget contained nothing of the sort. Bus and lorry owners, meeting efficiency criteria by converting to gas power by 1998 will see their vehicle excise levy reduced by up to £500 per annum. But bus and lorry owners were quick to point out that upgrading their vehicles may prove to be extremely expensive, and gas difficult to purchase, thus liquidating the incentive.

Coming very soon after the election, many of Labour's manifesto pledges were yet to take their exact shape before being costed into a formal budget. For example, the *Financial Times* dubbed 'transport' as 'the storm that never broke' (Batchelor and Griffiths 1997).

Measures were announced to increase the costs of motoring (increases in fuel duty and car tax). Despite expectations to the contrary, there were no reforms relating to company cars nor was there any reduction in VAT on energy-saving products. However it was indicated that EU law prevents this, at least on DIY products. This latter point, it was promised, would be pursued within the EU policy-making machinery with a view to change. In the run up to the 1998 budget the government will be looking at the possibility of introducing a quarrying levy, and discouraging water pollution.

The pledged cut in VAT on fuel to 5 per cent (Labour Party 1997: 12) was duly implemented. At first sight, this may look like an anti-environmental measure, going against the tenet that the polluter should pay. Seen in a broader context, it sits well with Labour's traditional concern with those with little income. The poorest fifth of households spend some 12 per cent of their income on fuel, the richest fifth, approximately 4 per cent (Tindale and Holtham 1996: iv). It also sits well with that part of the Green agenda keen to promote greater equity between people. As long as energy consumption is reduced by taking energy-efficiency seriously, greater equity between people and the environment may be achieved too.

Some in the Green movement expressed their disappointment with the first budget. Yet policy initiatives under review include the Common Agricultural Policy, eco-labelling and environmental taxes as well as transport, road building and pollution control.

In June 1997, the Labour Government ordered a review of the road programme, the outcome of which will tell us how far its approach will be different to that of their predecessors. If they decide that no new roads are necessary for the foreseeable future, it will go some way towards their earning green credibility. So too would measures to affect planning policy which should encourage the use of bicycles, public transport and at the same time ensure that built environments are safe and pleasant places to live and walk in.

The Labour government also said that it would not re-nationalise public transport. This would be a massive and expensive undertaking for which financial resources are lacking. A continuing concern, which it indicated it will deal with, is that of regulating private companies which operate public transport. Railtrack's record on underspending on its planned investment generated a good deal of controversy. According to Watson (1997), of the £450 million backlog on station work, just £50 million has been spent. Harper (1997c), reported on Railtrack's profits which were up by 60 per cent on last year, compounding the error of under-investment.

The new government also agreed to promote new green technologies and businesses (Labour Party 1997: 17), strengthen European cooperation on environmental issues and cut carbon dioxide emissions by 2010 (op. cit.: 39). The evidence suggests that cuts in emissions have mainly been achieved as a result of the run-down of our coal industry. It will therefore be interesting to see if the Government takes the expertise of the environmental movement on board as it develops policy. There is some indication that the precautionary principle, favoured by the EU, may find a place in policy, for example, Labour announced that it would ban the sale of pressurised drinks cans which release highly polluting gases. This was a radical change in approach since the precautionary principle was always resisted by the Conservatives, as it goes hand in hand with regulation and flies in the face of market forces.

Given that the Labour Party have not previously been guided by Green values, we now watch with interest to see if this becomes part of their way of operating in the world. The Chancellor's first budget speech underlined that sustainable development and, in particular valuing the environment will be put at the heart of future budgetary considerations. We have been promised a reformed welfare state. For the postwar years, Beveridge outlined five 'giant evils' which needed to be tackled: want, disease, ignorance, squalor and idleness. Current reforms might view our degraded environment as an additional giant evil.

THE FUTURE

Governmental framework for delivering Green policies

Looking ahead, let us assume for a moment that, true to its pre-election promise, the Labour government holds a referendum on proportional representation, (PR), and the electorate vote in favour of it. Along with other constitutional changes like devolution and decentralisation this might change our political culture. What might the effect on environmental policy be?

There are a number of issues at stake. On the one hand, the

proponents of PR believe that it could deliver a more representative democracy than the present system does and consequently political opinion in parliament. For example, the Green Party would probably become a mainstream, parliamentary party, with a significant number of MPs as would other minor parties. On the basis of manifesto positions of the major and significant minority parties (which in green terms means the Green Party, the Liberal Democrats and Plaid Cymru) we could say that we would have a greener system of government, and a different kind of democracy. However, there are caveats.

First, the quality of outcome would partly depend upon the kind of PR system chosen. Second, many warn against throwing out a system which works on the basis of opposition, such that a party with a clear electoral majority is both strong and able to deliver a coherent programme while at the same time responding to majority opinion. Third, the policy positions of the Greens are untried. In addition, the kind of democracy we have now has changed significantly over the postwar years, away from social democracy, towards something of a hybrid between this and a consumer 'democracy'. Some kinds of reform advocated by Greens, such as meaningful information to be given on the labelling of food and other consumables (which the Government signalled they would support via the European policy-making machinery) and the principle of the polluter pays, point towards consumer democracy. It would be a mistake, in my view for this definition of democracy to eclipse that based on notions of citizenship, but should rather be seen as complementary. Gender equity, across the whole range of welfare services, and in the outcome of how different people experience the human environment should also be paramount in building a new, practical democracy, but there is nothing intrinsic to PR that would automatically set such equity at its heart.

The Green Party manifesto, in setting a scene for 'real democracy' put issues such as PR (the additional member system), freedom of information, redistribution of power from central to local government, the end of unelected quangos and reform of the House of Commons (giving voters the right of recall to remove MPs from office who do not perform according to their mandates) at the centre of its concerns (Green Party 1997: 5). Social and economic justice are portrayed as necessary underpinnings to environmental integrity.

In a more immediate sense, we have a tangible commitment on the part of the government which is an example of integration, and of the high profile it seemingly means that environmental issues will have. The Deputy Prime Minister, John Prescott, is also Secretary of State for the Environment, Transport and the Regions. This signals a serious approach to integrating the work of departments which were previously conspicuous for their clashes in values.

A Freedom of Information Act and greater accountability would strengthen democracy. The new government appear committed to implementing this. In addition to the vote on the reform of the system to elect Members of Parliament, other issues which are to be reviewed include the reform of the House of Lords and devolution of power to Scotland and Wales. The government has also signalled that there will be a review of the way in which local government is constituted and funded. Given that many environmental issues appear at the local level such changes might provide a space in which radical change might follow. Labour has pledged to give local government a 'new duty ... to promote the economic, social and environmental well being of their area' (Labour Party 1997: 34). They will encourage 'democratic innovative local government, including pilot implementation of the idea of mayors with executive powers in cities' (ibid). We could hope that these innovations would improve the representation of poorer sections of society as well as bringing women more to the fore in local arenas (Quarrie 1992).

Environmental taxes

If a referendum on PR still seems a little far off, the development of environmental taxes has already begun. The Conservatives introduced a landfill levy (1996), and different rates of tax on leaded and unleaded petrol. These were but a small beginning.

The time may be right for using taxes and incentives judiciously. Opinion research commissioned by FOE/RSPB (1997) showed that over four-fifths of respondents endorsed the idea of environmental tax reforms.

The connection between raising environmental taxes and creating jobs, while at the same time curbing some of the worst excesses of pollution was an issue taken up in all the manifestos, but no clear strategies were outlined. The case for ecological tax reform was considered to be a worthwhile option by the authors of the Report of the Commission on Social Justice (1994: 393–5). The Government may look to this, as well as to a study carried out by the IPPR (Tindale and Holtham 1996: 98–107), on various ways in which taxes could be redrawn. Policies which increase taxes on pollution, and at the same time decrease employers National Insurance contributions have been mooted. This seems to go hand in hand with the belief that new jobs would be created. The Government may look at this in due course even though it was not mentioned in its first budget. There is no fundamental connection between raising environmental taxes, and creating jobs. This would have to be engineered, and would certainly take careful planning.

International Relations

Looked at as a whole, the government will also be concerned to play a cooperative role on the international scene. The control of climate change is just one issue where this is extremely important. Prime Minister Tony Blair reiterated the promise made in the Labour Party's manifesto to cut carbon dioxide (CO_2) emissions by 22 per cent by 2010 (Labour Party 1997: 39) at the Earth Summit II Conference held in New York in June 1997. Yet other issues relating to sustainable development were neglected at the conference which was meant to review the progress made since 1992 when the Convention on Climate Change *and* Agenda 21 were signed. Global injustices and poverty, gender equity, sustainable production and consumption were all issues remarkable for their relatively low key compared to the dominant issue of climate change.

Other pressing concerns include the legacy of nuclear weapons and waste, the abolition of unsafe pesticides and herbicides, the development and use of better technology to curb the use of incinerators which give off dangerous levels of pollutants such as dioxins, support for the production of safe and preferably organic food, support for the production and use of energy-efficient homes and appliances. Five years is not a long time in which to turn around fundamental aspects of our political economy, but a measure of this Government's success or otherwise will depend, to paraphrase what has become a green tenet, upon its delivering meaningful support to meet the needs of today's citizens, without jeopardising the well-being of tomorrow's.

REFERENCES

Batchelor, C. and Griffiths, J. (1997) 'The storm that never broke', *Financial Times* 3 July.

Carter, N. (1992) 'Whatever happened to the environment? The British General Election of 1992', *Environmental Politics* 1,3: 442–8.

Commission on Social Justice (1994) *Social Justice, Strategies for National Renewal*, London: Vintage.

Conservative Party (1997) *Leadership Abroad Responsibility at Home, The Conservative Green manifesto*, election manifesto, London: Conservative Party.

Conservative Party.(1997), *You Can Only be Sure with the Conservatives*, election manifesto, London: Conservative Party.

FOE/RSPB (Friends of the Earth/Royal Society for the Protection of Birds) (June 1997) *General Election 1997 Exit Poll – Key Findings*, London: FOE/RSPB.

Garner, R. (1996) *Environmental Politics*, London: Harvester Wheatsheaf.

Green Party (1997) *Green Party Manifesto*, election manifesto, London: Green Party.

Harper, Keith (1997a) 'Railtrack backtracks on subsidy', *Guardian* 27 July.

—— (1997b) 'A plan to transform the underground', *Guardian* 18 June.

—— (1997c) 'Fury over Railtrack profits', *Guardian* 5 June.

Labour Party (1997) *New Labour: because Britain deserves better*, election manifesto, London: Labour Party.

Liberal Democrats (1997) *Make the Difference*, election manifesto, London: Liberal Democrats.

Mayo, E., MacGillvray, A. and McLaren, D. (1997) *More Isn't Always Better, a special briefing on growth and quality of life in the UK*, London: New Economics Foundation.

MORI/Real World (1997) *Summary, Opinion Research*, April.

Quarrie, Joyce (ed.) (1992) *Earth Summit '92*, London: Regency Press.

Tindale, S. and Holtham, G. (1996) *Green Tax Reform, pollution payments and labour tax cuts*, London, Institute for Public Policy Research.

Watson, Ceilia (1997) '£450 million backlog on station work cut by just £50 million', *Guardian*, 6 June.

Women's Environmental Network (1995) Briefing on air pollution, London: Women's Environmental Network.

Chapter 13

The view from Scotland

Richard Parry

TWO SUPERIMPOSED CONTEXTS

Since 1974, General Election campaigns in Scotland have had two components: a United Kingdom aspect based on social and economic issues expressed by the policies of the Labour and Conservative parties, and a Scottish aspect about the policies of all parties to the 'national question' – the complex of questions about Scotland's identity and governance which are driven by the existence of an established, credible, pro-independence party, the Scottish National Party (SNP). There is a lack of articulation between these two components. The first is dominated by London-based media which remain the main supplier of information to the Scottish electorate and by the two main parties, whose Scottish activities are under the control of national headquarters. The second focuses on constitutional matters and neglects the Scottish dimension of policy issues. The SNP is a responsible, competitive and organised force which has had a double-figure electoral potential since its foundation in 1934 and a strong electoral threat since it won 30 per cent of the vote and 11 seats in the October 1974 General Election. The policies of the SNP have become more clearly left-wing over the years, but it remains a catch-all party whose parliamentary strength has been in the more rural, Conservative areas and which is available as a tactical option to put pressure on Labour and Conservative parties. It is much strengthened by not having as a principal purpose the defence of a minority language.

The Scottish party system going into the 1997 campaign took the form of a four-party system with a hegemonic Labour Party (dominating parliamentary representation and local authorities), a correspondingly weak Conservative Party, the SNP with 20–30 per cent of the vote but not enough local concentration to win it many seats, and the Liberal Democrats with a lesser aggregate vote than the SNP but a stronger parliamentary base (Brand *et al*. 1994). Table 13.1 summarises recent voting trends (for analysis see Brown *et al*. 1996: ch 7). In 1992 the Conservatives had done unexpectedly well in Scotland, increasing their vote share and gaining one seat from Labour. The 1994 European elections showed the Conservatives falling back and the SNP achieving their best-ever national vote. The 1995 council elections, the first under the reorganised single-tier authorities which were to assume responsibility in April 1996, were even more disastrous for the Conservatives as they failed to take control of any of the 29 new councils. This mid-term experience further undermined the legitimacy of Conservative government in Scotland and it posed the threat that at such a low vote level the Conservatives might lose most of their ten Scottish seats.

Table 13.1 Vote figures in Scotland, 1992–97

	Lab	Con	SNP	Lib Dem
1992 General Election (Turnout = 75%)				
Percentage of vote	39.0	25.6	21.5	13.1
Number of seats	49	11	3	9
Calculated number of seats based on 1997 boundaries	50	11	3	8
1994 European elections (Turnout = 38%)				
Percentage of vote	42.5	14.5	32.6	7.2
1995 council elections (Turnout = 45%)				
Percentage of vote	43.8	11.3	26.2	9.7
Percentage of vote in contests where all four parties participated	39.2	20.9	20.5	19.3

The other contextual variable is that of constitutional options, conventionally expressed as full independence (now accepted by the SNP as being enthusiastically within the European Union); some form of legislative devolution, now usually called a 'Scottish Parliament'; and no change from the status quo (see Table 13.2). Labour was anti-devolution until 1974, since then increasingly-strongly pro; the Conservatives supported it from 1968 to 1975 but since then have been increasingly strongly anti; the Liberal Democrats' (and predecessors) principled support has long been discounted. In the one explicit test – the referendum on 1 March 1979 about whether the Scotland Act 1978 should come into effect – the proposals were approved by 51.6 per cent of those voting on a rather low turnout,

Table 13.2 Polls of Scottish voters on constitutional options, 1997

Pollster	Published in:	Date of fieldwork	Options Ind.	Options Dev.	Options NC	Size Sample	Date of Publication
MARCH–APRIL 1997							
ICM	*Scotsman*	Tues 11–Fri 14	26	45	28	1000*	Mon 17 March
		Election called Monday 17 March					
ICM	*Scotsman*	Sat 29–Mon 31	26	48	24	1,000*	Wed 2 April
NOP	*Sunday Times*	Thurs 3 April	35	36	24	844	Sun 6 April
ICM	*Scotsman*	Fri 11–Sun 13	26	45	27	1,000*	Tues 15 April
ICM	*Scotsman*	Fri 18–Sun 20	27	40	30	1,000*	Tues 22 April
ICM	*Scotsman*	Fri 25–Sun 27	27	39	31	1,000*	Tues 29 April

Referendum voting intention: devolution – Yes 63%; tax-raising powers – Yes 53%

Notes: * Telephone poll
Ind. = Independence
Dev. = Devolution
NC = No change

but there was no parliamentary majority to override the provision in the Act that required a vote on its repeal if, as happened, less than 40 per cent of the electorate supported devolution. Polls before and after 1979 show a clear plurality in favour of devolution and a minority support for independence which in the 1990s has usually matched or exceeded support for the SNP. Opinions cut across voting allegiance: the 1992 Election survey suggested that 39 per cent of both Conservative and SNP supporters backed devolution rather than their parties' own positions (Brand *et al.* 1994: table 12.4). Support for the status quo did strengthen during the 1997 campaign and exceeds support for the Conservatives; polls during and after the election suggested a strong pro-devolution referendum vote and a lesser yes vote for tax-raising.

Social policy occupies an equivocal position in this pattern of electoral competition. The Scottish nation, as it survived after the Union with England in 1707, was defined by its separate and preserved legal, ecclesiastical and local government system. Some authors have suggested that this autonomy was more significant than the political authority that had been lost (Paterson 1994). Modern social policies – school education, hospitals and the Poor Law – sprang out of one or more of these traditions. The Scottish Office, founded in 1885 to assist the new ministerial post of Scottish Secretary, was integrated with other Scottish departments in 1939 and institutionalised the separate administration of Scottish social policy. Distinctive Scottish legislation and practice was generally preserved in the post-war welfare state, with the exception of social security and higher education. Certainly in education and social work, and to a lesser extent in housing and health, Scotland was different. In expenditure it was better off, reflecting a stronger tradition than England's of public sector activity in health, education and housing (on the latest 1995–96 figures identifiable public expenditure per head on these services was respectively 19 per cent, 28 per cent and 78 per cent greater in Scotland than in England (HM Treasury 1997: table 7.6B)).

This leaves us with a paradox. Social policy is the main dimension of Scottish civil society, and the main area of administrative devolution to the Scottish Office. It is accepted that all social policy apart from social security would be within the competence of a Scottish parliament. Pre-devolution, it constitutes the main element of substantive issue-based political debate in Scotland. But in electoral competition – even local elections – it becomes swamped by the two

campaigning variables discussed above, the all-Britain political context and positions on the national question. Social policy is made by
a combination of English-derived norms and of the consultative
process with professional and expert groups in Scotland. By 1997,
the two great post-war issues in Scottish social policy – unemployment and local authority housing – had both diminished in salience
and converged in scale with England.

PARTY ORGANISATION AND POLITICS GOING
INTO THE CAMPAIGN

Before the election the Scottish Labour Party (now so-called; until
the 1990s it was termed the Labour Party in Scotland to avoid
association with the now-defunct SLP formed by Jim Sillars in 1976)
was in the unusual position of not being ahead of the national party
in poll support. Since 1979 it had grown increasingly frustrated by
its unionist position that allowed the Conservatives to make laws for
Scotland despite Labour's dominant position. Many party activists,
allied to the trades unions, speculated about doomsday or breakaway
scenarios. In an effort to make progress in the domestic arena,
Labour agreed in 1989 to join an unofficial Scottish Constitutional
Convention which comprised trades unions, churches and pressure
groups as well as voluntary organisations, and was serviced by the
Convention of Scottish Local Authorities (Kellas 1992; Lynch 1996).
With the Conservatives and the SNP declining to take part, the
coalition aspect of the Convention depended on Labour and the
Liberal Democrats working together, which resulted in compromis-
es by Labour on the electoral system and on equal representation
of males and females in the Scottish Parliament. The result was that
Labour did not have full ownership of the devolution policy and was
saddled with proportional representation (an additional member
system similar to the German), income tax-raising powers for the
Parliament, and the notion of the 'claim of right' in which the
legitimacy of the Parliament was rooted in the wishes of the Scottish
people rather than in devolution to it by Westminster. The Convention's final document, 'Scotland's Parliament, Scotland's Right'
(1995) set out a lot of detail on the proposed responsibilities of the
Parliament while leaving much to be discussed before a workable bill
or White Paper could be drafted (for a helpful presentation, see
Constitution Unit 1996: 20–1).

Scottish Labour's position in the national party was reinforced during John Smith's leadership from 1992 to 1994. Smith was a figure of total Scottish authenticity who had emerged with credit as the junior minister in charge of devolution from 1975 to 1979. Gordon Brown as Shadow Chancellor also had a firm Scottish base as heir-apparent. After Smith's death, the election of Tony Blair put the Scottish party back on the defensive. Despite Blair's Scottish birth, parentage and secondary education, it has been the Englishness of his political understanding that has stood out. As an MP in the North-East, the area most critical of the privileges of Scottish devolution, Blair has been sensitive to the risk of the English backlash that undermined devolution in the 1970s. It is typical that Blair's legal mentor, Lord Irvine, was another Scot who had chosen to make his career at the English bar.

Labour's devolution policy was changed by the decision in June 1996 to have a pre-legislative referendum on the proposals, and, under jibes from Conservative Secretary of State Michael Forsyth about the 'tartan tax', to have a second referendum question on tax-varying powers (Jones 1997). It was only with difficulty that the Scottish Labour Executive was persuaded to back the proposals. After a bizarre interlude in which a second referendum to activate tax-raising powers was announced (embarrassingly endorsed by a statement of Blair's praising the sagacity of the Scottish Labour Executive which had been drafted before the event) and then dropped, the Scottish party and the Shadow Secretary of State George Robertson sullenly came to terms with the two-question referendum.

For the Conservatives, social policy had been derived from England and only unconvincingly related to presumed Scottish traditions of self-reliance. After 1987 the full complex of Thatcherite social policy had been imposed in Scotland: NHS trusts and GP fundholding; national testing in education; housing stock transfers and investment in housing associations; and competitive tendering in local government. In most cases these policies had been applied in a diminished and retarded way compared with England: there were only ever two opted-out schools (known as self-governing schools). Malcolm Rifkind's tenure as Secretary of State from 1986 to 1990 was not the happiest part of his career because it was dominated by the Poll Tax, introduced in Scotland a year earlier than in England. Ian Lang from 1990 to 1995 was courteous, amiable and ineffectual. Michael Forsyth was the real thing. A Conservative from the Scottish middle-class ambience that has produced so many Labour ministers, he asserted the advantages of Scotland's position in Whitehall and the risks of losing it. Although his right-wing positions were modified from his tenure as junior minister (1987–90), he accelerated the pace of market reforms in health, housing and education, and went on the attack on devolution.

THE SALIENCE OF ISSUES

A major theme in interpreting the salience of Scottish political issues is that no constitutional issue can outweigh in importance the main themes of social policy. Generally Scotland has been more left-wing than England on an active social policy, but the gap appeared to be narrowing in the early 1990s as the nations' economic fortunes became similar (Curtice 1992). For information about what was exercising the Scottish electorate in 1997, our best source, pending the results of the large Scottish Election Survey, is the poll taken by ICM in March, which showed that devolution was no more salient in 1997 than it had been in 1992. Health remained at the top, and education also failed to rise in salience despite the parties' emphasis on it; indeed, party lines on falling school standards had much more resonance in England than in Scotland, as an analysis of the manifestos shows (see Table 13.3).

Table 13.3 Most important issues in voting decisions of Scottish electorate

Percentage mentioning	April 1992	March 1997
National Health Service	53	46
Education	32	31
Welfare/pensions/help for the needy (financial)	13	23
Taxes	9	18
Unemployment/lack of industry	43	16
Economic situation/standard of living	16	14
Scottish Parliament/home rule/devolution	12	10

THE MANIFESTOS

Election manifestos are significant in setting out the policies of parties and claiming legitimacy for them. All the main parties now publish separate Scottish manifestos. Labour's was similar in Scotland and England and it would take a semanticist to distinguish the meanings of 'there are excellent schools in Britain's state education system' from 'there are many good schools in Scotland's state education system' or procedures to remove teachers 'who cannot do the job' (England) or are 'unsuited to the job' (Scotland). Even though most of the differences are editing changes and references to the powers of a future Scottish Parliament (and, of course, the omission in Scotland of the pledge to back the bid to host the 2006 football World Cup in England) there are some real differences. The education section in Scotland is distinctly softer, and does not include the phrase 'zero tolerance of underperformance' nor say that 'every school needs baseline assessment of pupils when they enter the school, and year-on-year target for improvement'. The rhetoric in the Scottish manifesto is much more of a partnership between parents, pupils and teachers and there is no chasing after the 'toughness' vote. Tony Blair's own foreword to the manifesto sheds for Scotland the talk of 'monolithic comprehensive schools' and of setting children by ability in each subject, saying blandly that 'we build on the best of the Scottish education system' (perhaps, charitably, we can put this down to saving space on the page for a paragraph on the Scottish parliament). On health, Scottish Labour promised to treble the savings on administration by halving the number of NHS trusts through mergers. The housing section does not mention housing associations as providers and is more bullish about giving new discretion and finance to local housing authorities. The wording on devolution is much the same in both (with the formula 'firmly based on the agreement reached in the Scottish Constitutional Convention'), and the Scottish manifesto goes no further in disclosing details about the proposals.

Education apart, Labour's policies could be applied without difficulty to a nation now facing much the same economic context as the rest of Britain, with similar levels of unemployment and an industrial structure which had moved away decisively from heavy industry. Welfare-to-work played well in Scotland because of its theme of diversion away from social security, the major non-devolved service. The health priority of more patient care was easier to push than in England because the starting-point was more favourable: the internal market was less developed and the pressure from waiting lists rather less marked.

The Liberal Democrats' approach was much the same as Labour's, with an only lightly edited version of the English manifesto (though the introduction is by Scottish leader Jim Wallace rather than Paddy Ashdown). The odd party out is the Conservative. They wrote what is basically a completely different manifesto for Scotland, including a different foreword by John Major. It is less verbose than the English one, with more bullet points and cutting of the preambles before the new policies are mentioned. The policies are generally the same ones, but there are some innovations for Scotland – like promises to allow nurses to take over some practising and prescribing duties from GPs, and making drug dealing a breach of housing tenancy agreements. Of course, a party so weak as the Conservatives in Scotland can be allowed to go its own way; but it does point to what many see as a possible resurgent role for the Scottish Tories as an opposition party in a Scottish Parliament.

The one distinctive Scottish manifesto is that of the Scottish National Party. Its main social policies are summarised in Table 13.4, and they are basically a throwback to the old style of election promises, with a catalogue of plans costing money. Improved cash

Table 13.4 The main social policies in the SNP manifesto

Social security

- Increase child benefit to £12.50 per week
- Restore benefit to 16- and 17-year-olds
- Increase state pension by £3 a week (single) and £5 (married)
- Cold Climate Allowance of £9.20 a week for pensioners and those on benefit
- Abolish means testing for residential care of elderly

Health

- Additional £35 million expenditure [about 0.8% more]
- Abolish internal market – have nationally planned integrated health system

Education

- An immediate 700 extra teachers [about 1.4% more]
- Free nursery education for 3–4-year-olds
- Return to full-value student grants
- £30 million more to training budget

Housing

- Transfer all local authority housing debt to central government within eight years
- Build up to 20,000 socially affordable homes in four years

Source: *Yes We Can* (manifesto of the Scottish National Party, 1997 General Election)

benefits are prominent. The SNP costed its social promises at £733 million in 1997/98 rising to £1,189 million in 2000/01, against about £19 billion currently spent on these services in Scotland. These would be financed by Scotland's alleged 'fiscal surplus' within the United Kingdom (partly oil revenues). With Labour so cautious, the SNP manifesto offered a more distinctive left-of-centre positioning than ever before, with a red-tartan message directed at young, urban Labour voters.

THE NATURE OF THE CAMPAIGN

The presentation of the campaign by the Scottish media was an essential defining element. The main tabloids are the strongly pro-Labour *Daily Record*, owned by the Mirror Group, with both a stronger and more respectable position in the Scottish market than has the *Mirror* in the English; and the *Sun* with its Scottish edition printed in Scotland and since 1992 pro-independence, a move regarded by many as an opportunistic one to position itself against the *Record*. The campaign started dramatically for the *Sun* and its Scottish readers. On 18 March 'The *Sun* backs Blair' was the headline in England, with a two-page editorial explaining why. None of this appeared in the Scottish edition, whose front page was 'Battle nations: Scotland's top of the poll agenda' with a Scottish flag, and whose editorial simply called for SNP leader Alex Salmond to be included in any leaders' TV debate. On 19 March another Scottish flag was the backdrop to the headline 'Bravehearts must wait . . . it's time for brave heads: why the Scottish *Sun* is backing Tony Blair'. In an editorial which lifted some phrases from the English one of a day previously, the Scottish *Sun* strained even their ingenuity to deploy the argument: 'only the SNP can deliver independence for Scotland in one go at the ballot box. But they will not win this election in Scotland . . . today the Scottish *Sun* says two things: Rise Now and Be A Nation Again – and get there using Labour as a stepping stone. We are throwing our weight behind the Labour Party at this election. Their plans for a Scottish parliament are far from ideal. But it's a start'. The SNP never quite recovered from this blow and reminder of the English roots of its main media supporter.

There are two main quality newspapers: The *Scotsman* of Edinburgh, which with *Scotland on Sunday* was taken over in 1996 by the Barclay brothers, the reclusive expatriate owners of *The European*. They installed Andrew Neil (the Scot who edited *The Sunday Times*) as Editor-in-Chief and weekly columnist, and he promoted some subtle changes in the paper's Lib–Lab pro-devolution stance. This was not exactly abandoned but right-wing writers were recruited. A significant move was to commission a poll just before the campaign started in which 75 per cent of respondents assented to the proposition that 'it is unfair for Scottish MPs to be able to vote on English and Welsh matters, when English and Welsh MPs cannot vote on Scottish matters'. This was the paper's basis for editorialising that Labour's scheme was 'grievously wounded' by not addressing this so-called 'West Lothian question', and proposing that post-devolution Scottish MPs should have no vote on purely English matters. *The Herald* in Glasgow was taken over in 1997 by Scottish Television and has over the years been rather more Conservative than *The Scotsman* though its columnists are now if anything more radical and it too backed a change of government.

Television is, put crudely, more regional than in England but basically not much different; additional effort goes on Scottish political stories rather than social policy ones. BBC Scotland ran its nightly campaign highlights programme and its own results broadcast, but carried all the main national news programmes. By the accident of its launch in the anti-devolution 1950s, ITV is not all-Scotland: north and east Scotland from Dundee to the Western Isles is served by Aberdeen-based Grampian Television, and the Scottish borders by Carlisle-based Borders Television. These latter two are vulnerable (and Grampian was indeed taken over by Scottish after the election) and tend to emphasise the local rather than all-Scotland aspect of politics.

We can get an idea of the campaign by analysing the stories covered in the two main quality newspapers, *The Scotsman* and *The Herald*. These papers have an uneasy relationship and tend to downplay stories generated by the other. They carried extensive election coverage – including profiles of all the Scottish constituencies in *The Herald* – but the main story was usually the British one. Table 13.5 picks out which on balance seemed the main Scottish election issue of the day, and the main British one if it were given more prominence. From this we can see how there was virtually no substantive Scottish social policy content to the campaign. What was Scottish was constitutional and personal; what was social was presented in all-Britain terms.

On only fifteen of the forty-five days of the campaign was election coverage in Scotland led by a Scottish issue, and eight of these were

Table 13.5 The main issues in Scotland

Date of press reports	Main UK issue if more prominent	Main Scottish issue
Week 1		
Tues 18 March	Major calls election	(none specific)
Wed 19 March	Windfall tax	Scottish *Sun* backs Labour
Thurs 20 March	Cash for questions	Unemployment figures
Fri 21 March	Cash for questions	SNP tax and spend proposals
Sat 22 March	Cash for questions	Michael Forsyth's absence from campaign
Week 2		
Sun 23 March	Cash for questions	Labour MP Norman Hogg stands down unexpectedly
		Allan Stewart's private life
Mon 24 March		Hogg standing down
Tues 25 March	TV debate argument	Allan Stewart stands down as Eastwood Conservative candidate
Wed 26 March		Blair in Aberdeen: promises drug supremo, rejects Church of Scotland's soft line
		Exclusion of left-wingers from shortlist to succeed Hogg
Thurs 27 March	Tim Smith stands down; allegations about Piers Merchant	
Fri 28 March		Hirst not running for Eastwood nomination; Allan Stewart taken to psychiatric hospital after nervous breakdown
Sat 29 March	Lab offer to stand down to oust Neil Hamilton	Shortlist for Eastwood Con nomination

Table 13.5 continued

Date of press reports	Main UK issue if more prominent	Main Scottish issue
Week 3		
Sun 30 March		Michael Hirst quits: 'Gay Sex Secrets Sink Top Tory' (*Sunday Mail*)
Mon 31 March		Hirst fallout and silence of Forsyth
Tues 1 April		Hirst fallout: Forsyth tries to get back to issues
Wed 2 April		Two Scottish polls with varying Con support
Thurs 3 April	Major launches Conservative manifesto	Forsyth launches Scottish Conservative manifesto
Fri 4 April		Blair travels to Scotland, interview with *Scotsman*
Sat 5 April		Blair in Scotland, testy press conference in Glasgow
Week 4		
Sun 6 April	Labour U-turns on unions and privatisation	*Observer* poll shows Conservatives behind in Eastwood
Mon 7 April	Martin Bell to take on Neil Hamilton	Labour MP Willie McKelvey to stand down after illness
Tues 8 April	Hamilton hangs in	SNP launches manifesto
Wed 9 April	Hamilton nominated, ambushes Bell	Scottish CBI disquiet on Conservative business rate plans
Thurs 10 April	Party insults over tax	Welsh Labour's Ron Davies implicitly attacks devolution tax powers
Fri 11 April	(little election news)	Scots Cabinet ministers meet, warn on devolution
Sat 12 April		Forsyth and Lord Mackay with different emphases on devolution

Week 5

Date		
Sun 13 April	Labour poll lead narrows	(little Scottish election news)
Mon 14 April	Blair relaunches in Milton Keynes rally	Blair does Scots radio phone-in
Tues 15 April	Major on Labour 'hypocrisy' on education	Labour fall in *Scotsman* poll
Wed 16 April	Tory Euro-divisions	Forsyth seems to back Euro-sceptics
Thurs 17 April	Major's emergency TV broadcast on Europe	Forsyth press conference clarifies Europe position
Fri 18 April		Blair's Edinburgh speech
Sat 19 April	Thatcher opposes EMU	Portillo in Scotland

Week 6

Date		
Sun 20 April	Tory infighting	Campaign to smear Sarwar in Govan
Mon 21 April		SNP poll boost
Tues 22 April	Jacques Santer's speech	Row over Brian Wilson's interview on Westminster rights after devolution
Wed 23 April		Police called in over alleged Govan voters' roll fraud
Fri 25 April	Row over state pensions	Scottish financial institutions' attitude to devolution
Sat 26 April	Major's election broadcast	SNP tops *Newsround* school election

Week 7

Date		
Sun 27 April		Scots Tories trailing in constituency poll
Mon 28 April	Major's tour round UK capitals	Govan Labour councillor joins SNP
Tues 29 April	Major's speeches on UK tour	Donald Dewar tipped as new Scots secretary
Wed 30 April		Forsyth warns of public spending cuts post-devolution
Thurs 1 May	Labour likely to win	Arguments over spending

Source: analysis of *The Scotsman, The Herald, Scotland on Sunday*

generated by three personal cases – the departures of Allan Stewart, former Conservative MP for Eastwood and Sir Michael Hirst, Scottish Conservative party chairman, and the controversial candidacy of Labour's Mohammad Sarwar in Glasgow Govan. For the media, it was the personalised election in which these stories provided a welcome alternative to weighty analytical pieces.

The party leaders approached Scotland in a paradoxical way. Major saw it as a safe haven where he could get the political agenda on to constitutional issues and claim political authority. Blair saw it as a trap where he would be exposed to what his entourage saw as the unsympathetic local media and where the vagueness of the devolution proposals would come under investigation. Blair indeed had his worst day of the campaign in Scotland. He unwisely spoke on-the-record to *The Scotsman* on the plane up when he said that (as reported verbatim by the paper):

> I would say to [my constituents] we are going to devolve these matters to a Scottish Parliament but as far as, you know, we are concerned, the sovereignty rests with me as an English MP and that's the way it will stay. . . . I mean it's like any local authority, powers which are constitutionally there, they can be used but the Scottish Labour Party has [no] plans to raise income tax rates . . . eh . . . and but no, of course, a Scottish Parliament once the power is given it's like a . . . the smallest English parish council, its got the right to exercise it.
>
> (*Scotsman*, 5 April 1997)

For his pains Blair had to endure a chilly press conference in which he was probed on devolution, and the phrases on 'sovereignty resting with English MPs' and 'parish council powers' entered into folklore. Happily for Blair he made his best speech of the campaign in Edinburgh on 17 April, when he commanded the stage of the Usher Hall, where he had attended pop concerts while at school at Fettes.

Election TV broadcasts added little. A soft-focus SNP broadcast with swirling mists, patriotic symbols and a call for 'a new spirit of love', directed by David Hayman, was aired on 14 April and later repeated. Labour stuck to rebroadcasts of the national message, with cosmetic mention of 'Scottish Labour' in the end titles. The Conservatives made the most comprehensive attempt at an issue-related Scotland-specific broadcast late in the campaign, arguing about devolution tax rises, a further sign that the London party machine was happy to let Scotland go its own way.

THE POLLS AND THE RESULT

In the end, the result was a Conservative wipe-out, a sensation and yet a predictable one. As in 1992, the Conservatives were vulnerable to a British-level swing against them, tactical voting by the opposition parties, and failure of their candidates' personal votes to compensate. In 1992, the tactical voting barely happened, but in 1997 the full application of these factors was evident. The Conservatives' two safest seats, Dumfries and Eastwood, were lost to swings large but not untypical in the national context, but in each case the former MP had stood down. Voting preferences did not change much during the campaign, except for a strengthening of the Liberal Democrat vote; Table 13.6 reports all the polls taken in Scotland. ICM's final poll taken 5–6 days before the vote mirrored the result almost precisely, a major achievement for a polling organisation.

THE OUTCOME AND THE FUTURE OF SOCIAL POLICY IN SCOTTISH POLITICS

The scale of the Conservative defeat was more important than Labour's victory. Even though Labour in Scotland just outpolled the British average, for the first time since 1979 the Scottish strength was no longer a deviant case in Labour's parliamentary profile. For the Conservatives, losing all their MPs denied them a legitimate Scottish role at Westminster. Their leading Cabinet ministers, Michael Forsyth (Stirling) and Malcolm Rifkind (Pentlands) held the swing to single figures but still lost easily. The SNP won three seats from the Conservatives but their overall vote was barely up and their long-run assault on Labour heartlands made no progress. The Liberal Democrats maintained local electoral success but did better than ever from tactical voting. The new MPs (Table 13.7) were mainly from the welfare state generation and seemed likely to reinforce the change in the Scottish parliamentary delegation away from male Tory grandees and Labour trades unionists.

Developments after the election reinforced the impression that an unusually favourable conjunction of opportunities for the implementation of devolution had occurred (Parry 1997). First, Donald Dewar became Secretary of State for Scotland rather than the Shadow Secretary George Robertson, whose reputation had suffered from the changes of course on devolution. Dewar had been so successful and respected as Chief Whip that his decision to resume the Scottish

Table 13.6 Scotland campaign polls, 1997

Pollster	Published in	Date of fieldwork	Lab	Con	SNP	Lib Dem	Don't know	Size of Sample	Date published
ICM	Scotsman	Tues 11–Fri 14	47	17	23	10		1,000[2]	Mon 17 March
		unadjusted[1]	53	14	23	8	18		
Election called Monday 17 March									
System 3	Herald	Thur 20–Mon 24	52	17	20	9	18	1,006	Wed 26 March
System 3	Herald	Thur 27–Sun 30	53	12	26	9		1,003	Wed 2 April
ICM	Scotsman	Sat 29–Mon 31	47	20	22	9		1,000[2]	Wed 2 April
		unadjusted[1]	51	18	19	9			
NOP	Sunday Times	Thurs 3	49	18	25	6		844	Sun 6 April
System 3	Herald	Sat 5–Sun 6	51	14	23	10	18	1,081	Wed 9 April
ICM	Scotsman	Fri 11–Sun 13	42	19	23	15		1,000[2]	Tues 15 April
		unadjusted[1]	43	17	24	15			
System 3	Herald	Sat 12–Mon14	52	13	24	14	20	1,080	Wed 16 April
NOP	Sunday Times	Thurs 17	47	15	28	8		950	Sun 20 April
Scottish Parliament voting intention			39	13	38	8			
ICM	Scotsman	Fri 18–Sun 20	47	18	21	11		1,000[2]	Tues 22 April
		unadjusted[1]	47	16	23	12	18		
System 3	Herald	Fri 18–Sun 20	47	15	24	12		1,080	Wed 23 April
NOP	Sunday Times	Thur 24	49	14	24	12		1,000	Sun 27 April
ICM	Scotsman	Fri 25–Sun 27	46	18	21	13		1,000[2]	Tues 29 April
		unadjusted[1]	46	15	22	14			
System 3	Herald	Sat 26–Sun 27	50	14	26	9	19	1,084	Wed 30 April
RESULT		THUR 1 MAY	45.6	17.5	21.9	13.0			

Notes
[1] For presumed underreporting of Con vote
[2] Telephone poll

Table 13.7 Conservative Scottish seat losses in 1997 General Election

Seat	Percentage fall in Conservative vote	New MP
Lost to Labour		
Ayr (notionally Lab in 1992)	−4.6	Sandra Osborne, community worker
Stirling	−6.7	Anne McGuire, voluntary sector administrator
Edinburgh Pentlands	−7.8	Lynda Clark, advocate
Aberdeen South	−10.1	Anne Begg, teacher
Eastwood	−13.1	Jim Murphy, party official
Dumfries	−15.1	Russell Brown, Councillor
Total Labour MPs: 56		
Lost to SNP		
Tayside North	−10.7	John Swinney, party official
Perth (by-election loss to SNP)	−11.1	Roseanna Cunningham, MP
Galloway and Upper Nithsdale	−11.5	Alasdair Morgan, computing officer
Total SNP MPs: 6		
Lost to Liberal Democrat		
Aberdeenshire W and Kincardine	−10.2	Sir Robert Smith, landowner
Edinburgh West	−10.2	Donald Gorrie, councillor
Gordon (notionally Con in 1992)	−21.9*	Malcolm Bruce, MP
Total Liberal Democrat MPs: 10		

Note: *Conservative notional majority in 1992 likely to have been overestimated because of differing structures of party competition in seats in the area

portfolio he held until 1992 was seen as a compliment to the office and an assurance that devolution implementation would be led by the Scottish Office. Second, the Conservative wipe-out made it impossible for them to mount a fully credible opposition to the devolution legislation. The formidable forensic debating skills of Michael Forsyth and Malcolm Rifkind were lost.

After a frantic period of planning, in which the lack of sufficient practical detail in the Convention's proposals was exposed, the devolution White Paper was published on 24 July. It confirmed that the major areas of social policy would be devolved. This led to the devolution referendum of 11 September. The issue here was not the likely majority for the policy, but the turnout (which would determine the long-term popular legitimacy of the proposals) and the vote on tax-varying powers (which would both determine the expenditure context of the Parliament and show the extent of bedrock support of the policy). The result, showing 74.3 per cent voting for devolution and 63.5 per cent voting for tax-varying powers, on a turnout of 60.4 per cent, set the stage for a move towards devolution that would allow social policy issues to be addressed within the Scottish political process.

CONCLUSION: THE END OF DISAFFECTION AND EXCLUSION?

The 1997 election campaign in Scotland was twice removed from the consideration of social policy issues. First, it was framed by the British campaign with its themes of competence to govern and avoidance of risk. With so few spending, building and employing promises in the areas with separate Scottish administration, there was no room for any debate on 'more resources to tackle social needs' lines. The Labour machine kept a grip on its potentially unreliable Scottish operation and so the message of advertising and TV election broadcasts was closely aligned. The Conservative campaign was if anything more home-grown, but an assertion of Scottish credentials was always doomed because of the long pattern of imposition of English social policies. The Liberal Democrats' main orientation was to maximise local appeal in areas where they were the main holders of or challengers to seats.

Second, the campaign detached the national question from policy and showed that voting for the SNP represented a choice, either principled or tactical, on the constitution rather than any verdict on the SNP's social policies (which have developed in a vacuum free from real political debate or tests of feasibility). As the main overarching issue, the national question displaced those of the inclusion or exclusion of economic and social groups which were addressed to some extent in England.

Whereas election results in Scotland from 1979 to 1992 threatened disaffection from a British political system that could not respect the political voice of the Scottish electorate, Labour's majority in 1997 brought Scotland back into the British political majority, a process made the easier by eighteen years of painful economic and social adjustment under the Conservatives. Scotland's welfare state remained more old-fashioned, better-resourced and less privatised than England's and those involved in it could see the way to a field of action in the Scottish Parliament. It is to there that the real social policy choices of the Scottish electorate will be deferred.

REFERENCES

Brand, Jack, Mitchell, James and Surridge, Paula (1994) 'Will Scotland come to the aid of the party?', in Anthony Heath, Roger Jowell and John Curtice (eds) *Labour's Last Chance?: The 1992 Election and Beyond*, (Aldershot: Dartmouth.

Brown, Alice, McCrone, David and Paterson, Lindsay (1996) *Politics and Society in Scotland*, London: Macmillan.

Constitution Unit (1996) *Scotland's Parliament: Fundamentals for a new Scotland Act*, London: Constitution Unit.

Curtice, John (1992) 'The North-South Divide', in Robert Jowell, Lindsay Brook, Gillian Prior and Bridget Taylor (eds) *British Social Attitudes: the Ninth Report*, Aldershot: Gower.

HM Treasury (1997) *Public Expenditure Statistical Analysis*, London: HMSO, Cm 3601.

Jones, Peter (1997) 'Labour's referendum plan', *Scottish Affairs*, no 18, Winter: 1–17.

Kellas, James (1992) 'The Scottish Constitutional Convention', in Lindsay Paterson and David McCrone (eds) *The Scottish Government Yearbook 1992*, Edinburgh: Unit for the Study of Government in Scotland.

Lynch, Peter (1996) 'The Scottish Constitutional Convention 1992–95', *Scottish Affairs* 15 spring: 1–16.

Parry, Richard (1997) 'The Scottish Parliament and Social Policy', *Scottish Affairs* 20, summer: 18–30.

Paterson, Lindsay (1994) *The Autonomy of Modern Scotland*, Edinburgh: Edinburgh University Press.

Chapter 14

The view from Northern Ireland

Eithne McLaughlin

The purpose of this chapter is not to discuss the politics of Northern Ireland *per se*. To understand discussion of social policy issues in the 1997 General Election, however, it is necessary to have some understanding of the historical impact of the politics of conflict and division on the development of, and debates around, social policy in Northern Ireland. For this reason, the first introductory section and the next historical background section, provide an outline of key dimensions of the relationship between the politics of conflict and social policy in Northern Ireland. The third section then focuses on how social policy issues featured in the 1997 General Election campaign.

A POLITICAL BACKGROUND

Northern Ireland was created in 1920 upon the partition of Ireland. It had its own 'domestic' parliament, with a restricted range of powers, until 1972. Between 1920 and 1972, the perceived need of the Unionist government to 'control' the minority nationalist population dominated politics and policies. The minority population were regarded as inherently suspect because their allegiance was to the ending of Northern Ireland and reunification with the rest of Ireland. This led to restricted entitlements to vote, 'gerrymandering' of electoral boundaries to ensure the return of as many Unionist politicians as possible to the Northern Ireland parliament and local government, and discrimination against nationalist/Catholic candidates in employment and in access to some public services (such as public housing) (see SACHR 1987, 1990; Whyte 1983).

A number of periods of violent unrest occurred in the five decades following partition. In 1969, an (initially peaceful) civil rights campaign attracted considerable international attention, especially in the USA. By 1972, however, violent political conflict had reached considerable proportions, and resulted in the decision of the British government to dissolve the Northern Ireland parliament and introduce 'Direct Rule'. This means that legislation for Northern Ireland is introduced as Orders-in-Council at Westminster, British ministers are responsible for the operation of the Northern Ireland government departments (Health and Social Services, Education, Environment, Finance and Personnel, Economic Development), and all departments and Ministers report to the Northern Ireland Office and the Secretary of State for Northern Ireland. In addition, 'Direct Rule' involved the removal of most of the public service functions of local councils. The most prominent responsibilities of local councils in Northern Ireland are now the public refuse system, graveyards and leisure centres, and building control approval (smaller scale responsibilities include some financial support for community groups).

For the last twenty-five years, then, the handful of Northern Ireland politicians who are or have been elected Members of (the Westminster) Parliament, have acquired experience of social policy through their participation in Westminster as well as through their constituency work (that is, bringing constituents' problems with education, social services, and so on, to the attention of the relevant public body and/or Minister). Those who have only participated in local government, however, have had much less opportunity, or need, to engage with social policy, at anything other than a superficial level. This alone would lead one to expect that social policy would not feature in the same way in general election campaigns in Northern Ireland as in Britain. However, there are also longer-term historical factors that have affected the way in which social policy is debated in Northern Ireland, and these are outlined in the next section.

THE HISTORICAL DEVELOPMENT OF SOCIAL POLICY IN NORTHERN IRELAND

Three particular features of social policy in Northern Ireland have made the development of, and debates around, social policy different from those in Great Britain (McLaughlin 1997). First, during the 1920–72 period, Unionism adopted a more residualist approach to social policy in Northern Ireland than was the case in Great Britain. Second, both before and after the introduction of

Direct Rule, non-departmental public bodies (NDPBs) or 'quangos', have been more important in Northern Ireland than in Britain, in delivering social policies and public provision. Third, the period following the introduction of Direct Rule has involved the introduction of social policy initiatives that differ substantively and ideologically from those in the rest of the UK, and which are directed at the politics of conflict, inequality and 'community relations'.

Residualism

Northern Ireland Unionism has been characterised as an inherently conservative/neo-liberal political ideology. The Ulster Unionist Party (the largest of the unionist parties) has been, and continues to be, affiliated to the Conservative Party in Britain. In the 1920–72 period, the possibilities for maintenance of conservative principles of minimal state intervention were historically greater in Northern Ireland than in Britain, partly because the trade union and labour organisations were weaker politically. In addition, the residualist approach to social welfare of the politically dominant Unionists accorded with that involved in Catholic social teaching, so there was little political challenge to residualism from the minority population.[1]

A further factor contributing to a more restrictive approach to social welfare in Northern Ireland than Britain was the problematic existence of the territory itself. The introduction into Northern Ireland of most of the post-war Beveridge welfare system was presented in symbolic terms as justifying the Union and partition, when contrasted with the less 'advanced' welfare system in the Republic (Ditch 1988; Connolly 1990). But the resulting political claim that Northern Ireland 'shared' the British welfare system over-simplified a complex situation. Entitlements to social security benefits carried more onerous residence conditions than in Britain, while parity was not achieved in levels of provision of health care, social care and nursery education. The former arose primarily from Unionism's desire to control population movement between the North and South of Ireland, and to influence the composition of the Northern Ireland population. For example, a residence qualification of five years out of the last ten was introduced to establish entitlement to unemployment benefit to 'safeguard against infiltration from Eire' (Ditch 1988: 92).[2] Family Allowances were one of the most contentious elements of the post-war welfare package. Debate around them embodied and expressed the (still present) Unionist fears of higher demographic growth among the nationalist compared with the unionist populations (and the threat to the continuation of the existence of Northern Ireland which that carries with it). Thus, the initial enabling Bill sought to give fourth and subsequent children less than the British benefits, partly in order to prevent Catholics in the north obtaining more benefit from this family policy than Protestants, and partly from a belief that generous Family Allowances would encourage 'undesirable' (i.e. Catholic) breeding. The outcome of these and other restrictions on the welfare system in Northern Ireland was a lower level of public expenditure than in Britain.[3]

'Quangoland'

The residualism inherent in Unionism as a political ideology had another aspect – the creation of special bodies to deliver public services. On the one hand, Unionist politicians, civil servants and professionals desired the (populist) benefits of the British welfare state but, on the other, they desired means which 'sought to achieve this end [but were] more in keeping with Unionist principles than those adopted in the system across the water. . . . These Unionist principles were seen as being the protection of freedom for the individual and minimal state intervention' (Ditch 1988: 99). A range of bodies was established between 1945 and 1950 which today would be characterised as quangos. They were: centralised (having mostly removed functions and responsibilities from local authorities); had members appointed by a Minister rather than elected by some appropriate constituency; were relatively autonomous from the sponsoring ministry; and were responsible for planning, policy, administration. These bodies facilitated a greater influence of professional and religious organisations on the shape and content of social policy, especially those on sexuality and family matters.[4]

The introduction of Direct Rule in 1972 increased the number of such bodies. Because local councils had had a poor record in terms of discrimination in the public services for which they were responsible (for example, social housing and social services), Direct Rule involved the removal of these functions from local government (Birrell and Murie 1980; Whyte 1983). New administrative bodies such as the Health and Social Services Boards and the Northern Ireland Housing Executive were established, so that the concentration of policy expertise shifted even further away from participants in representative politics. Direct Rule did, however, bring with it increased public expenditure.[5] By the end of the 1980s, however, nursery education (Hinds 1991) and social care (McLaughlin *et al.* 1997) provision, relative to need, continued to be lower than in Britain.

Social policies and 'community relations'

Sustained violent political conflict after 1969, together with international (especially USA) pressure and criticism, meant that in the immediate years following 1972, the British government introduced a series of reforms to politics and social policy geared to improving communal relations (SACHR 1987: 9–11; see also SACHR 1990). However, continued high levels of unemployment among Catholics, and its contribution to divisions and tensions in Northern Ireland, led to a focus on employment in the mid-1970s. The Northern Ireland-specific equality legislation introduced by the Fair Employment Act of 1976 was directed at ending direct discrimination in employment on the basis of religious or political identity. This 'isolationist' approach (that is, an approach predicated on legislative action rather than through broader equality measures, see Sheehan 1995) failed to alter the socio-economic differentials that had built up over time between the two communities in Northern Ireland. Neither the focus ('irrational' individual acts of discrimination), nor the scope (the field of employment), of this measure, could hope to make substantial inroads into these differentials.

By the end of the 1980s, pressure was mounting on the British government to look beyond the confines of this approach (Magill and Rose 1996; Wilford 1991). As a result, in 1989, fair employment legislation was reformed and enlarged in scope (SACHR 1987; Sheehan 1995; Osborne 1996).[6] The 1989 Act was also accompanied by a wider approach to equality involving an incremental series of non-legislative measures, aimed at securing greater equality of opportunity and equity. These measures included reforms in educational policy (Knox and Hughes 1993) and local government (Knox and Quirk 1994). But the two measures given most political importance by government were Targeting Social Need (TSN), announced in 1991, and Policy Appraisal and Fair Treatment (PAFT), launched in 1994, and previously known as 'equality proofing'.

TSN was directed at resource allocation decisions, and stated that public expenditure would be increasingly directed towards areas and people in the greatest social and economic need (predominantly but not exclusively Catholics). The policy was thus expected to indirectly address religious/political socio-economic inequalities and stimulate social and economic development in deprived areas. PAFT was directed at the policy-making process, requiring fairness, equity and disproportionate-impact assessments to be made in policy formulation and policy review. Both policies, but particularly the former, are remarkable for their introduction by a Conservative government, which in Britain favoured a 'trickle-down' approach to social and economic deprivation and inequality.

Both policies attracted considerable political attention in the 1993–96 period, and have been drawn on by voluntary organisations and some political representatives to challenge policy decisions. However, application of the policies has been weak. There is little evidence that TSN, as it was initially politically framed, influenced to any significant extent the spending patterns and decision-making of government departments and agencies between 1991 and 1996 (Quirk and McLaughlin 1996). This was partly because of a clash between the policy imperative of Conservatism of reducing public expenditure, and the public sector, as against the policy imperative of TSN – the direction of additional, or the skewing of existing, resources to deprived areas and groups. As a result, several government departments, including the 'exchequer' department of Finance and Personnel, operated on the basis that the general 'meeting need' function of all public expenditure was the same as Targeting Social Need, and did not alter their practices.

The PAFT guidelines were an enhanced and strengthened version of the 'equality proofing' guidelines which had been introduced in both Great Britain and Northern Ireland in 1990. Osborne *et al.* (1996) identified two views of the PAFT guidelines in Northern Ireland. As with TSN, the 'weak' view is held primarily by government departments, and holds that equity issues have to take their place alongside other policy imperatives, and cannot outrank principles such as parity with Britain, reductions in public expenditure and 'efficiency' requirements.[7] The 'strong' view, held primarily by voluntary sector and campaigning groups outside government, is that the PAFT guidelines set an overarching equity framework for policy making in Northern Ireland.

Policy inaction in relation to both TSN and PAFT was explained by civil servants in terms of the opposition between many of the policies adopted by the Conservative government in the UK and the objectives of social and economic equality, or at least equity, expressed in both the Northern Ireland-specific TSN and PAFT measures. This important political dynamic was, however, complicated and obscured by the intertwining of disadvantage, inequality and unionist/nationalist politics in Northern Ireland. In the year preceding the General Election, for instance, local politicians from the unionist family objected to resources being directed towards children from deprived areas through the various resource allocation formulae used to set school budgets. There were similar objections to what was described as the skewing of social housing resources to nationalist areas, such as West and North Belfast.

The basic principle of fair employment law and practices has now been accepted by the majority of unionist communities and politicians (see McVey and Hutson 1996), but there is strong opposition to 'going too far'. The latter includes measures like TSN because of its potential for a focus on equality of condition, or even outcome, rather than equality of opportunity. Meanwhile nationalist politicians have continued to press for more equality measures as an integral part of constitutional talks, and any settlement, on the future of Northern Ireland.

SOCIAL POLICY IN THE 1997 GENERAL ELECTION CAMPAIGN

In examining the presence of social policy in the 1997 General Election, it is not possible here to discuss all the political parties involved. What follows instead concentrates on those with the largest shares of votes. These are: the Ulster Unionist Party and the Democratic Unionist Party, on the unionist side, and the Social and Democratic Labour Party (SDLP) and Sinn Fein, on the nationalist side. It is also not possible to summarise every statement on every issue that could broadly be defined as social policy. Rather this section will, first, summarise the level of interest in social policy issues evident in media coverage and the parties' manifestos; second, look at party positions around public expenditure and the key public services of health and social security; and third, party positions around equality.

The level of exposure of social policy issues in the media

The first and most basic point to make is that journalistic analysis of parties and their manifesto positions did not include discussion of parties' stances on social policy issues at all. Constitutional questions, especially the parties' positions on who should be included in political talks on the future of Northern Ireland, dominated regional-level coverage of the election. However, from, and in, those constituencies where the competition was between candidates of similar constitutional orientation, there was some reported debate over social policy issues. The challenges and debates involved did not focus on broad social policy questions (such as the respective roles of the state, the market and the family) and rarely dealt with issues of social administration (for example, the internal market in the NHS).

Rather, candidates used social policy issues as a vehicle through which to remind the public of the social class orientation of the other party. Thus, some Democratic Unionist candidates attacked the records of their Ulster Unionist counterparts, claiming that their records showed Ulster Unionist candidates were not interested in the social and economic needs of people in the areas concerned. (The Democratic Unionists, though very far from being on the political Left, nevertheless draw more heavily on working-class Unionist voters than the Ulster Unionists). So class politics between candidates of the same broad constitutional hue brought social policy issues into the public arena in a very limited way.

A good example of this process was an exchange of letters in *The Irish News* (the main nationalist community daily). These letters concerned whether the SDLP or Sinn Fein could claim credit for bringing new inward investment into West Belfast. The SDLP asserted they were primarily responsible and that Sinn Fein's support for violence meant they had hampered rather than helped the disadvantaged of West Belfast ('what did Sinn Fein ever do to regenerate West Belfast?' queried Eamon Hanna, a local SDLP activist). Sinn Fein responded by detailing what they had done and stating that 'the approach to regenerating West Belfast pioneered by those in Eamon Hanna's wing of the SDLP [was] don't let the natives get involved but bus in highly paid "missionaries" from south Belfast.' (South Belfast is the richest and most middle-class area of Belfast) (*Irish News*, 17 April 1997; see also *Irish News*, 7 April 1997).

Social policy coverage in the party manifestos

While media coverage of social policy issues was slim, all but one of the parties' manifestos did cover social policy issues. The one that did not was that of the Democratic Unionists – their manifesto challenged the Ulster Unionists' record on protecting the union and the British government's co-operation with the Irish government in constitutional affairs. The manifesto ended by saying 'Other policy manifestos on each individual topic [unspecified] will be published separately on a daily basis during the election campaign' (DUP 1997: 5). However, none of these received any publicity, nor could they be obtained from the Party's head office during the election campaign.

In the other party manifestos too, constitutional issues took leading position, and a considerable proportion of the discussion of social and economic issues later in the Ulster Unionists, Sinn Fein and SDLP manifestos, tended towards broad, aspirational, social policy objectives, rather than systematic discussion of 'ways and means'. This may reflect the absence of a close involvement of those involved in representative politics in Northern Ireland in broad policy formulation at Westminster or in policy implementation in Northern Ireland, outlined in the second section of this chapter.

Public expenditure and taxation

Jim Prior, a former Secretary of State for Northern Ireland, once said 'In Northern Ireland, we're all Keynesians' (cited in O'Leary *et al.* 1988: 109) – that is, all the parties believe in the value of public sector investment. Certainly a common orientation across the parties, which cross-cut existing interplays of class and constitutional affiliations, was a desire to secure the largest possible share of UK public expenditure for Northern Ireland. However, there were also important differences between the parties which a simple reading of Jim Prior's comment obscures.

The SDLP's central values include 'social and economic rights as well as political rights' and therefore 'quality public services in health, education and housing and policies to create full employment'. The Party's approach to public expenditure is that 'A wealth generating economy will find the resources to fund its public services but where economic growth is slower there will be increased demands on welfare and the SDLP will pursue the case for those in need. Spending of this nature is clearly a form of public investment which provides for the very levels of existence and promotes social stability.' As a left-of-centre party, it was critical of the 'regressive Tory tax policies of driving down direct taxation which benefits the better off, whilst increasing indirect taxation, which penalises the poor and the less well off and leads to an increased demand on welfare'. On the other hand, the party did not directly call for higher direct tax rates for the better-off.

In contrast, the Ulster Unionists criticised the previous government for high levels of taxation overall and 'the follies which increased the Public Sector Borrowing Requirement, led to higher unemployment, reduced financial support for public services and dictated rises in taxation' (UUP 1997: 7). The cause of these follies appeared to be attributed to Britain's entry to the ERM and the gradual erosion of Westminster's control of its finances. Apart from this, the Ulster Unionists made no other analysis or comment on taxation. It may, however, be noteworthy that the party's limited tax and public expenditure statements were immediately followed by criticism of the proportion of GDP spent on social security benefits. In this regard, and in others (see below) the Ulster Unionists' 1997 position could be seen as a modern version of the earlier tradition of unionist residualism.

Although presenting itself as more to the Left than the SDLP, and with the 'principal political objective [of] the development of an economic democracy which tackles unemployment, bad housing and provides a proper health service and an open education system for all citizens' (Sinn Fein 1997: 2), the Sinn Fein manifesto contained nothing on the principles or practice of taxation. The implication was that if there was no spending on 'the war machine' (ibid.: 6) then appropriate public service levels could be either restored or developed. Thus, the party condemned 'cuts in spending on social services, health and education as funds are diverted to already substantial spending on maintaining Britain's military control of the Six Counties' (ibid.: 8).

The principal public services: social security

Much the same differences between the parties were evident in the specific policy areas chosen as a focus for this analysis. Turning first to social security, as noted above, the Ulster Unionist manifesto critiqued the proportion of GDP spent on social security payments, and how much these 'cost the UK taxpayer'. The Party's general position is that 'the time has come for a fundamental review of the whole social security system' (UUP 1997: 7), but it also called for greater spending in some areas. These were exclusively in relation to pensioners – the traditional deserving poor. Specifically, the Party called for: automatic supplementary pensions for pensioners who were too old to enter SERPS; exemption from electricity and telephone standing charges and TV licences for poorer pensioners living alone; travel concessions for pensioners equivalent to those in Britain; and improved statutory legal protection of occupation and pension funds. There were only three references to social security provision for other groups and none involved in the short-term at least increased spending on social security provision.[8]

The Sinn Fein policy position concentrated on unemployment, employment and economic development issues (see below) but did not present any analysis of, or prescription for, the social security system. This was also the case in relation to health care. Despite the Sinn Fein manifesto's dominance by issues of social exclusion and disadvantage, it was the SDLP manifesto which spelled out the implications of this type of analysis for the social security system.

The SDLP presented social security as one arm of an overall strategy to tackle poverty and promote social inclusion (the other arms being full employment and minimum wages).[9] Rather farther to the left than its sister party in Britain (Labour), the party's specific proposals included a number of reforms which would generally improve the incomes of those not in the labour market, across the whole age range: restoration of the value of Child Benefit and restoration of the right to Income Support of 16–17-year-olds; replacement of Social Fund loans with grants; an end to the Job-seeker's Allowance and to the capping of Housing Benefit, together with immediate access to help with mortgage payments when unemployed; the introduction of a comprehensive Disability Income Scheme, and an end to the points system used in assessment for Incapacity Benefit; an increase in the state retirement pension; and the reversal of any plans to privatise the Social Security Agency (the Northern Ireland equivalent of the Benefits Agency).

The principal public services: health care

While the Ulster Unionist manifesto appeared sceptical of the social and economic value to society of spending on social security, at least in relation to the non-retired population, it was considerably more fulsome in its commitment to the NHS. The Party argued that the NHS was experiencing three problems: inadequate funding levels; an over-elaborate system of administration; and an inability to prioritise. The Party noted and opposed the trend of reduced levels of health service funding and in particular the fact that the level of expenditure in Northern Ireland has fallen behind that of Scotland and Wales. Nonetheless the Party believed that problems with the effectiveness of the service itself, also reduced its ability to meet need. Thus, the Ulster Unionists proposed a re-examination of the effectiveness of what they saw as often overlapping administration structures, together with greater partnership between the various parts of the health service 'rather than what appears to be an increasing amount of competition between them'. The Party also argued that provision could be rationalised and hence made more efficient if professional expertise in the health service was harnessed to establish agreed priorities in the light of needs. Finally the Party wished to see reduced charges for prescriptions.

The SDLP's position accorded with a number of elements of the Labour Party's health care analysis, specifically that there should be a radical overhaul of the internal market, with three to five-year commissioning plans replacing the annual contracting cycle and with GPs and primary health and social care teams leading on these for local communities of around 100,000. The number of Health and Personal Social Services (HPSS) organisations, especially trusts, should also be reduced and the current plethora of small agencies should be incorporated into a reconstituted HPSS Common Services Agency. Of particular interest, was the Party's recognition that the distinctive feature of the NHS in Northern Ireland – its integration with social services and social care (following the establishment of Health and Social Services Boards in the early 1970s) – has not necessarily lived up to its potential. While this has probably been the case ever since the early 1970s, the possibilities of real integration were undermined by the establishment of trusts in the early 1990s. Most trusts in Northern Ireland are either acute health care providers, or community health and social services Trusts, and rarely cover both. Commissioners (Boards) have therefore had to operate as best they could by encouragement of co-operation across this provider divide. As a result, the party argued that trusts should be changed to become integrated providers of health and social care. In addition the Party expressed a commitment to obtaining increased funding for domiciliary service provision to bring this up to at least the level of the British average (see McLaughlin *et al.*, 1997, for a comparative analysis of social care services relative to need between Northern Ireland and Britain).

Equality issues and social policy

Discussion of economic development, fair employment and equality issues generally in the manifestos highlighted the different approaches taken to this by unionist and nationalist parties outlined at the end of the second section of this chapter. Sinn Fein called for strengthened Fair Employment legislation, including affirmative action, and a strengthening of the TSN policy. The SDLP called for the setting of targets for improvements in equality and strong implementation of TSN and PAFT, rather than strengthening of the Fair Employment legislation itself. The Ulster Unionists rejected any change to Fair Employment law on the grounds that this would shift the balance towards equality of outcome not of opportunity, and did not mention TSN or PAFT at all.

To tackle the 2.2:1 male Catholic/Protestant unemployment ratio, and the 1.7:1 female ratio, Sinn Fein particularly emphasised the potential of local economic regeneration, involving TSN and community-led regeneration programmes (Sinn Fein 1997: 9) together with strengthened fair employment legislation. Specifically, the party wanted: comprehensive preparation of disadvantaged areas for inward investment through increased co-operation between communities, government and the private sector; establishment of multi-agency/community-based jobs task forces; and greater support for Irish language economic development (ibid.). In terms of fair employment legislation, the party's specific proposals included: 'clear and comprehensible legal powers to end sectarian discrimination within a defined time'; 'affirmative action timetables for removing the imbalance in employment rates'; periodic reviews to assess the effect of fair employment legislation; support for the MacBride principles;[10] and repeal of the exemption of certain acts by government or its agents made on the grounds of public interest or public safety from anti-discrimination legislation (Sinn Fein 1997: 7).

The SDLP emphasised a 'social partnership' approach, incorporating the unemployed, trade unions and community groups into existing structures and agencies, rather than the 'bottom-up' approach of Sinn Fein. Economic development, the Party argued, requires 'a management framework' which 'includes the social partners – the unemployed, the trade unions and management', 'building on the social and intermediate economy' (SDLP 1997: 2–3). The latter means 'a systematic approach to the sector to match unmet need to unemployed people; working closely with the voluntary sector and the community sector' (ibid.). The Party argued there was a growing consensus around the need for attention to be focused more on equality-related measures than on the Fair Employment legislation itself, although the party was the only one which called for legal aid to be available to assist those who believed they had been discriminated against so that they could take their case to a tribunal. The Party attacked the government's record on the implementation of TSN, and called for the PAFT guidelines to be enshrined in law, to require policy-makers to assess the likely impact of laws and decisions on various groups in society (SDLP 1997: 15).

Neither 'bottom-up' nor 'social partnership' approaches to economic development and long-term unemployment were discussed by the Ulster Unionists. 'As a modern pluralist party', the party stated that it supported equality in employment, but argued 'it is essential that the highest value is placed on equality of opportunity irrespective of race, gender or creed. It must never be thought that equality of opportunity can be sacrificed in order to achieve a supposed equal outcome – the merit principle is crucial. For this reason we oppose so-called positive discrimination' (UUP 1997: 6).

There was, however, one similarity between the Ulster Unionists and Sinn Fein, not shared with the SDLP. This involved the placing of unemployment and lack of opportunity for young people into the context of emigration from Northern Ireland (Sinn Fein 1997: 8; UUP 1997: 6). Both claimed emigration was too high, and it seems reasonable to assume both are concerned that such emigration involves a loss of their actual or potential future voting population.

Again, reflecting the composition of their voting pools, the parties differed in how they discussed the non-urban sector. Both the SDLP and Sinn Fein emphasised the needs of rural populations and areas generally, while the Ulster Unionists concentrated on the needs and interests of farmers. Thus, Sinn Fein called for an 'integrated development programme' to stem the accelerating 'exodus from the land' (SF 1997: 11), prioritising job creation outside farming in rural areas, and with spending targeted at areas of greatest need (ibid.). The SDLP also emphasised rural development, and argued the need for measures to diversify the rural economy and resources to tackle poor rural housing conditions (SDLP 1997: 4).

The Ulster Unionists, on the other hand, eschewed the concept of rural development and instead emphasised the needs and interests of what the Party called 'the owner occupier farmer':

The owner occupier farmers of Northern Ireland are a hardy, self-reliant, industrious element of the population. The Ulster Unionists have a well established commitment to the continued existence of the Northern Ireland family farm. GATT and changes in the EU will have to be managed to keep intact the social structure of the rural population and we will promote policies which do so.

(UUP 1997: 19)

In addition to 'active management' of GATT, CAP, and so on, the party argued for special social policies for 'owner occupier farmers' such as the introduction of a special early retirement scheme in order to increase the proportion of younger farmers (ibid.).

CONCLUSIONS

Although the Ulster Unionists have been keen to emphasise the Party's cross-class nature ('We are a broadly based party, representative of every section of Ulster society', – Party leader, David Trimble's foreword to the manifesto), the approaches taken by the Party to a variety of social policies – social security, economic and rural development – would be likely to disproportionately benefit those on middle and higher incomes. The vestiges of unionism's historically residualist approach to social welfare, outlined in the first section of this chapter, remain evident. In contrast, and despite a class divide in the composition of voters for the two parties, both Sinn Fein and the SDLP advocate policies to decrease social exclusion, though they differ in terms of the mechanisms by which they believe this can be done.

Although none of the Northern Ireland parties have a direct say in, or responsibility for levels, of taxation, it is not the case that they are therefore identical in their approach to public spending. Rather, while all are concerned to ensure that Northern Ireland receives a share of UK public expenditure which reflects comparative levels of needs, the Ulster Unionists are unlikely to support higher rates of taxation in general in support of social objectives. This may partly reflect the reality of Northern Ireland – so long as the level of disadvantage remains higher among the nationalist/Catholic than the unionist/Protestant populations, policies which promote re-distribution from the better-off to the worse-off will, in unionist terms, 'disproportionately' benefit the minority population. Hence the Ulster Unionists' lack of enthusiasm for policies like Targeting

Social Need, and indeed measures to address (adult) long-term unemployment. Attempts to use social policies to improve 'community relations', such as those reviewed in the second section of this chapter, seem, therefore, unlikely to succeed in any immediate sense.

Historical political concerns about the demographic composition of Northern Ireland, and therefore the constitutional persuasions of the voting population, continue to influence approaches to social policy, among some parties at least, as they did before the introduction of Direct Rule, albeit in much less direct ways. Thus, both Sinn Fein and the Ulster Unionists wish to see improved prospects for young people in Northern Ireland in order to maintain or expand the size of their future potential voting pools. The intimate relationship between the politics of a contested state and social policies within it, with which this chapter began, is still relevant to analysis of the dynamics of approaches to social policy in the North.

NOTES

1 One of the interesting outcomes of such residualism was that the Poor Law continued in Northern Ireland after it had ended in Britain, so that by 1939, there were still more than 5,000 people being maintained in workhouses (Evason *et al.* 1976).

2 Similarly, the Family Allowances Act in Northern Ireland applied a residence test to British subjects not born in the UK, to aliens and to those from the rest of Ireland, with a stipulation that the family must have been resident in the UK in two out of the last three years (Ditch 1988: 90–1).

3 In 1962/3, for example, Northern Ireland's identifiable public expenditure was 8% lower than England's, 7% less than Wales' and 24% less than Scotland's (Connolly 1990).

4 The Orange Order and the main Churches all influenced education policy and laws on 'moral' issues such as homosexuality (Connolly 1990: 117–18).

5 Spend per head had become higher in Northern Ireland than Britain by the late 1970s. In 1977/8, for example, expenditure per head was 41% above that in England and Wales and 13% above Scotland (Connolly 1990). However, once migration, different administrative arrangements and higher levels of social and economic need are taken into account, the apparently higher figure reduces dramatically, if not completely. For example, in 1985/6, this apparent over-expenditure reduced from 39% to 5%, once such factors were taken into account (Connolly 1990).

6 There is a considerable literature on Fair Employment (most recently the three-volume series by The Standing Advisory Commission on Human Rights; Magill and Rose 1996; McLaughlin and Quirk 1996;

McVey and Hutson 1996) and it is not the intention to examine this in any detail here.

7 An example of this includes the government's recently reiterated position that, despite negative impacts on equality for women in employment found in a formal investigation by the EOC (EOC-NI 1996), the UK-wide policy of compulsory competitive tendering (CCT) in health and social services and education must continue, on the grounds that the 'public interest' is better served by cost-savings made through CCT than by gender equality in employment.

8 These were: adaptation of the National Insurance scheme to bring more temporary, casual and part-time workers into the scheme; a reduction of dependence on means-tested assistance during long-term unemployment on the grounds that this 'is destructive of family life', though no indications were given of how to effect this or what would replace means-tested assistance; and finally that the Job Seeker's Allowance should be reviewed after 12 months of operation (though no reason was given for why this was thought to be necessary).

9 'For the SDLP the social security system does not stand on its own. We believe it must be part of a package of policies designed to create wealth and jobs and ensure that people are in a position to take up employment' (SDLP 1997: 8).

10 These principles were launched in the United States in 1984 by Sean MacBride, John Robb, Inez McCormach and Fr Brian Brady. MacBride, a former IRA leader who had renounced violence, subsequently received both the Nobel and Lenin Peace Prizes, and held the post of Assistant General Secretary of the United Nations. The principles formed the basis of a campaign to require US corporations and other bodies investing in Northern Ireland to adopt a set of anti-discrimination measures. Some US states introduced the principles in legislation (see Rose and Magill 1996: 13–16).

REFERENCES

Birrell, D. and Murie, A. (1980) *Policy and Government in Northern Ireland*, Dublin: Gill and Macmillan.

Connolly, M. (1990) *Politics and Policy-making in Northern Ireland*, Hemel Hempstead: Philip Allan.

Ditch, J. (1988) *Social Policy in Northern Ireland Between 1939–1950*, Aldershot: Avebury.

DUP (Democratic Unionist Party) (1997) *Democracy – not Dublin rule!* election manifesto, Belfast: Democratic Unionists.

EOC-NI (Equal Opportunities Commission (NI)) (1996) *Report on the Formal Investigation into Competitive Tendering in the Health and Education Services in Northern Ireland*, Belfast: EOC (NI).

Evason, E., Darby, J. and Pearson, M. (1976) *Social Need and Social Provision in Northern Ireland*, NUU, Occasional Paper in Social Administration.

Hinds, B. (1991) 'Child care', in C. Davies and E. McLaughlin (eds) *Women,*

Employment and Social Policy in Northern Ireland: a Problem Post-poned?, Belfast: Policy Research Institute.

Knox, C. and Hughes, J. (1993) 'Equality and equity: an emerging government policy in Northern Ireland', *Ulster Papers in Public Policy and Management*, 22, Belfast: University of Ulster.

Knox, C. and Quirk, P. (1994) *Responsibility Sharing in Northern Ireland Local Government*, Belfast: Department of Public Administration and Legal Studies, University of Ulster.

McLaughlin, E. (1997) 'The development of social policy in Northern Ireland', paper presented in the 'Social Policy and Social Development in Complex Political Situations in Europe stream', EAASS conference, Cyprus, 19–23 March 1997.

McLaughlin, E. and Quirk, P. (eds) (1996) *Policy Aspects of Employment Equality in Northern Ireland*, Belfast: Standing Advisory Commission on Human Rights.

McLaughlin, E., Parker, G., Porter, S., Bernard, S. and Boyle, G. (1997) *The Determinants of Residential and Nursing Home Care among Older People in Northern Ireland*, Belfast: Department of Health and Social Services.

McVey, J. and Hutson, N. (eds) (1996) *Public Views and Experiences of Fair Employment and Equality Issues in Northern Ireland*, Belfast: Standing Advisory Commission on Human Rights

Magill, D. and Rose, S. (eds) (1996) *Fair Employment Law in Northern Ireland: Debates and Issues*, Belfast: Standing Advisory Commission on Human Rights.

O'Leary, C., Elliott, S. and Wilford, R. (1988) *The Northern Ireland Assembly 1982–1986: A Constitutional Experiment*, London: Hirst.

Osborne, R. (1996) 'Policy dilemmas in Belfast', *Journal of Social Policy*, 25, 2,: 181–99.

Osborne, R., Gallagher, A., Cormack, R. and Shortall, S. (1996) 'The implementation of policy appraisal and fair treatment guidelines in Northern Ireland', in E. McLaughlin and P. Quirk (eds) *Policy Aspects of Employment Equality in Northern Ireland*, Belfast: Standing Advisory Commission on Human Rights.

Quirk, P. and McLaughlin, E. (1996) 'Targeting social need', in E. McLaughlin, and P. Quirk (eds) *Policy Aspects of Employment Equality in Northern Ireland*, Belfast: Standing Advisory Commission on Human Rights.

Rose, S. and Magill, D. (1996) 'The development of fair employment legislation in Northern Ireland', in D. Magill and S. Rose (eds) *Fair Employment Law in Northern Ireland: Debates and Issues*, Belfast: Standing Advisary Commission on Human Rights.

Sheehan, M. (1995) 'Fair Employment: an issue for the peace process', *Race and Class*, 37: 71–82.

Sinn Fein (1997) *A New opportunity for peace*, election manifesto, Belfast: Sinn Fein.

Social Democratic and Labour Party (1997) *Real leadership, real peace*, election manifesto, Belfast: SDLP.

Standing Advisory Commission on Human Rights (1987) *Religious and Political Discrimination and Equality of Opportunity in Northern Ireland – Report on Fair Employment*, London: HMSO.

—— (1990) *Religious and Political Discrimination and Equality of Opportunity in Northern Ireland –Second Report*, London: HMSO.

UUP (Ulster Unionist Party) (1997) *Secure the Union, build your future*, election manifesto, Belfast: Ulster Unionists.

Whyte, J. (1983) 'How much discrimination was there under the Unionist regime 1921–68?', in T. Gallagher and J. O'Connell (eds) *Contemporary Irish Studies*, Manchester: Manchester University Press.

Wilford, R. (1991) 'Inverting consociationalism? Policy, pluralism and the post-modern', in B. Hadfield (ed.) *Northern Ireland Politics and Constitution*, Buckingham: Open University Press.

Chapter 15

The view from Wales

Michael Sullivan

Unlike Scotland, modern Wales is more or less wedded to the English state. It has no separate legislative system. Its education policy is, at the macro level at least, one that is shared by England. For these reasons, and others, the nature of the devolution package on offer in the 1997 Welsh referendum was for an Assembly without rights to make primary legislation or to vary levels of taxation in Wales from those levied in England. The Welsh assembly or *senedd* will to all extents and purposes act to mitigate the democratic deficit that is sometimes argued to exist in Wales.

Prior to the referendum, government policy in Wales has been overseen and implemented by the Welsh Office which, like its counterpart in Scotland, has acted as a super-ministry, performing the implementation functions of the Departments of Health, Education and Employment, Environment and so on, in relation to Wales. It has been assisted in these tasks by semi- or quasi-autonomous bodies like the Welsh Development Agency and the Development Board for Rural Wales.

The virtue of a *senedd*, as seen by pro-devolutionists, is that a direct level of accountability will be inserted into Welsh political and public life. This is nowhere more clearly seen than in relation to decisions made regarding economic and social policy, where the decisions of the Welsh Office and of existing or modified quangos will be subjected to scrutiny by a directly (and proportionally) elected assembly. But we get before ourselves. The purpose of this chapter is to consider those issues raised earlier in this book from the vantage point of Wales. It is concerned to plot, within the contexts already alluded to, the social policy prescriptions for Wales made by the political parties before the 1997 General Election. In doing so, it will of course expose the underlying political principles on which such prescriptions rely. It is equally influenced by a wish to unearth the way in which these issues developed outside the election and the further development of policy – as and if it has unfolded – since 1 May 1997.

LABOUR PLANS, WALES AND SOCIAL POLICY

As in England, Labour's election campaign in Wales was premised on a paucity of promises. In relation to social policy issues, as in other areas of policy, Labour's policy ideas were developed within parameters set by the Party's decision to retain the Conservatives' spending plans and a pledge not to increase rates of income tax. The context for the campaign in Wales, as much as in England, was cautious and careful. During the campaign, Ron Davies, the Shadow Secretary of State for Wales, echoed the Shadow Health Minister's commitment to make every pound count in the NHS (*Western Mail*, 20 April 1997), a fig-leaf formula agreed on to cover the Treasury team's decision to hold increases in expenditure on the NHS significantly below inflation for three years. Health managers in Wales saw such a strategy, as did their counterparts in England, as likely to lead to further bed shortages, hospital closures and a need to ration provision even more strictly. Already, Wales had seen what was feared to be the future as Wales's second largest district general hospital (DGH), *Ysbyty Treforys* (Morriston Hospital) ran into the buffers of competition, demand, reorganisation and resource scarcity. Situated in the north-east of the Swansea conurbation, Morriston – a 600-bedded DGH – found itself facing a deficit of around £3 million in the summer of 1996. Arguments raged between the NHS Trust and the Conservative-controlled Welsh Office about where blame should be apportioned for this significant problem. Ministers blamed bad management of resources and claimed that Morriston had been insufficiently vigilant to ensure that medical interventions matched resource allocation. Managers took the view that the transfer of a service to one of Swansea's other two DGHs, without reallocation of clinical and nursing staff, had led to the shortfall. Labour Shadow Ministers saw the Morriston crisis as illustrating the distortions introduced into health care by the internal market. Morriston's chief executive attempted to square the circle by terminating the employment of two consultants and fifteen nurses and was ultimately replaced as trust chief following a campaign orchestrated by the British Medical Association in Wales. The problem remained but the Labour critics of 1996 fought an election on policies that were seen as likely to create more and similar crises.

In the education field, Wales in 1997 continued to lag behind the *National Targets for Education and Training* (Istance and Rees 1995). Income levels in Wales remained, as the election was being fought, lower than Britain as a whole and when compared with its different regions: 'Wales [is] at the foot of the weekly earnings league with earnings for both manual and non-manual workers lower than in other regions' (Blackaby, Murphy and Thomas 1995: 211). In relation to economic inactivity the picture was similar. Census data reveals that of all 459 British local authority districts, nine out of the ten with lowest male economic activity levels were in Wales as were seven out of ten for women (ERES 1994). Proportions of one-parent families and of family violence are also disproportionately high in Wales (Sullivan and Istance 1996).

Viewed from Labour's perspective, then, Wales had been a prime victim of Conservative economic and social policy since 1979 and Labour's general commitment to social amelioration along with specific and tight economic targets were likely to have particular salience in the Welsh situation.

What in detail, then, can we glean from the Welsh manifesto about Labour's social policy prescriptions for Wales? First, the Welsh manifesto – 'New Labour because Wales deserves better' (Labour Party 1997) – addresses the NHS in Wales. In the contexts described above, it makes interesting reading. In the health field the manifesto commits Labour to:

- Reduce Welsh waiting lists;
- End the internal market in health;
- Set tough quality targets for hospitals;
- Develop a new public health drive, particularly in relation to tobacco use;
- Raise spending in real terms every year.

On the face of it, the last promise appears odd, given the Shadow Chancellor's decisions on resources. If we read a little further, however, we see an attempt at the circle being squared. In Wales, as elsewhere, an incoming Labour government would increase spending on direct patient care by diminishing the number of managers employed in the system. Put crudely, the internal market had generated the need for increased numbers of managers at NHS trust and District Health Authority level in order to service the formal agreements and transfers of resources inherent in the reorganised system. Labour's plans were to liberate £85 million in NHS Wales by cutting through what it saw as 'red tape'. This commitment, when distilled, is to address the equation whereby the internal market was seen as creating over 1,000 extra managers and diminishing the nursing workforce by 3,000. The intention was to create a new funding calculus by ending the Welsh internal market and GP fund holding and moving towards primary care-led purchasing of services.

Given levels of economic inactivity in Wales, Labour's welfare-to-work initiative might be seen as having particular salience. The initiative was seen by the Party as aimed at halting the growth of an 'underclass' and as providing effective help for lone parents. Its goal in Wales was to reverse the trend towards greater unemployment and underemployment and, as elsewhere, also to reverse a perceived dependency culture.

The Party leader's first priority of 'education, education, education', delivered during the campaign with his customary disdain for the indefinite article, looms large in the Welsh manifesto as it does in the master document. Along with its general UK commitments, it commits a Labour government to increase provision of education through the medium of the Welsh language. It promises to enhance provision at the pre-school stage and to make Welsh a compulsory subject for 14–16-year-olds by 1999. The Welsh manifesto promises zero-tolerance of failing schools.

Some reflections

A reading of the Welsh manifesto proves an interesting exercise. A Welsh dimension in relation to social or economic policy is substantially absent. Imported into the text of the British (or is it English) manifesto are Wales-specific statistics. Do we have here something of a political contradiction? Labour's manifesto sees devolution for Wales as an important policy plank, yet, in relation to other policies, Wales is seen as demanding little that is specifically Welsh. Or is this perhaps evidence of consistency rather than policy conflict? Wales is successfully, for the most part, incorporated into the British state. Its political practices and political culture are, as some would argue, indistinguishable from those in England. From such a perspective, the Welsh devolution project is easily seen as merely one of the first initiatives to ameliorate a democratic deficit.

PLAID CYMRU: A WELSH SOCIAL POLICY PLATFORM?

Plaid Cymru – in English, 'the party of Wales' – has, like the SNP, developed into a socialist, pro-European political party. Its aspirations are for Wales to be a member state of a federal Europe and its policy concerns are primarily aimed at greater self-determination for Wales. Though accepting the political inevitability that Plaid would remain a minority party in Wales after the general election, its manifesto and so-called White Papers on health and employment provide a radically different view of the future to that of Labour. In relation to health, Plaid's White Paper calls for an increase in taxation and public expenditure to create a substantially un-rationed health service in which GPs and hospital doctors become salaried employees of a Welsh ministry of health, which in turn would relate to a Welsh parliament. As a first step to a federal Europe, Plaid argued for a devolved *senedd* with primary legislative and tax-raising powers (Plaid Cymru 1997a). Its employment White Paper (Plaid Cymru 1997b) again sees increased public expenditure as the only feasible route to creating 100,000 jobs and thus full employment in Wales. If Labour's Welsh manifesto is short on specificity, then Plaid's election documents are admirably clear in their proposals. The prescriptions in relation to social policy are quintessentially 'old Labour' – a sort of Welsh Bennery – while its national aspirations are for a federal rather than devolved UK constitution.

THE LIBERAL DEMOCRATS AND SOCIAL POLICY IN WALES

Like the Labour Party's, the Liberal Democrats' Welsh manifesto is apparently a cut-and-paste job of the UK manifesto with some Welsh or Wales-related issues inserted. Unlike Labour, however, the Liberal Democrats are specific in their social policy prescriptions. In Wales, as elsewhere the Party campaigned on a platform that argued for:

- Increased funding for the NHS to halt hospital closures, reintroduction of free optical and dental services, reduced waiting lists and raised standards in the NHS;
- Increased and hypothecated income tax to provide one penny in the pound for increased education spending;
- The encouragement of fuller employment by allowing employers to top up benefits to get the unemployed back to work.

CONSERVATIVES AND SOCIAL POLICY AND WALES?

A glance at the Welsh Conservative manifesto provides us with no real surprises. In general the message of this anti-devolution party was the UK-wide advice of 'steady as she goes'. Like Labour, the Conservatives promised in Wales, as elsewhere, to cut management costs in the NHS. In education, the manifesto holds firm on the division of the school system into conventional state schooling and direct grant provision. The promise for Wales and the rest of the UK in relation to social policy was to continue the Thatcher/Major restructuring of the welfare state.

Social policy spending

When Major succeeded Thatcher in 1990, social policy spending accounted for 22 per cent of GDP. This rose by 1993 to nearly 27 per cent, considerably higher than in 1979. Consequently the then Chancellor, Kenneth Clarke decided to use the new autumn budget to raise taxes. More than this, his deputy, Michael Portillo, announced a fundamental review of spending on the welfare state. The 1997 Conservative manifesto with its emphasis on halting the further development of a British underclass also picks up themes from the outgoing administration's morality armoury. Here right-wing ministers were given their head on social issues. As a result the old concerns about social security fraud and lone parents and public housing re-surfaced. This led to the reintroduction of a distinctly Thatcherite tone on issues of the family and the responsibilities of individuals. This was no more obvious than in relation to social security policy where the Party went into the election with the inheritance bequeathed by three right-wing Cabinet ministers in the early 1990s. These ministers attempted to turn public opinion against certain classes of benefit claimants. In August 1992, Peter Lilley, the Secretary of State for Social Security, had revived the dependency-culture debate, expressing concern about teenage pregnancies and the cost of single parents to the state. These remarks were echoed in September 1993 by the then Treasury minister Michael Portillo who feared that single teenage parents could be led into a life of poverty-stricken dependency by the state's provision of what he called over-generous benefits. Later, on a visit to a housing estate in south Wales, John Redwood (Secretary of State for Wales until his leadership challenge to John Major in 1995) returned to the lone-parent debate, suggesting that young women were becoming pregnant with no intention of living with the father of their child. In such a situation, they knew, Redwood argued, that the state would take care of their social security and housing needs. He therefore called for changes to policy and attitudes.

The extent to which these interventions were made with the then Prime Minister's support is unclear. Though he was to refer to three ministers, when he thought he was off-air, as 'the bastards', the epithet was earned for their anti-European stance rather than their views on social policy. Be that as it may, the Welsh electorate, together with the rest of the British electorate was faced with more of the same in relation both to the substance, tone and ideology of Conservative social policy prescriptions.

THE DEVELOPMENT OF THEMES: THE GENERAL ELECTION CAMPAIGN IN WALES

From the start of the general election campaign in Wales, the prospect of an electoral wipe out for the Conservatives appeared a distinct possibility. Holding four parliamentary seats when the campaign commenced, the Conservatives were to emerge from the election with no Welsh MPs. It was anticipated that the Liberal Democrats would hold on to the Montgomery seat they had held in the last parliament and that they might reclaim Brecon and Radnor. In the event they won both seats. Plaid Cymru were expected to hold on to the four seats they held before the election but the apparent electoral strength of Labour meant that they made no further inroads into Labour territory. From early on in the campaign, then, attention was focused on the Labour Party. On the face of it, there was much of interest. Blair's 'New Labour' Party had, in the previous two years or so, redefined the nature of Labour social democracy. Gone, or at least buried for the most part, was the language of egalitarianism. The 'Old Labour' truth that the poor could climb out of poverty only with the mildly redistributive help of ameliorative social democratic social policy had been replaced by an increasing belief in the existence of a dependency culture in which the poor remained poor because they lacked the personal qualities necessary to climb out of poverty (Sullivan 1997a). Spending promises of the sort made by Labour in previous elections (including the ones that they won) were replaced by a promise to be economically prudent. The welfare state, not only

Labour's political property but also the essence of Welsh Labourism, appeared to be one of the areas in line for review if Labour were to win the UK election. Superficially then, the ground was set for a conflict of political cultures between the New Labour model army of Millbank and Walworth Road on the one hand and unreconstructed old Welsh Labourism on the other. That cultural conflict, however, hardly simmered, much less boiled over, and Labour's apparently conservative social policy programme raised little political heat in the Welsh election. There appear to be a number of reasons for this.

THE NEW LABOUR TURKS

Since Blair's election as Labour leader in 1994, New Labourism had made some inroads into constituency Labour parties in Wales and had led to the adoption of Blair sympathisers in some of the few remaining seats which Labour wished to win from the Conservatives or wished to retain. An extreme example of this was the resignation of Roy Hughes (the distinctly Old Labour MP for Newport West) to make way for the adoption of Alan Howarth, who had in the previous year abandoned the Conservative Party and crossed the floor of the House of Commons to join Labour. To the ranks of New Labour were added political retreads such as the one that saw Kim Howells, the erstwhile research officer for the Welsh NUM and old-style socialist renounce socialism as anachronistic and join the New Labour campaign. Decisions, made for a variety of reasons, by right-leaning but Old Labour MPs (a sort of Hattersley tendency) to keep their disagreements with the leadership as a matter for consenting adults in private, contributed to a relatively smooth run for Blair's redesigned social democracy in Wales.

AN OLD LABOUR SPIN

Welsh social democracy is likely to have been helped by the spearheading of the Welsh campaign by Labour politicians with a distinctly Old Labour whiff about them. This too helps explain the relative quiescence of Old Labour. The then Shadow Secretary of State for Wales, Ron Davies, is infamous in New Labour circles for three main reasons: he is alleged to have moved the motion for the deselection of Neil Kinnock in the early 1980s following the latter's failure to support Tony Benn for the deputy leadership of the Labour

Party; he recently expressed his republican views in an attack on the Royal Family, which he was prevailed upon to withdraw; and his views on the welfare state appeared to owe more to the inspiration of the Tredegar Medical Society and Aneurin Bevan than they did to New Labour spin doctors. In leading the Welsh campaign, he was ably assisted by Peter Hain, the MP for Neath (and now Parliamentary Under-Secretary at the Welsh Office) who is more famous for his leadership of the campaign against apartheid in the late 1960s, while still a Liberal and his leadership of the Tribune Group. The political appearance during the campaign was of a relatively autonomous Welsh Labour Party, a trick first successfully carried out for the Conservatives by Peter Walker when the non-Thatcherite Conservative Secretary of State for Wales.

AN APPETITE TO WIN, A FEAR OF LOSING

In each General Election since, and including, the one in 1979, Wales has returned a significant majority of Labour MPs and, even at its lowest electoral point in 1983, Labour garnered a significant majority of the votes cast in the election. A growing perception of both democratic deficit and of the illegitimacy of Conservative governments to hold sway in Wales has played a significant part in the decisions of New Labour to put its weight behind devolution and a *senedd* for Wales. It seems also to have produced an unusual discipline and a will to win the electoral battle at all costs. This, in itself, has been a significant factor in legitimising, in Wales at least, rather alien notions about the welfare state. Put simply, the Welsh Labour Party, Labour supporters and perhaps the Welsh people as a whole have acquiesced in the forging of a post-social democratic Labourism. Welsh Labourism has traditionally been collectivist and communitarian. Support for a comprehensive and universal welfare state has been based on the ideas of social solidarity and community support. The post-war welfare state has also loomed large in the enhancement of opportunity for many ordinary citizens of Wales in the post-war period. When Kinnock asked 'why am I the first Kinnock to go to university and why is Glenys [Kinnock] the first woman from her family to go to university' during the 1987 General Election campaign and when he answered his own question by arguing that it was because they were children of the welfare state, he was observing the litany of old-style Welsh social democracy. The idea was not only that the welfare state increased individual opportunity and enhanced citizen rights (Marshall 1963) but also that it was the very essence of socialism. It was so because it enshrined the idea that the state had a responsibility to care for all its citizens and the vision that individuals had a responsibility for each other. During the election campaign the Party considered reconfiguring welfare provision, embraced the idea of an underclass, and apparently accepted the concept of a dependency culture. These shifts in presentation constitute major changes in the Party's vision of social democracy (and perhaps its abandonment). The acceptance of these seismic shifts by the Welsh Labour Party was helped and maybe determined by a desperate will to win and fear of losing.

RESONATING WITH A MODERN ELECTORATE

These major changes and these emerging new themes, together with the political conversion of some and the retirement or silence of others, may well of course have been influenced by a perception of value shifts within the Welsh electorate in relation to some areas of policy. They may also be a reasonably faithful reflection of some of the subterranean values held by supporters of Old Labourism as well as by devotees of Blairism.

In Wales, as elsewhere, the social and economic policy changes of the years since 1979 had created winners as well as losers. People's capitalism (as Mrs Thatcher had described it) had facilitated home ownership for many council house tenants and made shareholders of ordinary as well as extraordinary citizens. Labour, while retaining majority representation in Wales had seen its vote fluctuate and more importantly had seen it fall away across the border. The idea that value shifts had occurred within the Welsh electorate were confirmed by the Party's own polling and, as in England, it wished to capture middle Wales in the way that Clinton had managed to capture middle America.

Additionally, however, some of Labour's policy prescriptions were consistent with views held by pro-Labour voters in Wales as elsewhere. Throughout the 1980s and 1990s, the Party's own polling and academic studies confirmed that support for heartland services of the welfare state was accompanied by victim-blaming ideologies in relation to other sectors. The most obvious of these services are those to do with social security and income maintenance where public perception includes the prominent view that many claimants are work-shy members of a dependency culture or underclass.

Perceptions of the welfare state also came, during the 1980s, to include the view that a vibrant private sector was necessary to parallel the public sector in welfare so that 'voice, choice and exit' might be ensured (Papadakis and Taylor-Gooby 1991). It would be a mistake, then to see the roots of New Labour social policies as reaching only as far back as the election of Blair as Party leader.

Labour's thinking on social policy has moved, over the last decade, from old-style social democracy to a less-than-grudging acceptance of some of the changes introduced by Conservative governments. During this process a sort of citizenship theory has re-emerged. If we look at Labour's social policy agenda in the late 1980s and early 1990s the following trains of thought emerge. First, there are certainly elements of the old social democratic approach in its strategy for social policy. In its 1991 strategy document on health it sideswipes at the Conservatives' emphasis on efficiency strategies in the NHS. It declares that 'most of what appears as inefficiency [in the NHS] is the product of underfunding'. Second, and notwith-standing this standard response, even here there is substantial recog-nition of the durability and acceptability of some elements of the Conservatives' health service reforms. Of most significance, perhaps, is Labour's intention, despite earlier ambivalence, to retain the split between the commissioner and provider in the NHS and personal social services, a crucial element in the emerging welfare pluralism. This is clearly an acknowledgement of the potential success of this mechanism in improving service. Its clear acceptance of the commissioner/provider strategy as a mechanism to improve effect-iveness and efficiency suggests, though it does not ensure, that managed competition, perhaps in a more restricted form, is as attractive to the policy elite in the Labour Party as it was to the last government. This, alongside other acknowledgements of Con-servative social policy, might suggest that Labour, like the Con-servatives, sees a degree of competition in welfare as likely to assist not only its commitment to peg direct taxation at its present level but also a commitment to meet need.

Labour had moved a great distance, even before the 1992 election. Its policy aspirations in the 1990s appear to take account of the shifts in public opinion documented in recent commentaries on welfare provision. Labour may, in crude terms, have become more aware in the late 1980s of the complexities contained within public attitudes to welfare. Those complexities embrace not only the strong support for heartland welfare state services, which – or so I have argued elsewhere (Sullivan 1992) – have acted as a brake on Conservative social policy plans, but also ambivalence to social security provision and some universal benefits (see also Papadakis and Taylor-Gooby 1991).

What appears to be emerging is a fusion between Beveridgian welfare state concepts and ideas about a so-called 'opportunity state' (Sullivan 1990). This move was reflected in many of Labour's policy documents in the late 1980s. During this period, the Party carried out a policy review as part of the process of rehabilitating the Party in the eyes of the electorate, after a period in the early 1980s when it had appeared to be controlled by its left wing. Those documents that concentrate on welfare issues are noteworthy because they stress the concern of the Party with individual issues such as liberty, freedom of choice and consumerism which appeared to be the property, through much of the 1980s, of right-wing Conservatism in government. Labour's former deputy leader, Roy Hattersley, expressed the task addressed in these documents. In a short essay written at the end of the 1980s, he argued that the responsibility of a future Labour government would be to 'provide and popularise an acceptable theory of distribution that is both consistent with egalitarian principles of socialism and with a modern economy'. This could amount to an acceptance not only of much of the change wrought in methods of economic management in the 1980s but also of some of the directions in social policy followed during this decade. It is also a re-working of Marshall in new conditions. The aim of the new social democracy is to create a sort of equality that is consistent both with its political past and with the retention and development of market capitalism. It is this project that spawned Labour's 'Social Justice Commission' and it is a concern with equality of accord rather than material equality that appears to have been the engine driving Labour social policy development in the 1990s.

In important respects, then, old-style social democracy is dead. New Conservatism, influenced, though not fully determined, by the radical Right, has – in welfare as elsewhere – transformed the debate about and the practice of welfare provision. In doing so, it has not only created a new sort of Conservatism. It has also forced Labour into a new Labourist position. That position is one in which 'citizenship' serves as a conceptual bridge from Fabian social democracy to a sort of market socialism.

So much, then for the reasons lying at the heart of Labour's transformation and its culmination in the 1997 election campaign in

Wales and the UK. Having successfully negotiated the electoral hurdle, what happened after 1 May?

THE REFERENDUM

On 18 September 1997, the referendum on Welsh devolution took place. Despite earlier optimistic projections, the Welsh electorate, or to be more accurate, around half of it, delivered a resounding political 'maybe'. Unlike the result in Scotland, the majority in favour of a Welsh assembly was wafer thin: when the final results were counted the 'yes option' attracted 50.4 per cent of the vote, with 49 per cent of the voters dissenting. Victories for the *le dros Gymru* ([Vote] Yes for Wales) campaign were registered in the central industrial (or post-industrial) valleys of south Wales, in the industrial–rural coastal plain of south west Wales, in west Wales and in north west and central north Wales. Mid-Wales, many of the south-eastern and north-eastern areas of Wales, Newport and Cardiff, the capital city, swelled the vote for the 'just say no' campaign. It is much too early to conduct a satisfactory analysis of the reasons for this result, though once the data are available such an analysis will be fascinating. A number of provisional but striking features seem to emerge from the result and reports of the campaign. First, support for the assembly was markedly weaker in border areas and in those areas of Wales that have benefited most from inward investment or regeneration. Cardiff is a particularly embarrassing example here. As a corollary, support for the government's policy was strongest not only in areas where political nationalism was also strong (the rural heartlands of west and north Wales) but also in those areas of south and south west Wales which have benefited less from economic regeneration. Second, in the eastern extremities of the country, strong anecdotal and opinion evidence appear to suggest that voters elided the idea of devolution for Wales with strengthening of the claims of the Welsh language and of cultural nationalism. In doing so, they may well have exposed the fault line that often characterises discussions of Welshness and to have indicated the lack of resolution in Wales of the question: 'what is a Welsh identity?' Finally, campaigners on both sides have pointed to the difficulty of promoting devolution and an assembly in a society that has no recent tradition of separate social, political and legislative institutions from England. What, the question goes, would such an assembly do?

The response of the government and of the Secretary of State for

Wales has been to accept the referendum result as support for Labour's devolution policy but to commit the government to be inclusive in its choice of membership of the commission which will decide on the exact model of the assembly and the particular form of proportional representation used to elect it. In other words, the immediate political reaction has included considerations of ways in which the dissenters, and particularly the Conservative Party in Wales might best be guaranteed representation in the assembly in order to ensure that they participate in the administration of a partly devolved Wales.

SOME CONCLUDING REMARKS

The Labour government appears to have embarked on a process which may lead to a radical restructuring of the welfare state and the principles which underlie it. Those issues differ little whether we are looking at them from a Welsh or English perspective. In the future those issues might develop a Welsh spin as a result of the establishment and further development of the *senedd*, a possibility grasped – but only just – by the Welsh people.

REFERENCES

Blackaby, D., Murphy, P. and Thomas, E. (1995) 'Wales: an economic survey', *Contemporary Wales* 7: 209–23.

ERES (1994) *A Study of the Economically Inactive and their role in the Labour Market*, Cardiff: ERES and Welsh Office.

Hattersley, R. (1989) 'Afterword' in K. Hoover and R. Plant (eds) *Conservative Capitalism*, London: Routledge.

Istance, D. and Rees, G. (1995) 'Education and training in Wales: problems and paradoxes revisited', Contemporary Wales, 7, Cardiff: University of Wales Press.

Labour Party (1997) *New Labour because Wales deserves better*, election manifesto, Cardiff: Wales Labour Party.

Marshall, T. H. (1963) 'Citizenship and social class', in his *Sociology at the Crossroads*, London: Heinemann.

Papadakis, E. and Taylor-Gooby, P. (1991) *The Private Provision of Public Welfare*, Hemel Hempstead: Harvester Wheatsheaf.

Plaid Cymru (1997a) Manifesto, Cardiff: Plaid Cymru.

—— (1997b) Employment White Paper, Cardiff: Plaid Cymru.

—— (1997c) Health White Paper, Cardiff: Plaid Cymru.

Sullivan, M. (1990) 'Communities and social policy', in R. Jenkins (ed.) *One Step Forward?*, Llandysnl: Gower.

—— (1992) *The Politics of Social Policy*, Hemel Hempstead: Harvester Wheatsheaf.

—— (1997a) 'Democratic socialism and social policy', in R. Page and R. Silburn (eds) *British Social Policy in the Twentieth Century*, London: Macmillan.

—— (1997b) 'The social democratic perspective', in P. Alcock, A. Erskine and M. May (eds) *The Social Policy Companion*, Oxford: Blackwell.

Sullivan, M. and Istance, D. (1996) *Children and Social Exclusion*, Swansea: University of Wales Swansea.

Chapter 16

A new deal for Britain?

Susanne MacGregor

INTRODUCTION

After the 1997 election, the pollsters congratulated themselves that, on the whole, they got it right this time. Use of telephone interviews and random digital dialling (RDD) delivered the goods (perhaps partly because this meant their samples were more representative of those who actually went out to vote than interviews with people in the street had been). Interestingly, they found the Labour lead to be stronger among ex-Directory voters than among more ordinary folk. They concluded that the campaign itself had been boring and went on too long and that the key movement was the anti-Tory 'time for a change' mood (SRA 1997).

The main issues which concerned people, so polls reported, were education, health, and Europe. Labour picked up on a vague feeling that things could be better and offered precise, limited targets regarding such things as class sizes and getting young people back to work.

The Major government had lost because of its divisions over Europe and especially because of its association with sleaze. In electoral democracies, the key questions have to do with issues of competence and trust. If they are to survive, governments have to be able to combine efficiency with legitimacy. After four terms in office, the Conservatives had lost control on both fronts. The election of a New Labour government offered the opportunity to restore people's faith in democracy.

Labour was firmly elected as the legitimate government and its rhetoric and image had won strong support. Now the question would be could it deliver – could it run the country efficiently and effectively? The dominant opinion of expert commentators on the New Labour government was that the devil would be in the detail.

Yet, long after the first one hundred days were over, Blair and Brown were receiving record popular support.

END OF THE WELFARE STATE

In this election campaign, the language of the old welfare state disappeared. Discredited words like redistribution and socialism vanished from the lexicon. Purple and yellow took the place of red, and the Union Jack and the British bulldog were key images. Both the main parties claimed the one-nation mantle and fought over values like patriotism, discipline, prudence, duty and law and order.

So with Labour's victory must it now be accepted that the old welfare state (the post-war social settlement found in most advanced industrial societies) has finally gone? The question for the turn of the century would then be what will take its place? The dream of the free marketeers that the welfare state could simply be abolished has proved false. Some needs have to be met, some functions performed, some system of regulation brought in. What form should this take?

The chapters in this book have analysed the deep problems that have built up in key areas of governance, human services and social infrastructure in the past ten years and more. Poverty and inequality remain blots on British society, ones to which, perhaps, society is now less willing to turn a blind eye. The social and personal pressures that face a large impoverished and disaffected group of people, the result of years of underprovision and failings of key services (especially in education, health, youth justice, social security, employment policy and housing) cannot be dealt with through easy quick-fix solutions. Change will take longer than a day, one or even two terms of office. The first step to solving these serious social questions is to recognise the sheer size of the task that confronts the government. Nothing less than determined social reconstruction will do. As Beveridge, fifty years ago, argued for an integrated, comprehensive, universal strategy that would co-ordinate key policy areas – health, housing, social security, employment and education – so as the year 2000 approaches, what is needed once again is to look at problems as a whole – a holistic approach – extending also to include social and environmental regeneration and the criminal justice system. Such co-ordination, in a complex, diverse society, to be effective, needs to be implemented through devolved structures operating at local or regional levels but with co-ordination at national level paralleling these developments. Leadership from the top is needed to generate the political will to face up to these challenges and to place both economic success *and* social justice at the top of everyone's agenda.

The argument of this final chapter is that such a truly radical programme would need to go beyond and be distinctly different from the American-inspired social policies which appear to influence some New Labour thinking.

MAY 1 1997

Words like landslide were used to describe the results of the 1997 General Election. Modern electorates are increasingly volatile, focusing on specific interests and issues, and in 1997 almost a third didn't vote at all. Does this provide the ground on which radical reform can be built?

The most significant aspect of the election result was the collapse of support for the Conservatives, their lowest since 1929. The Conservatives received 9.6 million votes (compared with 14 million in 1992). Their share of the vote at 31 per cent was their lowest since 1832. Their 165 seats represented their lowest share since 1906.

Votes cast for Labour totalled 13.5 million, 2 million more than in 1992 but less than their total in 1951. Labour won 43 per cent of the votes cast (compared to 35 per cent in 1992). This was the highest proportion they had won since 1966. From this they took 418 seats out of a possible 659 (compared to 393 out of a possible 640 in 1945). Overall Labour gained 146 seats.

The Liberal Democrats won 46 seats and attracted 5.2 million votes.

Was this a new dawn? How much did the landslide of seats (the first-past-the-post system exaggerating the swing to Labour) just show that people wanted to get the Tories out and how much did it represent genuine support for Labour? Could Labour have won with a more radical programme, even with an old Labour programme? (Brittan 1997).

There is little doubt that Labour's tight control of images and messages, and the tight discipline it exerted over its troops, helped in the run up to and during the election campaign. These features of New Labour continued well after the election as the new government saw the need to control its backbenchers and aimed to avoid the problems of discord and argument that had disfigured previous Labour administrations.

But this was to be no simple change of administration. The election of New Labour, it was claimed, represented a changed political culture from which would flow new political alliances. Nothing less than a fundamental realignment of British politics and reform of British institutions and constitution were now on the agenda. One-Nation politics would be the government's theme, building a new consensus in which key words were co-ordination, partnership and integration.

The aim through proposals for devolution was to encourage greater empowerment and deliver a slimmer, less intrusive state. With the new philosophy of decentralisation and devolution comes more stress on the rights and duties of all members of society. Such a centre-left realignment would, it was hoped, lead to the dominance for a generation of the new radical centre. The end of the old politics meant the end of Old Labour, old policies and old welfarism. Instead we would see the arrival of all things bright and beautiful. Quite what would be beneath the glitter remained to be seen.

In this successful repositioning of Labour, the Blair project had followed the lead of US President Clinton, who had successfully turned round the attack that the Democrats were soft on crime, welfare dependency and family values. The line to take was to be aggressively populist and anti-liberal – tough not tender – tough on inflation, tough on public expenditure and public sector pay, tough on crime and drugs, and tough on failing schools.

THE FIRST 100 DAYS

After one hundred days, New Labour's mentor President Clinton offered congratulations. The *Guardian* welcomed the checks on central power, including a directly-elected Mayor for London, devolution proposals for Wales and Scotland, and the incorporation of the European Convention of Human Rights. However, it expressed concern in an editorial (9 August 1997) about the new government's 'puritanical, almost Cromwellian streak' involving proposals about how much homework children should do and what time they should be off the streets. The editorial also commented that not everyone seemed included in the in-group – the glitterati were there at the Downing Street parties but not party activists and trade unionists.

Another group who seemed to be particular favourites of the new government were business representatives. One election slogan had been 'Labour Means Business'. Businessmen were recruited to help the new government tackle the difficult issues of social policy: to reform the tax system, Martin Taylor of Barclays Bank was brought in; to head the welfare-to-work task force – Sir Peter Davis, Chief Executive of the Prudential.

The Economist's verdict on Labour's early days was that 'there have been some encouragingly brave and even radical moves', citing the passing of control over monetary policy to an independent Bank of England and a big shake-up in financial regulation (9 August 1997: 17). It praised the new government's resolve on Northern Ireland and the decision to invite the Liberal Democrats to join a cabinet committee on constitutional reform.

The Economist was less impressed by the tendency to act as though in a permanent election campaign, the setting up of focus groups to evaluate policy ideas and what seemed at times like an exaggerated fear of criticism. Did this indicate 'an unwillingness to lead or to take unpopular decisions? . . . the permanent campaign, the media manipulation, the excessive interest, at times, in symbols rather than substance, are more worrying', concluding 'if this government does such things when life is easy, how will it be when things get tough?'(ibid).

As the political season resumed in autumn 1997, the Liberal Democrats robustly criticised Labour's policies on health and education, arguing that shortage of funds would prevent them delivering. The Conservatives' disarray led some Liberal Democrats to aim at becoming the main Opposition party.

EVALUATING LABOUR'S PERFORMANCE IN OFFICE

How will the new government be judged and how would they like to be judged? The long-term aim is the creation of a modern, meritocratic society (Brown 1997). The new government would tackle inequality from first principles: 'starting from an understanding of the modern economy and based on a realistic programme', they were 'committed to tackling the causes of poverty – unemployment, low skills and low wages – and not simply the consequences'. The key would be to ensure 'continuous and accessible equality of opportunity . . . the denial of opportunity has become an unacceptable inefficiency, a barrier to prosperity'(ibid.).

In his election address, when competing for leadership of the Labour Party, Tony Blair had signalled his concern about the growth of a dependency culture. Not only his style and campaign, and party management, derive from the lessons learnt by President Clinton but many of his social policies seem also to have American roots.

Reform of welfare is to be a high priority for the new Labour government – welfare understood as social security, especially pensions and provision for the unemployed and lone parent families. The government aims to 'act speedily to achieve welfare state and employment reform' (Gordon Brown, speech to the IMF, 23 September 1997). At the Labour Party conference in Brighton in late September 1997, Gordon Brown set out his reforming policies, claiming these indicated a return to a commitment to a high and stable level of employment. There would be a radical shake-up of the tax and benefit system, introducing an American-style earned income tax credit (partly or wholly to replace, even enhance, the current family credit scheme). This would be part of a three-pronged approach along with a minimum wage and job creation. The aim was to reform the system, to 'modernise' it, so that it would help people back to work. The advantage of the tax-credit system is that it can increase the take-home pay of the working poor without increasing the overt size of the social security budget. Implementation will not be easy, partly because of Britain's system of independent rather than household tax assessment.

The New Deal for the unemployed, running alongside these changes, would offer, from May 1998, every young person under 25 years of age who had been unemployed over six months, one of four possibilities (presented as 'options' but not in fact offering much choice to an individual claimant) – a job, education, voluntary work, or a place on an environmental task force (later a fifth option of self-employment was added). From June 1998, those long-term unemployed out of work for over two years, would be helped back to work by a government subsidy to employers who took them on, of £75 a week. The welfare-to-work programme would be extended from autumn 1998 to single parents, who would be offered advice in finding work and training, and to the disabled, for whom new job opportunities would be created. 'This is a genuine national crusade against unemployment and poverty' he said, in an exclusive interview with the *Guardian* (27 September 1997) in advance of his speech to the party conference the following Monday.

The principles on which Brown's decisions rest are to encourage work, savings and fairness. The aspiration for a 10p to 40p tax range would be very progressive once it had been achieved, he has argued.

Raising the ceiling for National Insurance contributions is ruled out – it was ruled out in 1992 when he took over as Shadow Chancellor. The approach he will adopt will be one aiming to create jobs. Lack of work and lack of skills are the key problems for Britain which it will be the government's priority to tackle. The principles which guide his approach, and which are central to business too, are: stability; investment; education; reform of the welfare state; and a constructive engagement with Europe. As regards the public finances, the first task is to control the PSBR. Because this had been allowed to rise too high, tough decisions had to be made about public expenditure. A fundamental review of spending would be conducted which would inform decisions to be made after the first two-year freeze on ceilings. But there is room for choices to be made about expenditure within existing budgets (e.g. phasing out assisted places scheme; student loans to replace grants), (*On the Record*, BBC1 TV, 23 March 1997).

These reforms follow similar trends in other English-speaking social economies, principally in USA, Canada, New Zealand and Australia, sometimes introduced by Labour governments.

The current war on 'welfare as we know it' in the United States has been seen by Fran Piven as being about 're-encoding the "poor" as the marginal "other"' (Piven 1995: xii). But this is not how it is presented. It is presented as being about creating opportunity and healing divisions. Which is it in fact?

These symbolic constructions and what they represent are at the heart of the contemporary welfare policy debate. A key concept is that of the underclass, a term which, in spite of much critical comment (cf Katz 1993; Alcock *et al.* 1994; Morris 1994), has now entered the everyday language of politicians and broadcasters.

WELFARE-TO-WORK: A NEW PATERNALISM IN SOCIAL POLICY

There is a general tendency in both Europe and America to place more stress now on welfare-to-work programmes. But these vary greatly depending on how they are introduced and how much they cost. Key issues have to do with what degree of compulsion is required, how much punitiveness is built into procedures, what level of remuneration is paid, what is the quality of the experience and the training available, and how much general support is given, especially with regard to child-care arrangements. These are crucial differences distinguishing the programmes found in Sweden, Denmark, France, Australia, Canada, USA and Britain.

In his book *The New Politics of Poverty*, the conservative American sociologist Lawrence Mead argued that '[d]ependency at the bottom of society, not economic equality, is the issue of the day (Mead 1992: ix). He believes that 'this shift has occurred not because the country has become more conservative, but because traditional approaches to social reform have been exhausted. Government has failed to overcome poverty simply by expanding opportunity, the traditional American solution to social problems' (ibid.). The problem lies with the welfare state which did not set behavioural standards for the dependent. 'The focus of politics is now conduct rather than class' (op. cit: 2). Employment is essential to effective citizenship and it is non-work which, apart from crime, is the behaviour of the poor that most offends the non-poor, he claims. 'The shift from the working class to the underclass as the main social issue is a watershed in America's experience and increasingly that of the West as a whole' (op. cit.: 16).

American moves towards workfare began in the 1980s. Great stress was given to the critical issue of chronic poverty. Declining schools were seen as the main barrier to producing 'a world-class workforce'. Requirements that employable Aid for Families with Dependent Children recipients work or look for work were first legislated in 1967 and they have become steadily more stringent (op. cit.: 167). The original purpose of workfare was to deter employable people from going on welfare at all and this seems to be effective as mandatory work requirements cause almost a third to give up on assistance.

The shift in language which has taken place more recently in American policy is seen in the increasing stress on obligation. The public wants to see clients doing something to help themselves, it is argued. A requirement to work is helpful to the dependent poor, it is claimed, as they have become locked into passivity and withdrawn from normal life.

Mead sees the US 1988 Family Support Act 'as the leading monument to the new paternalism in social policy' (op. cit.: 200). The aim was to prepare people for self-reliance and enforce mainstream social values. The issue was the balance between opportunity and obligation (op. cit.: 204). Ordinary people place great stress on restoring order – it is the elites who have doubts about this – and they generally are not the ones who have to live with the consequences – a point frequently made by Jack Straw, Britain's Home Secretary. Maintaining social discipline has strong appeal to ordinary voters.

The eminent urban policy analyst, Nat Glazer, has explained these trends in terms of the importance of symbolic politics. He has argued that Clinton needed a welfare reform mainly for symbolic reasons not because there is really a welfare crisis. The costs involved are actually quite minor. The problem being addressed is not the needs of the poor but the undermining of the work ethic and the need to maintain the discipline of labour and avoid social unrest.

'Welfare' he says 'has come to stand for the rise of a permanent dependent population cut off from the mainstream of American life and expectations, for the decay of inner cities, for the problem of homelessness, for the increase in crime and disorder, for the problems of the inner city black poor ... ending "welfare as we know it" seems to promise some relief from these social disorders' (Glazer 1995: 21). A number of other commentators agree that the welfare debate is principally a diversionary one distracting from the real debate about political economy needed in the United States where real incomes of ordinary people have been steadily falling. 'Welfare women' are being blamed for the declining standards of living. The actual cost of 'welfare women' is quite small but the issue holds a large place in the public imagination and in debate.

American social policy analysts have concluded that workfare cannot be an effective solution to unemployment in the absence of enough steady, decent-paying, full-time jobs to go around. The administrative costs of operating these programmes outweigh any savings gained by cuts in welfare payments. The argument that somehow these schemes would improve the social fabric is even more hotly disputed, since removing the women from their fragile communities removes its most stable element. It is the women who have contributed actively to community-based activity in crime and drugs prevention, for example. This unpaid caring work of women in poor communities, not least in child-rearing itself but also in neighbourly activity, is consistently under-recognised and under-valued by those in authority – a similar point is made by Bea Campbell in her descriptions of life on poor estates in England (Campbell 1993).

Desmond King, a British historian of comparative policy, has pointed out that work-welfare 'denotes three sorts of government policy for the unemployed: first, placement policies to marry jobseekers with vacancies; second, training schemes intended to augment jobseekers' skills; and third, workfare programs sometimes imposed upon jobseekers as a condition of receiving benefits' (King 1995: xi). The British and the American approaches to work-welfare share some characteristics deriving from their shared liberal traditions. The principal elements of these schemes are 'the priorities of excluding the undeserving from public assistance, distinguishing them from worthy recipients, and imposing work requirements on beneficiaries' (op. cit.: xiii).

What is crucial is the wider social policy context in which such schemes are introduced, especially 'whether benefits are linked to work requirements; whether registration at labor exchanges is compulsory or voluntary; whether participation in training programs is compulsory or optional; whether benefits are provided as cash or in-kind; and whether programs are designed to complement, supplant or support market processes' (op. cit.: xiv). The resurgence of workfare in the 1980s and 1990s illustrates the dominance and resilience of liberal values. Modern British work-welfare rests in part on programmes whose design is borrowed directly and uncritically from the United States (op. cit.: xv). King reminds us that in October 1993, the Tory Party's endorsement of the New Jersey work-welfare scheme, which penalised mothers who had additional children while receiving public benefits, was a crowd winner at the annual conference. And in 1997, Harriet Harman was reported to have sent advisors over to Wisconsin to observe their schemes as possible models for the New Deal.

A survey of evidence conducted by the Ontario Network of Employment Skills Training Projects has concluded that Canadian studies have shown that workfare works when it is voluntary; when there is an accurate initial assessment of the participants' needs; when the needs identified in the assessment are supported by the appropriate services; when there are multi-tiered services and support, such as job search support, job training and education; when safe, quality child care is available; and when income supplements are available for clothes, haircuts and transportation. Workfare does not work, they conclude, where the community is suffering from high unemployment (people cannot move into permanent jobs if the jobs do not exist); they do not work where there is low government investment in the programme; where the programme is mandatory with strict guidelines and enforcement; where the workfare jobs displace people currently holding jobs; where there is no initial assessment or that assessment is inaccurate; where the programme consists only of job search support; and where there is no support for training or child care (21 February 1996 Irykert@web.UUCP).

Will British reforms be simply a copycat version of north American ideas? Or might they instead build on British respectable working-class traditions and values? In the UK, Frank Field the new Social Security Minister began to formulate ways of 'freeing the underclass' in his 1989 book *Losing Out*. The political aim of such reforms, he argued then, should be a 'programme that combines an appeal to self-interest with one of altruism' (op. cit.: 17) or, as Tony Blair said on the steps of 10 Downing Street on 2 May 1997, that the aim was to create one Britain, one nation 'in which our ambition for ourselves is matched by our sense of compassion and decency and duty for others'.

The focus of the new politics of social policy, Field has argued, should be on reasserting the old ethical tradition of the Labour Party, appealing to common decencies. Practical proposals for getting people back to work would include the relocation of civil service jobs, targeting government purchasing, and raising skills levels. Long-term unemployment should be attacked by guaranteeing a place on employment training or other training, education or a pre-employment course, local compacts between employers and youth training schemes, and a temporary work safety-net. Personal needs assessment, job search advice and, as a final fall-back, a temporary work scheme were also proposed by Field in 1989. Training and Enterprise Councils (TECs), he said, might play a role in developing these programmes and incentives to employers would be needed to encourage them to take on these workers.

Changes in tax and benefit, especially child benefit, would be needed to increase the incentive to work and deal with the unemployment and poverty traps. Changes in National Insurance and improved rights for part-time workers might also form part of the picture.

Since his time at the Child Poverty Action Group and at the Low Pay Unit, when he stressed the need to use the sharp elbows of the middle class to improve the lot of the poor, Frank Field has always stressed the need to link the better-off and the poor to win political support for reform. Appeals to the poor alone will never get anywhere in an electoral democracy, he has argued – and this is even more the case now when the majority are well-off, comfortable and contented, though they may be increasingly insecure and worried about what the future holds for their children.

The need to combine self-interest with altruism is a key message from New Labour as it works to create a modern, fair and strong new Britain.

THE NEW DEAL

Gordon Brown first used the term New Deal in 1992 and his economic policies became a central part of Labour's manifesto commitments. The stress was on investing in growth and infrastructure. In his 22 May 1995 Mais lecture, Tony Blair similarly committed New Labour to a combination of low inflation and supply-side measures.

On crude figures, the welfare-to-work initiative could be expected to be a sure winner since it was being introduced when unemployment was falling anyway and when skill shortages were appearing (for example, in computing to prepare for the millenium reprogramming). In summer 1997, unemployment fell to a seventeen-year low at 1.5 million. Vacancies were at a peak. The Conservatives claimed that this showed they had left the economy in a very healthy state and that the welfare-to-work initiative would be a needless waste of taxpayers' money.

But the country will need another 1.4 million new jobs, 900,000 for men and 500,000 for women, to meet the projected increase in the UK's working population over the next eleven years (Trinder and Worsley 1997). And beneath the global figures, there remain disturbing trends which would need to be addressed by a dedicated unemployment policy. Two-fifths of the unemployed have been out of work for more than a year; one-fifth of working-age households have nobody working.

Labour's New Deal focuses on the long-term unemployed and the young. Pathfinder areas would begin the initiative in January 1998 with other areas following three months later. Partnership arrangements at local level, usually led by the Employment Agency, would seek to develop the most appropriate response for that locality. In areas of high unemployment, it was recognised that the public sector, notably local authorities, would need to be involved actively since these are often the main providers of jobs in those areas and have the infrastructure to develop new initiatives. Doubts remained about the willingness of business to get involved: some businesses, both large and small, expressed concern about the quality of some of the claimants who might be referred to them for work. In some areas, 30 per cent were said to have a criminal record or history of drug use (not at all surprising when the prevalence of these conditions in the age-group is considered). Employers were reluctant to take on the burden of training such workers, even with a job subsidy.

Dennis Snower commented that the New Deal policies play for high stakes. 'In a few years time these measures may have paid for themselves or turned out to be disastrously expensive; they may have reduced unemployment or spawned endless schemes that keep people out of the unemployment statistics without giving them jobs' (*Guardian*, 11 August 1997). The final assessment will depend on whether the New Deal is able to avoid what he labels 'three savage economic diseases'. These are 'public sector bulge' (increased public expenditure to create jobs); 'labyrinthitis' (too many small-scale overlapping or duplicating schemes adding up to very little); and 'labour compulsion' (forcing people into jobs for which they are unsuitable, unproductive and unmotivated).

But there are also doubts about relying on supply-side measures alone. Workless households are clustered in unemployment black-spots, like Tyne and Wear (29.5 per cent of households without work) Merseyside (28.9 per cent) Strathclyde (28.1 per cent) inner London (23.4 per cent) and South Yorkshire (23.3 per cent). Peter Robinson of the Centre for Economic Performance at LSE found that Britain's unemployed are increasingly better-skilled: their problem is that they live in areas where there is no demand for their labour (Hutton 1997: 30). And since high proportions in some areas may be lone mothers, however skilled they are, the need for child-care and flexible work arrangements coupled with housing costs, limit the opportunities to escape the unemployment trap.

'The point is that in a Tyne and Wear or Strathclyde, unemployment cannot be analysed in terms of labour market failure that can be addressed by job subsidies or training palliatives; such is the economic structure there are no jobs at any wage – and the price mechanism alone is not going to jump-start the area out of its decline' (ibid.). More wide-ranging and comprehensive policies are needed linking social policies across welfare reform, education, health, housing, social services, employment policy, environment, low pay and minimum wage legislation, incorporation of EU directives, urban and regional regeneration, and law and order, as the chapters in this book have made clear. The new government may be open to taking on this greater challenge as it attempts to deliver on its promise to make Britain a better place to live.

SOCIAL EXCLUSION

It is now common to talk about social exclusion rather than poverty in the welfare debate. At its best, this term reflects the republican, social solidaristic notions of French social philosophy, familiar to sociologists reared on Durkheim. Social exclusion has been seen by some writers as a term which can act as a counterweight to the underclass concept, with its assumptions about an associated tangle of behavioural pathologies promoted in frequent references to lone parents, crime and drugs. The difference is in the focus on structure and process rather than individual pathology and on the activities of those who do the excluding rather than on the excluded alone.

In European discourse the emphasis now 'is on the structural nature of a process which excludes part of the population from economic and social opportunities. The problem is not only one of disparities between the top and bottom of the social scale but also between those who have a place in society and those who are excluded' (CEC 1993).

Here, the replacement of poverty with exclusion is primarily a switch from static to dynamic analysis, focusing not merely on counting the poor but highlighting the processes which lead to exclusion. It directs attention away from the faults of the poor themselves – blaming the victim – towards the rest of society – we who are doing the excluding.

To attack social exclusion and worklessness, the 'Government will need to start thinking strategically about a range of policies that interlock at local and national level and whose aim is nothing less than rebuilding the structure of local economic activity and community life' (Will Hutton, writing in the *Observer* 21 September 1997).

The spatial dimension to social exclusion, the disconnection and growing gap between the mainstream and the discarded, requires intervention programmes to address wider issues than merely the personal characteristics of poor and unemployed individuals. The quality of the social environment in which people live their lives must form part of the focus of holistic, multi-sectoral, interconnected policies if real impact is to be seen. This requires new ways of working, cutting across the old single sectors through networking and forming alliances, co-ordinated at local level by one lead authority – most usefully probably this should be the local authority.

The taboo about talking about poverty and inequality, and thus perhaps opening a real debate about taxation and public finances, may have been lifted after the new government was stung by criticism led by Roy Hattersley (for example, writing in the *Guardian* 6 August 1997: 'Why Labour is wrong about income tax'). It was announced that a Cabinet Committee on Social Exclusion would be set up in autumn 1997, chaired by Tony Blair himself. It would consist of civil servants and representatives of business and charities but would decidedly not have any extra government money to spend.

The Unit would target action against poverty and social exclusion. Peter Mandelson, announcing this initiative in a Fabian Society lecture in August 1997, said that the exclusion of millions of citizens from mainstream economic and social life is 'the greatest challenge we face'. The new unit would co-ordinate policies across departments and develop a new anti-poverty programme, involving senior staff and ministers along with representatives of local authorities and voluntary organisations. This unit would build on the themes signalled in Mr Blair's first speech outside Parliament as Prime Minister when he visited the Aylesbury estate in south London in June 1997. Then he had promised empowerment not punishment, and a new bargain between us all as members of society.

It was not clear whether this new Social Exclusion Unit would be adequate to the scale of the problem to be addressed. There were hints that some saw exclusion as a marginal issue, represented only by the grossest forms of homelessness and long-term unemployment. There are problems with such an approach, principally that it ignores all the evidence of rising poverty and inequality over the 1980s, a result of changes in employment but also of cuts in the welfare state. Part of the problem is the inadequacy of levels of income support and the reduced range and standard of provision in many public (or semi-public) services. It ignores the situation of the working poor, resulting from low pay and casualisation of employment. Class as much if not more than behaviour lies at the root of many of these problems (Adonis and Pollard 1997). And in addition what happens is that if you deal generously with defined 'excluded groups', you risk alienating the hard-working not-quite-poor, who see it as inequitable that preferential treatment goes to their neighbours, whom they may see as unworthy of such care and attention. To offset such criticism and political backlash, programmes then have to include punitive elements so that the treatment the excluded receive remains less favourable than that of those poor and not well-off who are included (to use contemporary parlance) – that is, the old problem of the Poor Law in welfare continues to cast its long shadow.

To really recognise that prevention is better than cure would require attention not only to the *individual* at-risk factors that lead to poverty and exclusion but also to the *systematic* factors that lead to exclusion, like housing allocation policies, employment and education policies and health and social service differentials. In the longer term, the test of the new government will be whether it can tackle these. In much 'market social-ism' rhetoric, New Labour has accepted the le Grand thesis that public services replicate or exacerbate inequalities rather than reduce them (le Grand 1982). The strategy of attacking inequality through a redistribution of resources, through progressive taxation and public expenditure, has been discredited.

Now, there is some sense in New Labour's decision not to increase public expenditure thoughtlessly but to delay decisions until a comprehensive review of spending has been conducted. If the aim were to redistribute within existing budgets through radical shifts in priorities, much could be done to tackle poverty, inequality and unfairness. But this would require strong and bold government. Already by summer 1997, it was evident that attempts to shift resources from higher to further education and schools would run into resistance. Shifting resources from shires to cities, from teaching hospitals to public health, from Oxford and Cambridge to the ex-polytechnics, any such proposals would create a furious storm of opposition. What the government does not seem to have taken into account, however, in accepting the le Grand argument, is that his analysis omitted to consider the one area of social expenditure which emphatically does redistribute directly from better-off to badly-off – social security. Unless the social exclusion strategy includes an immediate review of the adequacy of income-support levels, the lives of the poor, especially those left untouched by welfare-to-work proposals – children, older persons, the disabled and sick – will continue to be a shaming indictment of an affluent society.

The question for a government aiming at a second term is, however, will people vote for this? Will enough of the electorate see it as in their interest to invest in the future, to make provision for old age and infirmity and insure against the risks of modern life, encourage social cohesion, reducing disaffection, crime and disorderly behaviour, and be prompted by compassion, by altruism, to help those worse off than themselves? In the war years, it was the way classes were thrown together in bomb shelters and in the London Underground, and through the evacuation policies and armed service, that made the middle and working classes aware of the deprivations of their fellow citizens. But in late twentieth-century Britain, the biggest divide of all is between the ordinary people in the middle and the poor. This divide has been exacerbated and consolidated by spatial segregation and broken any alliance there might have been. The alliance which supported Labour and the welfare state settlement for many postwar years was between the professional middle-classes and the organised labour movement. Public sector union militancy (among other things) damaged the alliance between these groups in the 1970s. The poor had benefited only if they could appear to be linked to either of these groups, as clients and culturally or socio-economically. Deindustrialisation and the collapse of the old manual working-class broke the bridge between the poor and these groups socially and politically. Labour could choose to represent the poor and a few of their liberal middle class advocates (and lose elections) or it had to opt to represent the new 'hard-working, ordinary people', made up of the children of the old respectable working class, who through social mobility and educational opportunity, and a general increase in material income, had become comfortably off. Social policy was the glue which had welded together the old social contract. The reshaping of the class structure undermined this politial alliance and called for a new one to be invented. This was what the New Labour project aimed to do.

The potential to deal with social problems has never been greater. Since the Second World war, global economic wealth has increased sevenfold and average incomes have tripled (Watkins 1995: 1). When we compare childhoods of the 1940s and 1950s with the comforts (and waste) of today, there is simply no comparison. As the Institute for Fiscal Studies has pointed out, there is no inevitability about the conclusion that we cannot afford better public services – this is primarily a matter of political choice. But it is a choice which needs to be introduced into public debate through a period of education and dialogue.

The New Deal idea is important. It represents a new bargain, a new arrangement or agreement between government and people and between groups in society. A new political settlement is being constructed. The spoils will be shared out differently in future. New partnerships will include business at the centre and all parties will have new rights and duties.

In this new contract, the economy will be left to run itself with minimal interference from government. Government's focus is on education and welfare reform, making people more employable and suited to the new jobs that the free economy will generate. A middle way which is neither old Left nor new Right is the ambition.

The aim is to conquer unemployment with active supply-side measures and to transform the welfare state to make it both more effective and more affordable. It is accepted that it is no longer possible to have Keynesianism in one country. To aim at full employment is over-ambitious. Rather the stress is on long-term investment and improving workers' skills.

SOCIAL JUSTICE AND A FLEXIBLE MARKET – RECONCILING THE IRRECONCILABLE?

The new Labour government quickly moved to promote, at home, in Europe and beyond, its belief that all countries need the flexibility without which a dynamic market cannot function well and stimulate new jobs. But in addition, they said, it was the responsibility of government to guarantee 'flexibility-plus' i.e. flexibility plus higher skills and higher standards in schools and colleges; plus partnership with business to raise investment in infrastructure, science and research and to back small firms; plus an imaginative welfare-to-work programme to put the long-term unemployed back to work; plus minimum standards of fair treatment at the workplace; plus new leadership in Europe (Peter Mandelson, Minister without Portfolio in the new Labour government writing in the *Guardian*, 15 August 1997).

Tony Blair has said that the basic principles of New Labour are those that have always been those of the Labour Party – justice and progress. But these will be applied in a different way for the modern world – stressing education, skills, technology, design and invention, and the role of small business. This will require different attitudes and a different role for the state. The aim is to extend educational opportunity to all young people. This is at the heart of modern radicalism (*Channel 4 News* 29 April, interview with Jon Snow). New Labour, he said, is born of conviction. But you don't put eighteen years right in eighteen days. The new government would restore faith in politics and the idea that government can do something to assist people. There would be a fresh start characterised by decency, purpose and vision.

Had red-blooded socialism been watered down too much? Not at all said Lord Callaghan (the last Old Labour Prime Minister). The very thinness of the promises is an advantage. If Labour can deliver on these, it will restore trust in the system – this is the crucial first step. Once people are convinced that they can trust the Labour Party, then this will colour the experience of a generation for the rest of their lives (BBC1 *Election Report* 2 May 1997).

It is true that if Labour can restore respect for democratically-elected government, they will have performed an important service for the country. Distrust of the Conservatives had spread from that one party to the whole of government and authority in general in an alarming way throughout the late 1980s and 1990s. In 1991, in *The Poll Tax: Flagship or Folly?* I argued that the poll tax was seen as arbitrary, chaotic and unjust, and that this was part of its political purpose. 'Those adversely affected by it, especially the swathe of new young voters, were to be completely turned away from the idea that it is possible to have fair, decent, well-organised responsible public services, and from the idea that it is possible to influence government through following the normal procedures of discussion and complaint' (MacGregor 1991: 126). As Neal Ascherson remarked, 'the poll tax was part of an invitation to stay out of politics and riot instead – as an "underclass" should' (*The Independent on Sunday*, 26 July 1992). The campaign against the poll tax united the poor and the prosperous against a bad law and was a key moment in the turning away of British people from the road down which Thatcherism was leading. It marked the turning of the tide which New Labour recognised and responded to.

Restoring trust is essential but welfare is Labour's big social policy test. New Labour believes that if it can crack the welfare problem, it will divest itself once and for all of its tag as the party of the underdog and establish control of the political centre-ground, ushering in at least a second and maybe a third term in office.

Labour has now successfully re-presented itself as the party of the majority not the party of minorities. Its task in government will be to maintain this image if it is to win its much coveted second term and establish itself as the natural party of government for a generation of voters. Tony Blair's success has been to put into practice what had long been argued as necessary since *Must Labour Lose* was published in the late 1950s (Abrams and Rose 1960). New Labour's advisor, Philip Gould extended this analysis in the mid-1980s.

Gould's account argued that, in the 1980s, Labour had lost the allegiance of skilled workers, particularly in the South and Midlands, partly as a result of Mrs Thatcher's popular policies of tax cuts and sale of council houses. The Labour party was seen as old-fashioned, a party of minorities and the poor, and out of touch with ordinary people's aspirations, dominated by the trade unions and vulnerable to extremists. The test and the key to success was to represent Labour as modern, competent, responsible and representative of the aspirations of the upwardly mobile (Anderson and Mann 1997).

The collapse of the old working-class and its divide into those who have escaped to relatively comfortable surroundings (albeit hanging on by their fingernails to this security and through dint of hard work and wives' earnings) and those left behind in the decaying areas of social housing is the key fact of contemporary social politics.

Social problems concentrate in areas to which a previous generation of working-class residents had been displaced in the slum clearance programmes of the post-war years. Now with changes in housing policy, which have led to seven in ten houses being owner-occupied or being bought with a mortgage, the remaining 30 per cent of the population, living in what is now known as social housing, are where many social problems appear to be found. These disadvantaged include lone mothers with children, rehoused homeless families, mentally ill people resettled in the community, migrants and refugees, all living in close proximity in areas with high rates of unemployment and poverty.

In the United States, liberal (social democratic) sociologists like Elliott Currie and especially William Julius Wilson have analysed the collapse of communities like these. Lack of jobs is fundamental. Currie identified shrinking employment opportunities and blasted prospects for young people with the destruction of the cohesion of entire neighbourhoods (Currie 1993: 97). In his recent book *When Work Disappears*, W.J. Wilson describes, from detailed studies conducted in Chicago, how the drugs economy moves into the vacuum left by the disappearance of regular formal employment (Wilson 1996). The central co-ordinates of social life – time and space – are patterned differently in jobless neighbourhoods compared to those more closely linked into the dominant capitalist-industrial economy. In describing how these jobless neighbourhoods had gone down, increases in drug trafficking and drug consumption figured large in residents' narratives. Wilson comments 'the decline in legitimate employment opportunities among inner-city residents has increased incentives to sell drugs' (op. cit.: 21). He argues that it is not poverty *per se* which causes these social problems but the changes in social organisation (values and habits) that go along with extensive joblessness (long-term and high rates of unemployment in a given neighbourhood).

Surely this is a specifically American problem? Could Britain inherit the American nightmare? At one point it was thought not, because of the existence of our more extensive welfare state. But now people are beginning to wonder. If moves to restrict income support to young men are extended further, the driving out into the underground economy seen in American cities could be replicated here.

It is trends like these which have led to a change in language from talking about poverty to talking about social exclusion. The stress is on the growing gap between the poor and the rest – no longer simply a smooth hierarchy of disadvantage and a shared if contested social order.

Galbraith has characterised the culture which allows gross poverty and alienation to co-exist with unprecendented levels of affluence as the culture of contentment (Galbraith 1992). The economically and socially fortunate are now a majority of those who actually vote. They are the contented *electoral* majority (in Britain, as in America, the disaffected don't vote). They have developed a shared view that the state is a burden but not in those areas from which they benefit, like medical care, or which they support, like expenditure on police or the military. They are no longer shocked by recitations of the numbers living in poverty or of growing inequality of income and wealth. Monetary policy has replaced fiscal policy as the main means of regulating the economy.

But taken-for-granted assumptions about progress and economic success have been proved wrong. It cannot be assumed that economic growth will naturally and easily eliminate poverty, preventable disease and urban squalor. Charity and growth are not enough. The existing processes of economic development cause poverty at the same time that they generate wealth. A new social policy is needed to counter the shared assumption of post-war social policy – of both Right and Left – that economic growth is the unchallenged priority of all governments and that social problems may be dealt with in a simple way either through the trickle-down effect or by redistributing the fruits of economic growth. Growth *per se* does not achieve social objectives. Current patterns of growth generate many of the most severe problems, including severe threats to the environment: this raises questions about how long such growth is sustainable. Growth alone has not reduced poverty and inequality. Growth alone has not cut unemployment (Jacobs 1996).

Labour have identified the key groups who are in poverty, lacking the means to participate in the economic, social, cultural and political life of Britain: these they see as, in particular, the five million people in workless homes; the three million on the nation's 1,300 worst council estates; the 150,000 homeless families and the 100,000 children not attending school. These are to be the priority groups on whom the new Social Exclusion Unit will focus its attention. The bottom-line measure of the government's performance then in the area of social policy will be its ability to improve the quality of life of these people, the poorest of the poor. More money would be available – but only 'when economic circumstances and the re-ordering of public expenditure make this possible'. The danger with Labour's policies is that they are at once too timid and too optimistic: they exaggerate 'the numbers that can be taken off welfare, exaggerating the savings that such programmes will make, and ignoring the importance of social security as a strategy for combating poverty' (*Guardian* editorial, 15 August 1997). Without a commitment to realistically adequate levels of income support, especially for those who cannot work (children, the sick, disabled and pensioners) and without restoring a commitment to redistribution as part of its *raison d'être*, New Labour's endeavour to produce a socially just and caring society will be drowned by the contradictory goal to create a modern meritocratic society.

'In a modern welfare state' said the Christian Socialist Tony Blair in his speech to the TUC annual conference in 1997, 'the role of government is not necessarily to provide all social provision but to organise and regulate it most efficiently and fairly'. Some feared this indicated that the hidden plan was to replace state provision by private or other forms of insurance. And with what consequences for inequality and poverty?

At the same conference, the Archbishop of Canterbury spoke of the rights of workers, evoking memories of a previous Archbishop, the 'people's Archbishop' – William Temple, who had played a large part in the construction of the postwar welfare state, (Temple was the author of *Christianity and the Social Order*, a Penguin Special which sold 139,000 copies in 1942, setting out Christian Socialist ideas). In a not quite so revolutionary (but in context a surprisingly radical) speech, Carey argued that in 1997 workers should have a say in the decisions that affect their lives. They have a right to be represented. Bitter experience has taught us, he said, that market forces make good servants but bad masters. Power has shifted too far towards the employers in current arrangements, he said. Much has been made of the importance of restraining taxation and public spending, he added, but these are not necessities but choices that we have made. The key point is that there is a choice.

The 1997 TUC conference exemplified the new politics of partnership, the new alliances and consensus which is being built up. The TUC was addressed by Tony Blair as Prime Minister, the Archbishop of Canterbury, and by Adair Turner of the CBI. The new inclusivity was fully embraced by the new unionism of TUC General Secretary John Monks – would it be reciprocated?

FULFILLING THE ASPIRATIONS OF THE MAJORITY OF PEOPLE IN A MODERN WORLD?

In May 1997, the rhetoric of economic success and social cohesion appealed to many people genuinely wanting a change. The election victory was won on a wave of good will towards New Labour. Many people want to see improved public services, especially in education and health, a society whose culture is restored with moves towards life-long learning, enhanced opportunities and more equitable distribution of resources, more supportive community structures and renewed concern for the development of young people, caring for the vulnerable and a revived sense of responsibility among all citizens. Labour has a great opportunity here which it must not squander. Many want them to succeed and want to be able to join in this new challenge and to make their contribution. They don't want to be blamed, belittled, chastised and locked out of the very social partnership which is supposed to be the hallmark of New Labour. They don't want genuinely well-meant constructive criticism to be read as cynicism and 'not being one of us'. Labour's ability to build a genuinely participative and inclusive society, in which opportunities are equitably distributed and in which a revived sense of the value of public service and the public good flows from greater empowerment and decentralisation, will be the core test of their achievement and on which they will be judged at the next election. Facing up to the huge problems which they have inherited, and which are mapped out in the chapters of this book, will be a great task. A few mistakes will be forgiven but real change will be expected. The public services have decayed and the social infrastructure weakened (even collapsed) in some places. These problems cannot be solved by warm words alone.

The government began well with enthusiasm and a responsiveness to the wellsprings of shared, commonsense, sometimes radical, proposals, which had been suppressed for so many years under the dogmatic Thatcher–Major governments. The civil service were energetic in their support and willing to help in putting these ideas into practice. But at some point, the difficult issue of resourcing the key human services will have to be addressed. Raiding the social security budget may turn out not to be the answer. Other sources of revenue will need to be identified, in addition to the National Lottery and one-off windfall taxes. The government will need to develop a project of political education to match its projects of renewal and reorganisation, one which encourages the British people as a whole to face up to the issue of how to pay for welfare and the tough choices they have to make between ever-more private consumption and better services and more security.

> Labour in 1945 combined idealism and practicality in equal measure to lead a national crusade for a Britain based on social justice, equality of opportunity and social solidarity ... it set up the pride and joy of British socialism – the National Health Service. What is more, at the end of its period in office, the Labour government secured the largest vote ever achieved by the Party ... The lesson of 1945 should be clear: democratic socialism can be both practical and popular.

So wrote Tony Blair in the foreword to Austin Mitchell's *Election '45* (Mitchell 1995). These principles guide hopes for a new Labour government fifty years later. And at the next General Election, these old principles will be the ones by which Labour in office will be judged, when the people come once again to make their choice.

REFERENCES

Abrams, M. and Rose, R. (1960) *Must Labour Lose*, Harmondsworth: Penguin.
Adonis, A. and Pollard, S. (1997) *A Class Act*, London: Hamish Hamilton.
Alcock, P., David, M., Phillips, M., and Slipman, S. (1994) 'Commentaries', in *Underclass: the Crisis Deepens*, by C. Murray, London: IEA.

Anderson, P. and Mann, N. (1997) *Safety First*, London: Granta.

Brittan, S. (1997) 'Better than you deserve', *Financial Times*, May 3.

Brown, G. (1997) 'Why Labour is still loyal to the poor', *Guardian*, 2 August.

Campbell, B. (1993) *Goliath: Britain's Dangerous Places*, London: Methuen.

CEC (Commission of the European Community) (1993) *European Green Paper on Social Policy*, CE 81 93 292 EN C.

Currie, E. (1993) *Reckoning: Drugs, the Cities and the American Future*, New York: Hill and Wang.

Field, F. (1989) *Losing Out: The Emergence of Britain's Underclass*, Oxford: Basil Blackwell.

Galbraith, J. K. (1992) *The Culture of Contentment*, London: Penguin.

Glazer, N. (1995) 'Making work work: welfare reform in the 1990s', in D.S. Nightingale and R.H.Haveman (eds) *The Work Alternative: Welfare Reform and the Realities of the Job Market*, Washington: Urban Institute Press.

Hutton, W. (1997) 'Spend to save welfare and to make work', *Observer*, 21 September.

Katz, M.B. (ed.) (1993) *The 'Underclass' Debate: views from history*, Princeton, NJ: Princeton University Press.

Jacobs, M. (1996) *The Politics of the Real World*, written and edited for The Real World Coalition, London: Earthscan.

King, D. (1995) *Actively Seeking Work? The Politics of Unemployment and Welfare Policy in the United States and Great Britain*, Chicago and London: University of Chicago Press.

le Grand, J. (1982) *The Strategy of Equality*, London: George Allen and Unwin.

MacGregor, S. (1991) *The Poll Tax: Flagship or Folly?*, Manchester: Centre for Local Economic Strategies.

Mead, L. (1992) *The New Politics of Poverty: the Nonworking Poor in America*, New York: Basic Books.

Mitchell, A. (1995) *Election '45: reflections on the revolution in Britain*, London: Fabian Society.

Morris, L. (1994) *Dangerous Classes: the Underclass and Social Citizenship*, London and New York: Routledge.

Piven, F. (1995) 'Foreword' to *Words of Welfare*, by S.F. Schram, Minneapolis/London: University of Minnesota Press.

SRA (Social Research Association) (1997) 'Polls and the General Election' Seminar 10 July, London.

Trinder, C. and Worsley, R. (1997) *Carnegie UK Trust Report*, London: Carnegie Trust.

Watkins, K. (1995) *The Oxfam Poverty Report*, Oxford: Oxfam, UK and Ireland.

Wilson, W. J. (1996) *When Work Disappears: the World of the New Urban Poor*, New York: Alfred A Knopf.

Index

Abrams, M. 266–7
accountability 30–1, 35, 36, 187, 191; Wales 233
Adam Smith Institute 157–8
Adelman, P. 20
Adonis, A. 262
ADSS 113, 117
advance corporation tax 52
Agenda 21 186, 192
air-traffic control 9
Aitken, Jonathan 131
Alcock, P. 254
Allied Medicare 106
Analysis 49
Anderson, P. 267
Annual Tax Contract 47–8
Apple, M. 76
Appropriate Personal Pension (APP) 156, 163, 164, 165, 166
Archbishops' Commission 149
Armstrong, Hilary 36
Ascherson, Neal 266
Ashdown, Paddy 2, 7, 49
Ashley, Lord 114
Association of Directors of Social Services 113, 117
asthma 185
Audit Commission 31, 35; criminal justice 170, 175, 176; performance indicators 25; residential homes 108–9
Australia 150, 254, 255

Baker, Kenneth 78
Balchin, B. 30

Baldwin, P. 40
Ball, S.J. 75
Balloch, S. 112, 117
Balls, Ed 13
Bank of England 51, 71
Bar-Hillel, M. 134
Barber, Michael 85
Barclay brothers 203
Basic Pension Guarantee 157, 158
Basic Pension Plus 157–8, 163
Batchelor, C. 188
Bayley, Hugh 95, 101
BBC Scotland 204
Bebbington, A.C. 108
Beckett, Margaret 158
Bell, Martin 2, 8, 9, 12
benefits *see* social security benefits
Benefits Agency 25, 26, 27
Benn, Tony 240
Beresford, P. 116
Beyond Pension Plus (Butler) 158
Birmingham Six 174
Birrell, D. 217
Black Report 96
Blackaby, D. 235
Blacks: and social services 118
Blackstone, Baroness Tessa 81, 85
Blair, Tony: criminal justice 170, 171; dependency culture 252–3; economic policy 259; education 74, 236; election as leader 199; employment 64–5, 66, 67, 69–70; environmental issues 191–2; General Election campaign 1–2, 5, 7, 11–12, 14; justice and

progress 265–6; Labour Party reforms 19–20, 21; lessons of 1945 271; modernisation 94–5; NHS 99, 100; one nation 9–10, 258; pensions 158, 163; poverty and social security 148; Scotland 8, 201, 208; social exclusion 262; at TUC conference 269, 270; United States contacts 13
Blunkett, David 66, 85–6
BNA 106
Boateng, Paul 101, 113, 114, 115
Booth, Cherie 2, 6
Borders Television 204
Borrie, Sir Gordon 81
Bottomley, Virginia 93
Bow Group 158
Bowden, Sir Anthony 4–5
BPG 157, 158
BPP 157–8, 163
Brake, M. 171
Brand, D. 116
Brand, Jack 195, 197
Bridgewater case 174
Brindle, D. 99
Britain Divided (Child Poverty Action Group) 149
British Social Attitudes Survey 137, 140, 141
Brittan, S. 53, 250
Brook, L. 140, 141
Brown, Alice 195
Brown, Gordon: Bank of England 71; employment 65–6, 67; enabling state 20–1; equality of opportunity 145, 252; local government funding 112; modernisation 94–5; New Deal 259; NHS 103, 104; public expenditure 49; Scottish base 199; taxation 3, 9, 45, 51, 53, 67, 253–4; television debate 50; United States contacts 13
Brown, Michael 4–5
Bruce, Malcolm 50
Brummer, Alex 52
BSE 184, 185
budget: environmental issues 187–8, 189; pensions 164–5;

poverty and social security 150, 151; taxation 51–2
Building Societies Act 1986 123
Bulger, Jamie 171, 174
Burchardt, T. 54
bureaucracy 25, 27; education 76; NHS 99, 100, 102, 103
Busch, A. 14
Bush, George 178
businessmen 251–2
Butcher, T. 24, 34
Butler, D. 16, 92
Butler, Eamonn 157–8
Bynoe, I. 34

Cabinet Committee on Social Exclusion 262
Caesar, J. 14
Callaghan, James 78, 266
Calpin, D. 36
Campbell, Bea 256
Campbell, K. 165
Canada 254, 255, 257
CAP 185, 188, 228
capital receipts 135, 136
Care Alternatives 106
care in the community *see* community care
carers 111, 115, 159
Carey, George 269–70
Carlile, Alex 176
cars 181–2, 185, 187
Carter, Jimmy 255
Carter, N. 183
Castle, Barbara 161, 162
Catholic Bishops' Report on poverty and educational failure 149
CCBI 9, 49–50, 139, 148–9, 152
CCETSW 116
CCT 26, 31–2, 35, 136, 199
CEC 261
Central Statistical Office 110
centralisation: education 79–80
Channel 4 News 265
Charter of Local Self-Government 36
Charter Mark 33
charterism *see* Citizen's Charter

child benefit 224, 258
Child Poverty Action Group 149
Child Support Act 142
Child Support Agency 26, 27
childcare 145, 147
children: social exclusion 262;
    social services 107, 109, 111, 113
Children Act 1989 109
Children's Services Plans 109
choice 21, 244; education 79, 83;
    NHS 100; pensions 156; social
    services 111
Chomsky, N. 71
Christian Socialism 269–70
Christianity and the Social Order
    (Temple) 269–70
Chubb, J. 75
Church, C.H. 60
Church Action on Poverty 149
churches 66–7, 198
Citizen's Charter 17, 25, 26–7; and
    education 79; party policies 33–4
citizens' juries 34
citizenship 34, 36, 190, 243, 244
citizenship pension 159
Clarke, Kenneth 43, 50, 92, 238
Clarke, M. 30
class 221, 262, 264
class sizes 85, 88
Clifton-Brown, Geoffrey 158
climate change 192
Clinton, Bill 13–14, 251, 253, 255
closed circuit TV 169
Clynes, J.R. 15
Commission of the European
    Community 261
Commission on Social Justice
    81–2, 244; criminal justice 171;
    environmental issues 191; equal
    opportunities 118; health policy
    93–4; pensions 159–60, 161,
    162–3; poverty and social
    security 143–4, 145, 151; social
    services 111–12
Common Agricultural Policy 185,
    188, 228
communitarianism 21
community care 92–3, 100, 107,
    111; funding 113–14

Community Care Alliance 112
Community Care (Direct
    Payments) Act 1996 111, 116
community initiative 30
Community Programme 72
community relations 216, 218–20
community safety orders 169
competition 21, 25, 31–2, 75–6
compulsory competitive tendering
    26, 31–2, 35, 136, 199
conflict 216, 218
Connolly, M. 216
Conservative Party: criminal
    justice 168, 169–70, 171, 172,
    172–5, 177–8; customer
    orientation 33–4; distrust 266;
    education 74–5, 77–80, 83–4, 88;
    election campaign 1–13, 248;
    election results 12–13, 15–16,
    250; employment 57, 58–9, 60–4,
    66–9, 70–1; environmental issues
    181–3, 185–6, 191; Europe 60;
    health 95, 243; housing 122, 123,
    125–35; local authorities 28–31;
    management and efficiency
    31–2; mental health 118; NHS
    91–3, 96, 98–100; Northern
    Ireland 219; pensions 155–8,
    163, 164, 165; poverty and social
    security 142–3, 146, 147–8;
    problems 18–19; Scotland 194–5,
    197, 198, 199–200, 201–2, 208,
    209, 211, 212; social policy
    17–18; social services 106–11;
    taxation 46–7, 48–9, 53; Ulster
    Unionist Party 216; values 21,
    244; Wales 238–9, 245; welfare
    delivery 24–8, 34; welfare-to-
    work 257, 259
Constitution Unit 198
constitutional issues 195–7, 198,
    252; Northern Ireland 221, 222;
    see also decentralisation;
    devolution; proportional
    representation
consumer democracy 190
consumerism 21, 24, 34, 35, 244
contract culture 31
contracting-out 25–6, 91

The Convention on Climate Change 192
Convention of Scottish Local Authorities 198
Cook, Robin 66
corruption *see* sleaze
Council of Churches for Britain and Ireland 9, 49–50, 139, 148–9, 152
Council of Europe 36
council housing *see* social housing
Cowell, D. 176
Cowling, M. 15
Crawford, M. 162
criminal justice 168–9, 177–9; Conservative Party 172–5; election campaign 170–2; party policies 169–70; stakeholder debates 175–7
Criminal Justice Acts 175
Crosland, Anthony 44, 77, 80
CSJ *see* Commission on Social Justice
Currie, Edwina 163
Currie, Elliott 267
Curtice, John 200
customer orientation 25, 26–7, 28; party policies 33–4
Cutler, T. 35

Dahrendorf Report 40, 43
Daily Express 8, 163
Daily Mail 8, 174
Daily Record 203
Daily Telegraph 5, 8, 13; health 91, 98, 99, 104; pensions 163
Dale, R. 76
David, M.E. 76, 77, 78
Davies, A.J. 20
Davies, B. 164
Davies, Sir Peter 150, 252
Davies, Ron 234, 240–1
Deakin, N. 43
Dearing report 86–7, 88
Dearing, Sir Ron 83
decentralisation 36, 189, 190, 251
Deem, R. 76
democracy 181, 190–1
democratic deficit 36

democratic renewal 36
Democratic Unionist Party 220, 221, 222
demographic timebomb 161–2
Denmark 255
Department for Education and Employment (DfEE) 27, 83, 86, 88
Department of the Environment 103, 130
Department of Health 32, 95–6, 101, 106, 108, 109, 118
Department of Health and Social Security 161
Department of Social Security 27, 131, 139, 164
dependency 152; Conservative Party 142, 238; Labour Party 144, 146, 239, 242, 252–3
deregulation 21; education 75; financial sector 123, 124; labour market 57, 63–5
Development Board for Rural Wales 233
devolution 189, 191, 251; Scotland 195, 197, 198, 199, 200, 201, 208, 209, 212; Wales 233, 236, 237, 241, 245–6
Dewar, Donald 209, 212
Diana, Princess of Wales 6
Dilnot, Andrew 44, 48, 49–50, 53
Disability Income Scheme 224
disabled people: social exclusion 262; social services 114, 118; welfare-to-work 150, 253
discrimination 218
Ditch, J. 216, 217
divorce: pension sharing 163, 164
Dobbs, Michael 1
Dobson, Frank 101–2, 103
Dorrell, Stephen 98, 106
Downes, D. 168–9, 173
Downey, R. 114
Downey report 65
Downey, Sir Gordon 4
drugs 202, 267–8
DSS 27, 131, 139, 164
DUP 220, 221, 222
Dwelly, T. 136

E coli 185
Eaglesham, J. 164
Earth Summit II Conference 192
eco-labelling 188, 190
Economist, The 252
economy 3, 4, 47; Conservative
  policy 17; and environmental
  issues 187; growth 268–9;
  Labour policy 152, 259;
  Northern Ireland 224, 226–7;
  Wales 235
education 74–5, 88; consensus
  politics 77–8; Conservative
  government 78–80; in election
  campaign 83–4; expenditure 263;
  funding 51; international context
  75–7; Labour policy 80–3, 252,
  254; Liberal Democrats 47; local
  authority role 27, 29–30;
  Northern Ireland 218, 220;
  performance indicators 33–4, 35;
  public attitudes 140, 248;
  Scotland 197, 200, 201; Scottish
  National Party policy 202;
  Wales 235, 236, 238
Education Act 1944 77, 78
Education Act 1992 79, 82
Education Action Zones 86
Education Development Plans 86
Education Reform Act 1988 26, 77,
  78–9
Education Standards Commission
  35
effectiveness: criminal justice 175
efficiency 21, 31–2, 219; criminal
  justice 175; NHS 100
EFILWC 72
elderly: burden on working
  population 156, 157, 161–2; fear
  of crime 172; social exclusion
  262; social security 223–4; social
  services 109–11, 113, 114
Election '45 (Mitchell) 271
election campaign 1–13; American
  influences 13–14; Labour Party
  control 250; Scotland 203–8,
  212–13; Wales 239–40
election manifestos *see* manifestos
Elliott, Larry 126

employment 56; and education
  81–3; in election campaign 68;
  and environmental taxation 191;
  Labour policy 253, 254;
  Northern Ireland 218, 220, 224;
  party policies 57, 58; Plaid
  Cymru plans 237; *see also*
  unemployment
Employment Agency 259
Employment Service 25, 26, 27
empowerment 116
energy policy 181, 183–4, 192;
  Labour Party 185, 187–8
enterprise culture 156
Environment Agency 181, 182, 183
environmental issues 181; the
  future 189–92; Labour Party in
  government 187–9; party
  policies 184–7; and privatisation
  181–3
equality 21, 244; on Green agenda
  188; Northern Ireland 218–20,
  226–8; *see also* inequality
equality of opportunity 145, 152,
  252; education 77–8, 80–3, 88;
  Northern Ireland 218; social
  services 118
equality proofing 218, 219
ERA 26, 77, 78–9
ERES 235
ERM 171, 223
ethnicity 77, 78, 80
European Convention of Human
  Rights 251
European Foundation for the
  Improvement of Living and
  Working Conditions 72
European Monetary Union 10,
  70–1
European, The 203
European Union 58–60, 64–9;
  Commission 261; Conservative
  Party 4, 10–11, 63, 71, 248;
  environmental issues 187, 188;
  Labour Party 62, 69–70, 254;
  Plaid Cymru 237; Scottish
  National Party 195
Evans, B. 19
Evening Standard 8

Excellence in Schools (Department for Education and Employment) 85–6
Exchange Rate Mechanism 171, 223

Fabian Society 94
fair employment 220, 226–7
Fair Employment Act 1976 218
Faith in the City (Church of England Archbishops' Commission) 149
Family Allowances 216–17
farmers 227–8
Farnham, D. 24
Fayed al Mohamed 4
federalism 237
Field, Frank 144–5, 149–50, 258–9; pensions 160–1, 162–3, 164, 166
Financial Management Initiative 25
Financial Times 6; Budget 151; health 101, 102; pensions 162, 164, 165; taxation 9; transport 187
Finch, J. 108
Finn, D. 150
Fitz, J. 76
flexibility 21, 265; labour market 62, 64–5, 69–70
flexibility plus 62, 66, 265
food labelling 190
food safety 181, 183–4, 185, 192
Foote, G. 20–1
Ford, Gerald 255
Ford, J. 126
Forrest, R. 128
Forsyth, Frederick 8
Forsyth, Michael 199–200, 209, 212
Fortune Account, The (Adam Smith Institute) 157–8
Foster, Derek 31, 36
foundation schools 29
France 58, 59, 255
fraud 62, 102–3, 148, 238
freedom of information 191
Friends of the Earth (FOE) 184, 191
fuel: VAT 188

funded pension schemes 156, 160, 162
funding *see* private sector; public expenditure
Funding Agency for Schools 29
further education 83, 86–7
Further and Higher Education Act 1992 79

Galbraith, J.K. 58, 268
Gardiner, George 7
Garner, R. 182
gazumping 132, 134
gender issues 80, 190, 192; education 74–5, 77, 78; Scottish Parliament 198
General Elections 15–16; Scotland 194–5, 209, 210–11; Wales 239
General Social Services Council 115–16
Germany 58, 59
Gewirtz, S. 76
Glatter, R. 76
Glazer, Nat 256
Glennerster, H. 42
globalisation 140
Gloucestershire 114
Golsborough 106
Goodman, A. 139
Gould, Philip 13, 267
Governance of Britain Act 36
GP fundholding 32, 92, 98, 102, 199, 236
Grampian Television 204
grant-maintained schools (GMS) 29, 31, 79
Green Party 189, 190
green perspective *see* environmental issues
Greenberg, Stan 13
Greer, Ian 4
Greer, P. 26
Griffiths, J. 188
Griffiths, R. 28
GSSC 115–16
Guardian: Conservative Party 11; criminal justice 173, 176, 177, 178; equality of opportunity debate 145; flexibility plus 265;

health 91, 98, 99, 102, 103, 104;
home care services 114; home
ownership 126; Labour's first
100 days 251; Media Watch 170;
New Deal 253, 260; opinion
polls 22; poverty and social
security 148, 151; social
exclusion 262, 269
Guildford Four 174
Gummer, John 186
Guthrie, J. 165

Hain, Peter 241
Hale, C. 171
Hamilton, Christine 6
Hamilton, Neil 2, 4–5, 7–9, 12
Hamilton, Thomas 174
Hanna, Eamon 221
Hanna, Vincent 50
Harden, I. 26
Harding, T. 116
Harman, Harriet 257
Harper, K. 182, 183
Hattersley, Roy 145, 244, 262
Hayek, Friedrich von 158
Hayman, David 208
HBAI 139
health 184, 185; inequality 94,
95–6, 104; public attitudes 140,
248; see also National Health
Service
Health Action Zones 103
Health Education Council 96
Health of the Nation, The
(Department of Health) 95–6
Health Quality Commission 35
Herald, The 204
herbicides 192
Herman, E. 71
Hewitt, Patricia 81
higher education 79, 80, 83, 87–8
Higher Education in the Learning
Society (Dearing Report) 87
Hills, J. 54, 107, 139
Hinchcliffe, David 112
Hinds, B. 218
Hirst, Sir Michael 7, 208
Hobsbawm, Eric 49
Holtham, G. 188, 191

home care services 106, 114
Home Office 175
home ownership 122–7, 132, 133–4
homelessness 135, 136, 262; and
crime 170, 177
Hood, C. 25
Hoover, K. 142
Horam, John 10
Horton, S. 24
Hough, Mike 178
house building 125
house prices 123, 124
Households Below Average
Income 139
housing 16, 121–2, 140, 267; green
perspective 181, 183–4, 185;
party policies 132–7, 202;
Scotland 197, 199, 200, 201; see
also social housing
Housing Act 1980 123, 127
Housing Act 1988 26, 128–9
Housing Action Trusts 27, 31
Housing Association Grants 130
housing associations 27, 31, 130, 199
housing benefit 122, 129–32, 224
Howard, Michael 173, 176, 178
Howarth, Alan 240
Howells, David 85
Howells, Kim 240
Hughes, J. 218
Hughes, M. 76
Hughes, Roy 240
hunting 184
Hutson, N. 220
Hutson, S. 131
Hutton, Will 40, 260, 261
hypothecation 47

identity cards 169
IFS see Institute for Fiscal
Studies
income support 262, 263, 269
income tax 45–6, 57
independence: Scotland 195,
197, 203
Independent 3, 5, 64, 66, 99, 100
Independent on Sunday 68, 266
individual responsibility 21, 107,
108, 142, 186

Inequalities in Health (Health Education Council) 96
inequality 17, 49, 139–46, 152–3, 249; Council of Churches report 9; and crime 170; health 94, 95–6, 104; Northern Ireland 216, 220; and public transport 183; and social exclusion 262, 263, *see also* equality
Institute of Economic Affairs 177
Institute for Fiscal Studies: budget analysis 151; choice 264; in election campaign 9, 49–50; income tax 47; NHS funding 102; public expenditure crisis 43
Institute for Public Policy Research (IPPR) 34, 81, 112, 191
Institute for Study and Treatment of Delinquency (ISTD) 175, 176
internal market 32, 92, 93, 95, 102; Wales 234, 235–6
Irish News, The 221
Irvine, Lord 1, 199
Istance, D. 235
Italy 59
ITV 204

Jacobs, M. 39, 269
Jenkins, Roy 173
Jobseeker's Allowance 58, 63, 224
Johnson, P. 49–50
Jones, G. 163
Jones, H. 18
Jones, Nicholas 4, 21
Jones, Peter 199
Joseph Rowntree Foundation 39, 110
Jowell, Tessa 101, 104

Katz, M.B. 254
Kavanagh, D. 16, 92
Kellas, James 198
Kellner, P. 134, 136
Kelly, A. 108
Kelly, G. 146
Kempson, E. 107, 139
Kennedy, Helena 83
Kennedy report 86–7

King, Anthony 12, 16
King, Desmond 256–7
Kinnock, Neil 19, 20, 240–1
Kirkwood, Archie 150
Knox, C. 218

labour market 57, 60, 70, 140; and Commission on Social Justice 81–2
Labour Party: criminal justice 168, 169–70, 171–2, 177–8, 179; customer orientation 33–4; education 74, 78, 80–3, 84–8; election campaign 1–14, 248; election results 12–13, 15–16, 250; employment 57, 58, 59, 60–4, 65–71, 258; environmental issues 182–3, 183, 184–5, 187–92; equal opportunities 118; fit to govern 3, 15, 91, 97, 98; in government 251–4, 270–1; housing 132–7; local authorities 28–31, 190–1; management and efficiency 31–2; New Deal 259–61; NHS 91–2, 93, 93–5, 97–100, 101–5; pensions 158–66; poverty and social security 143–52; reform 19–22, 91; Scotland 194–5, 197, 198–9, 200–1, 208, 209, 212; social exclusion 261–5; social justice 265–70; social services 107, 111–12; taxation 44–9, 51, 53–4; Wales 234–6, 239–45; welfare delivery 35–6
landfill levy 181, 191
Lang, Ian 68–9, 199
language 194, 236, 245
law and order *see* criminal justice
Lawrence, Sir Ivan 176
Lawrence, Philip 174
Lawrence, Stephen 174
Lawson, Nigel 124
le Grand, J. 263
leadership 186
Leadership Abroad, Responsibility at Home (Conservative Party) 185–6
Leathley, A. 161

Lewis, Derek 173, 175
Lewis, J. 115
LGA 113, 117
LGMB 117
Liberal Democrats: criminal justice
   169, 177, 178; education 84;
   election campaign 2, 3, 10;
   election results 12–13, 250;
   employment 64; environmental
   issues 183, 184, 187, 189;
   health 104; housing 133; and
   Labour government 252; NHS
   96–7; popular support 50;
   poverty and social security
   147–8; Scotland 195, 197, 198,
   201, 209, 212; social services 111;
   taxation 43, 47–8, 49, 53; Wales
   237, 239
Liddell, Helen 164
Liddiard, M. 131, 136
lifelong learning 82, 84
Lilley, Peter 6, 67, 142, 157, 238
Lister, R. 142
local authorities 36; CCT 31–2;
   Citizen's Charter 25;
   compulsory competitive
   tendering 26, 35, 199; education
   79; funding 190–1; housing 125,
   127; Northern Ireland 217, 218;
   party policies 28–31; social
   services 27–8, 108–9, 113–15
local authority housing see social
   housing
local education authorities 27,
   29–30
Local Government Association
   113, 117
Local Government Management
   Board 117
local management of schools
   (LMS) 79
locally maintained schools 29
London School of Economics 176
London Underground 183
lone parents 145, 260; Labour
   policy 61–2, 88, 150, 253; Wales
   235, 236, 238–9
long-term unemployment: Labour
   policy 61, 253, 259; Liberal

Democrat policy 64; Northern
   Ireland 228–9; and social
   exclusion 262
Losing Out (Field) 258
Lynch, Peter 198
Lynes, Tony 161–2
Maastricht Treaty see Treaty of
   European Union

McCrae, Jo 101
McFate, K. 39
MacGregor, John 163
MacGregor, S. 266
McLaughlin, E. 215, 218, 219, 225
McVey, J. 220
Magill, D. 218
Major, John: and bastards 239;
   election campaign 1–2, 4, 5,
   8–10, 11, 12; Europe and
   unemployment 67–8, 69; and
   housing 126; image 18; on
   Labour Party 51; pensions 157,
   163; Scotland 202, 208; Social
   Chapter 57, 59, 64; social policy
   17
Major, Norma 2, 6
Maltese, J.A. 14
managerialism 24, 34, 35
Manchester airport 184
Mandelson, Peter 1, 151, 262, 265
manifestos 8, 60–1; criminal justice
   168, 169–70; education 83–4;
   employment 61–4;
   environmental issues 184–7, 190;
   health 96–7; housing 132;
   Northern Ireland 221–2;
   pensions 159; poverty and social
   security 146–8; Scotland 200–3;
   social services 111–12; taxation
   46–8; Wales 235–9
Mann, N. 267
manufacturing industry 56
Maples, John 93
market-type mechanisms 25–6; see
   also competition; contracting-out
marketisation: education 75–6
markets 71
Marshall, T.H. 242
Mawhinney, Brian 1, 8–9

Maximum Working Time
Directive 59–60, 63
Mayo, E. 187
Mead, Lawrence 255
Meadows, P. 151
media: criminal justice 174–5, 178;
election campaigns 2, 14, 15;
Northern Ireland 220–1;
Scotland 194, 203–4; *see also*
television
mental health 111, 118
Merchant, Piers 7, 8
Milburn, Alan 101, 102, 107
Millard, M. 43
MIND 112, 118
minimum wage 60, 62, 147
Mirza, Heidi 85
miscarriages of justice 173, 174
Mishra, R. 77
Misspent Youth (Audit
Commission) 170, 175
Mitchell, Austin 271
modernisation 21, 94–5, 101
Moe, T. 75
money purchase schemes 156, 162,
165, 166
Monks, John 270
Moore, John 92, 142
Morgan, R. 168–9, 173
MORI 182, 184
Morris, Estelle 85
Morris, L. 254
Morriston Hospital 234
Moss, P. 82
Murie, A. 128, 217
Murphy, P. 235
Murray, Charles 142
Must Labour Lose (Abrams and
Rose) 266–7

National Grid for Learning 86
National Health Service:
compulsory competitive
tendering 26; Conservative
policy 91–3; efficiency 32;
funding 51; Labour policy 93–5,
101–5, 243; Northern Ireland
216, 224–5; party policies
96–100; performance indicators

25, 33, 34, 35, 36; Plaid Cymru
policy 237; popular concern 91;
purchaser–provider split 35;
reforms 25, 28; Scotland 197,
200, 201; Scottish National
Party policy 202; and social
services 117–18; Wales 234,
235–6, 237, 238
National Health Service and
Community Care Act 1990 92
National Institute of Economic
and Social Research 68
National Institute for Social Work
116
National Insurance 254; and
pensions 156, 157, 158; and
pollution taxes 192
National Lottery 48; after-school
places 150; NHS 98, 99
National Policy Forum 44
National Savings Pension Plan 160
NDPBs *see* quangos
Neil, Andrew 203–4
Netherlands 59
New Deal 150, 253, 259–61
New Economics Foundation 187
New Labour 248, 250–1, 270;
criminal justice 171; inequality
263, 264; justice and progress
265–6; pensions 158–61, 166;
Wales 239–41, 243
'New Labour because Wales
deserves better' (Labour Party)
235
New Politics of Poverty, The
(Mead) 255
new public management 24, 25–8,
34, 35, 36
New Statesman 158
New Zealand 254
newspapers 203–4
Next Steps agencies 25, 26, 27, 31,
35
NHS *see* National Health Service
NHS trusts 26, 31, 92, 199
NICs *see* National Insurance
NIESR 52
Nine O'Clock News 67
No Turning Back Group 157

non-departmental public bodies
   see quangos
Northern Ireland 214, 228–9, 252;
   election campaign 220–8;
   political background 214–15;
   social policy 215–20
NSPP 160
nuclear industry 192
nursery education: Northern
   Ireland 216, 218; vouchers 79, 85
nurses 202

Observer 12, 102, 148, 261
occupational pensions 155–6, 159,
   164
Ofsted 79, 83, 86
Ofwat 183
old age pensions *see* pensions
Old Labour: pensions 161–3, 166;
   Wales 239–41
older people *see* elderly
O'Leary, C. 222
On the Record 66, 254
one nation 2, 10
one-parent families *see* lone parents
Ontario Network of Employment
   Skills Training Projects 257–8
Onyett, S. 116
Oppenheim, C. 139, 140, 142, 151,
   152
opportunity 21; *see also* equality of
   opportunity
Osborne, R. 218, 219
Ouseley, Sir Herman 118
owner occupation 122–7, 132,
   133–4

PAFT 218–20, 226, 227
Pannell, B. 126
Papadakis, E. 243, 244
Parent Plus 146
parental responsibility orders 169
Parry, Richard 43, 209
part-time workers 258
partnership 21
partnership insurance plans 108,
   109–10
Paterson, Lindsay 197
Patient's Charter 34

Pay-As-You-Go (PAYG) scheme
   156, 160, 161, 162, 166
Penn, H. 82
pensioners *see* elderly
pensions 108, 155–6, 165–6, 224;
   Conservative policy 157–8, 163;
   Labour policy 158–65
Pensions Act 1995 164, 165
Pensions Guarantee 159, 160
performance measurement 25,
   35–6; education 75, 83–4; *see
   also* Citizen's Charter
personal pensions 156, 159
personal responsibility 21, 107,
   108, 142, 186
personal social services *see* social
   services
pesticides 192
PFI 94, 95, 99, 101
Phinnemore, D. 60
Pirie, Madsen 157–8
Piven, Fran 254
Plaid Cymru 190, 237, 239
Plant, R. 142
Plender, John 158
PM 65
police 17, 176–7
Policy Appraisal and Fair
   Treatment 218–20, 226, 227
Politeia 107
Poll Tax 199, 266
Poll Tax, The (MacGregor) 266
Pollard, Charles 177
Pollard, S. 262
pollution 181, 182, 183, 187, 188;
   Green Party 190; and health 185;
   taxes 192
pollution inspectorates 181
popular capitalism 156
Portillo, Michael 238
poverty 139–46, 152–3, 249; in
   election campaign 148–9; global
   192; and health 184, 185; Labour
   Party in government 149–52;
   Northern Ireland 224; party
   policies 146–8; public attitudes
   140–2; and social exclusion 261,
   262–3, 268; United States 255
Power to the People 50

PR 189–90, 198
precautionary principle 188–9
Prescott, John 3, 10, 191
Prior, G. 164
Prior, Jim 222
Prison Service Agency 175
prisons 173, 175
Private Finance Initiative 94, 95, 99, 101
private health insurance 104
private sector 39, 40, 150, 243; environmental issues 182–3; housing 30, 128–9
privatisation: central government departments 26, 27, 224; education 75–6; and environmental issues 181–3; social services 106–7, 115, 119
Project Work 58, 63, 146
proportional representation 189–90, 198
PSBR see public sector borrowing requirement
public administration model 24–5
public expenditure 39–41; controlling 42–3; employment 70; housing 129–30, 135; Labour policy 44, 45, 49–50, 254, 263; Northern Ireland 217, 218–19, 222–3, 225, 228–9; public transport 183; Scotland 197; social security 147–8; social services 113–15, 119; Wales 237, 238
public health 101, 185
public housing see social housing
public sector borrowing requirement 42, 43, 223; Labour policy 70, 135, 254; and public transport 182
public services see welfare delivery
public transport 182–3, 188
purchaser–provider split 28, 32, 35, 92

Quality Commission 33, 35
quangos 36; Northern Ireland 216, 217–18; Wales 233

Quarrie, Joyce 191
quarrying levy 188
Quirk, P. 218, 219

RADAR 114
Railtrack 189
Rao, N. 33
Rayner scrutinies 25
Real World Coalition 182
Redwood, John 5, 7, 238–9
Rees, G. 235
referenda: proportional representation 189; Scotland 195, 196, 197, 199, 212; Wales 233, 245–6
regulation: environmental issues 182, 183, 186, 188–9; social services 109, 115–16
Reich, Robert 13
Renewing the NHS (Labour Party) 93, 95, 96, 99
residential homes 106
Residential Homes Act 1984 106
residualism 215, 216–17, 223, 228
Resource Management Initiative 25
retirement pensions see pensions
Reynolds, David 85
Ridley, F.F. 34
Rifkind, Malcolm 66, 199, 209, 212
Right to Buy 16, 17, 127–8; and home ownership 122, 123–4, 133; and local authority role 27, 125
roads 182, 184, 188
Robertson, George 199, 209
Robinson, P. 57
Robinson, Peter 260
Roof 136
Rose, R. 16, 266–7
Rose, S. 218
Rowlatt, J. 30
Royal Association for Disability and Rehabilitation 114
Royal Commission on Criminal Justice 174
Royal Society for the Protection of Birds (RSPB) 184, 191
Rumbold, Angela 10
rural development 227–8

SACHR 214, 218
Santer, Jacques 10–11
Sarwar, Mohammad 208
Saunders, P. 122, 123
schools 25; *see also* grant-
    maintained schools; self-
    governing schools
Scotland 194–8, 212–13; devolution
    191, 251; election campaign
    203–8; election results 209,
    210–11; future of social policy
    209, 212; issues 200; party
    manifestos 200–3; party
    organisation and politics 198–200
Scotland Act 1978 195, 197
Scotland on Sunday 203
'Scotland's Parliament, Scotland's
    Right' (Scottish Constitutional
    Convention) 198
Scotsman 203–4
Scottish Constitutional
    Convention 198, 212
Scottish Labour Party *see* Labour
    Party
Scottish National Party 194–5, 197,
    212–13, 237; election broadcasts
    208; election results 209;
    manifesto 202–3; and Scottish
    Constitutional Convention 198;
    and *Sun* 203
Scottish Office 197
Scottish Television 204
SDLP *see* Social and Democratic
    Labour Party
Securities and Investments Board
    164
Security in Retirement (Labour
    Party) 160
Sefton 113–14
self-governing schools 199
senedd 233, 237, 241, 245
SERPS *see* State Earnings Related
    Pension Scheme
Setting the Pace (Labour Party) 170
Sheehan, M. 218
Sheeley, Nick 67
Shepherd, Gillian 66
Sherman, J. 161
Shrimsby, R. 163

Silcott, Winston 174
single parents *see* lone parents
Sinn Fein 220, 222; class politics
    221; demographic concerns 229;
    equality issues 226, 227; social
    exclusion 228; social security
    224; taxation 223
sleaze 7, 65, 169, 170; Conservative
    Party 3–5, 18, 22, 248; Tatton
    constituency 2, 8–9
Smith, C. 44
Smith, John 19, 81, 198–9
Smith, Tim 4–5, 7
Snower, Dennis 260
SNP *see* Scottish National Party
social breakdown 40, 267–8
Social Chapter 57, 59–60, 64, 66;
    Labour policy 62, 147
Social and Democratic Labour
    Party 220; class politics 221;
    equality and social partnership
    226–7; health 225; social
    exclusion 228; social security
    224; taxation and spending 222–3
social exclusion 40, 261–5, 268;
    Labour policy 21; Northern
    Ireland 224, 228
Social Exclusion Unit 151, 262, 269
social housing 127–8, 238;
    Citizen's Charter 25; Northern
    Ireland 220; party policies 30;
    Scotland 198; social problems
    267; *see also* Right to Buy
social justice 81, 152, 265–70
Social Justice Commission *see*
    Commission on Social Justice
Social Justice (Commission on
    Social Justice) 81
Social Loans 224
Social Research Association 248
social security: Conservative policy
    142–3; in election campaign
    148–9; Labour policy 143–6,
    149–52, 253; Northern Ireland
    223–4; party policies 146–8;
    public attitudes 140–2; Scottish
    National Party policy 202
Social Security Act 1986 155–6,
    158, 159

social security benefits 141, 148, 216–17; *see also* child benefit; income support; state pension
social services 27–8, 119; Citizen's Charter 25; education and training 116–17; Northern Ireland 216, 218; party policies 30, 111–12; under Conservative government 106–11; under Labour government 113–18
social services departments: care in the community 92–3; purchaser–provider split 32
Social Services Inspectorate 109
social workers 111, 112
Sopel, J. 93, 95
sovereignty 60
SRA 248
stakeholder pensions 159, 160, 162, 166
Stakeholder Welfare (Field) 144
stakeholding 11, 21; criminal justice 169, 175–7
standards 21, 25; education 79–80, 86; social services 107, 116
Standards Inspectorate 33
Standing Advisory Commission on Human Rights 214, 218
State Earnings Related Pension Scheme 155, 166; Conservative policy 155–6, 165; Labour policy 158–9, 160, 161, 162
state pension 155, 159, 161, 165–6
Stenson, K. 176
Stewart, Allan 7, 208
Stewart, J. 30
Straw, Jack 31, 172, 175, 176, 256
Strong, S. 112
Sullivan, M. 235, 239, 244
Sun 2, 7, 203
Sunday Times 10
sustainable development 181, 186, 189, 192
Sweden 255
Symes, V. 57

Tackling the causes of crime (Labour Party) 170

Tackling Crime Effectively (Audit Commission) 176
Targeting Social Need 218–20, 226, 227, 228–9
tartan tax 48, 199
tax-credit system 151, 253
taxation 42–3, 53–4; election campaign 49–50, 67, 170; environmental 181, 184, 188, 192; Labour policy 44–9, 51–2, 70, 243, 253–4, 262; Liberal Democrats 84, 147, 239; Northern Ireland 222–3; party policies 45–9; and pensions 156; Plaid Cymru 237; Scottish Parliament 199, 212
Taylor, A. 19
Taylor, Lord Chief Justice 176
Taylor, Martin 150, 252
Taylor Committee 151
Taylor-Gooby, P. 137, 140, 141, 243, 244
television 204, 208; debates 1–2, 50
Temple, William 269–70
Thatcher, Margaret 6, 16–18, 242; education 78; NHS 91, 92; and Tony Blair 5
Thomas, E. 235
Times, The 8, 9, 75, 158, 161
Tindale, S. 188, 191
tobacco advertising 104
Today 45, 65, 66, 67, 69, 163
Tonge, J. 70
Townsend, Peter 161, 162
Trade Union and Employment Rights Act 1993 57
trade unions 264; erosion of powers 57, 58–9; and Labour Party 2, 20, 68–9, 71; Northern Ireland 216; Scottish Constitutional Convention 198; TUC conference 270
training 70, 72
Training and Enterprise Councils (TECs) 63, 258
transparency 36
transport 181–3; Labour policy 185, 188
Travis, Alan 172

Treasury Committee 162, 164
Treaty of European Union 57; *see also* Social Chapter
trickle-down theory 142, 219
Trimble, David 228
Trinder, C. 259
tripartite model 56, 59
Tritter, J. 79
trust: Conservative Party 2–3, 248; Labour Party 4, 21–2, 266; and NHS 99, 100; and taxation 46, 47–8
TSN 218–20, 226, 227, 228–9
Tumim, Stephen 178
Turner, Adair 270

Ulster Unionist Party 220, 222, 228–9; class politics 221; equality issues 226, 227–8; health 224–5; residualism 216–17; social security 223–4; taxation and spending 223
underclass 152, 254, 261, 266; Labour policy 170, 242
unemployment 56, 57–9, 70–2; and crime 170; election campaign 64–9; figures 60, 68, 71; and health 185; and housing 124–5, 126; Labour policy 69–70, 253, 259–61; Northern Ireland 218, 224, 227; Scotland 198; Wales 236; *see also* employment; long-term unemployment
Unemployment and the Future of Work (Council of Churches for Britain and Ireland) 66–7, 139, 148–9
Unionism 214, 215, 216–17, 220; *see also* Democratic Unionist Party; Ulster Unionist Party
United Nations Conference on Environment and Development 1992 186
United States: presidential campaigns 1–2, 13–14; social housing 267–8; tax credits 151, 253; unemployment 58; welfare-to-work 254, 255–7
Utting, D. 108

UUP *see* Ulster Unionist Party

value for money 21, 25, 114
values 22
VAT 45, 46, 187–8
vehicle excise levy 187
voluntary action: environmental issues 186
voluntary organisations: social services 112
Voters Can't Be Choosers 50

Waine, B. 35, 156
Waldegrave, William 162
Wales 233–4, 246; Conservative policy 238–9; devolution 191, 245–6, 251; election campaign 239–42; Labour policy 234–6, 242–5; Liberal Democrats 237; Plaid Cymru 237
Walker, Alan 161, 162
Walker, Peter 241
Wallace, Jim 201
Walsh, F. 97
Ward, Judith 174
Ward, S. 164
waste 185, 192
water: pollution 188; privatisation 183
Watkins, K. 264
Watson, Ceilia 189
Weale, M. 52
Webb, S. 139
Webster, P. 161
welfare delivery 24; Conservative Party 24–8; customer orientation 33–4; and local authorities 28–31; management and efficiency 31–2; party policies 34–6; *see also* National Health Service; Next Steps agencies; social services
welfare dependency *see* dependency
welfare-to-work 52, 58, 60, 107, 254–9; and crime 170; disabled 253; election campaign 65, 67, 68; environmental awareness 185; European experience 71–2; Liberal Democrats 146;

manifesto commitment 69, 146;
Scotland 201; single parents 253;
social care workforce 117; Wales
236; and women 88; young
people 61, 62, 64, 150–1
Welsh Development Agency 233
Welsh Office 233
West, A. 76
West, Rosemary 174
West Lothian question 204
Western Mail 234
When Work Disappears (Wilson)
267–8
White, S. 152
Whitty, G. 75, 76
Whyte, J. 214
Wilford, R. 218
Wilkinson, Richard 96
Wilson, Harold 20
Wilson, William Julius 267–8
windfall tax 45, 48, 65, 70;
disagreements 9; and welfare-to-
work 52, 61, 62, 107
Wistow, G. 106
Wolf 162
women: care in the community
92–3; education and
employment 88; election
campaign 6; independence 140;
local government 191; minimum
wage 62; as MPs 13, 85; pensions
164; social services 118; welfare-to-
work 256
Women's Environmental Network
185
Woodhead, Chris 75
Woolf Report 173, 176
workfare *see* welfare-to-work
Working Time Directive 59–60, 63
World at One 48, 67
Worsley, R. 259

Young, G. 52
Young, Hugo 172
Young, R. 106
young people: crime 170, 175;
housing 131; Labour policy 253
youth unemployment 68, 259;
Northern Ireland 227; public
expenditure 65–6; rebate scheme
67; welfare-to-work 61, 62, 64,
69, 71–2, 150–1
Ysbyty Treforys 234

zero tolerance 169, 172